Mechanisms of Cortical Development

Monographs of the Physiological Society

Mechanisms of Cortical Development

David J. Price and David J. Willshaw
University of Edinburgh,
Edinburgh, UK

OXFORD UNIVERSITY PRESS

OXFORD

UNIVERSITY PRESS

Great Clarendon Street, Oxford OX2 6DP

Oxford University Press is a department of the University of Oxford.
It furthers the University's aim of excellence in research, scholarship,
and education by publishing worldwide in

Oxford New York

Athens Auckland Bangkok Bogotá Buenos Aires Calcutta
Cape Town Chennai Dar es Salaam Delhi Florence Hong Kong Istanbul
Karachi Kuala Lumpur Madrid Melbourne Mexico City Mumbai
Nairobi Paris São Paulo Singapore Taipei Tokyo Toronto Warsaw

with associated companies in Berlin Ibadan

Oxford is a registered trade mark of Oxford University Press
in the UK and in certain other countries

Published in the United States
by Oxford University Press Inc., New York

Library of Congress Cataloging-in-Publication Data

Price, David, 1957 Dec. 20–
Mechanisms of cortical development / David J. Price and David J. Willshaw.
p. cm. — (Monographs of the Physiological Society; 47)
Includes bibliographical references.
1. Cerebral cortex—Growth. 2. Developmental neurophysiology.
I. Willshaw, David. II. Title. III. Series: Monographs of the Physiological Society; no. 47.
[DNLM: 1. Cerebral Cortex—physiology. W1 M0569QW no. 47 2000]
QP383.P74   2000   612.8'25—dc21   99-39684
ISBN 0–19–262427–X

Typeset by
Newgen Imaging Systems (P) Ltd., Chennai, India
Printed in Great Britain by
Bookcraft (Bath) Ltd,
Midsomer Norton, Avon

Preface

The last hundred years have seen rapid advances in our understanding of the human brain. Just over a hundred years ago it was first established that nerve cells are independently functioning elements. Fifty years ago the propagation of the nerve impulse and the nature of chemical synaptic transmission were first described. Twenty-five years ago the first evidence for a biochemical basis for synaptic modification was established.

Fifty years after the discovery of the structure of DNA, and with the rapid advance in our knowledge of the genome and its effects, it is no surprise that current investigations of what determines the development of the brain is focused sharply on the instructions controlling development that are contained in the genome, how these instructions are expressed in biochemical terms, and how their expression is reflected in the development of brain structures themselves and ultimately the functioning of the adult nervous system. Notwithstanding, a proper understanding of the development of the nervous system will require knowledge about a variety of processes, ranging from the development of specific nerve cell types, the formation of specific neural structures, and the development of patterns of interconnectivity at the subcellular, cellular, systems and psychological levels.

We have attempted to describe a multidisciplinary, multilevel approach to the development of the cerebral cortex, drawing on information from other parts of the nervous system where appropriate. Scientific knowledge is accumulating at an alarming rate and there is a danger that a book of this type will be out of date before it becomes printed. We have tried to concentrate on those aspects of the development of the cortex which will still be true in the years to come. Perhaps details will alter, certain experimental results that we cite will be found to be wrong or will have to be modified but we hope that the broad principles that we describe will remain the same.

We would like to thank all those who have helped and encouraged us finally to complete this book: in particular, Tamsin Pearson, Tim Hely, Volker Steuber, and Geoff Goodhill for help with the content; Rosanna Maccagnano, Fiona Jamieson, Stephen Felderhof, Emma Black, Rachel Ellaway, and Teresa Levers for assistance in preparing the manuscript, and Norah Spears and Jon Butt for comments on the text. David Willshaw thanks Mike Gaze for guiding him along the MRC career path and he is deeply grateful to many colleagues, particularly Christopher Longuet-Higgins, Christoph von der Malsburg, and colleagues at NIMR, Mill Hill; most importantly to Mike Gaze and the late Martin Prestige, both of whom inspired him to work on neurobiology. David Price would like to thank all those who have guided his scientific career, in particular his father, William Price, and advisors John Russell, Bill Watson, Colin Blakemore, and David Weisblat, his numerous co-workers in Oxford, Berkeley, and Edinburgh and his collaborators in Edinburgh, the UK, and abroad.

April 2000   D.J.P.
                                                                                                             D.J.W.

Contents

Previous Volumes in this Series

All these volumes are now out of print.

Volumes 43–48, published by Oxford University Press, are listed on p. ii.

1

Introduction

1   THE EVOLUTION OF THE CEREBRAL CORTEX

Life on earth began several thousand million years ago. The cerebral cortex of mammals probably arose from the primordial cortex of amphibians and reptiles (Herrick, 1948; Kruger, 1969; Riss *et al.*, 1969; Bayer and Altman, 1991) some 300 million years ago (Novacek, 1992). Until 1–2 million years ago, there were no species with brain sizes similar to those of modern man, *Homo sapiens*. To gain an impression of the relative rapidity with which the brain has evolved, we could equate the time that life has existed on earth to a year, with the origin of life on the 1st January and the present day being midnight on the 31st December. Mammals would appear at around the beginning of December, and *Homo sapiens* would appear a few hours before midnight on the last day of the year (Fig. 1.1).

As is illustrated in Fig. 1.2, the evolution of the mammalian brain has involved the disproportionate enlargement of the cortex and, in particular, the rapid development of the neocortex. This region has characteristic cell types arranged around its outer edge in layers (the cortical grey matter) and it dominates the brain of more advanced mammals. Its extreme folding in primates and man gives it a very large surface area (Fig. 1.2). If the cortex were to be laid out flat, a rat's would occupy the surface area of a postage stamp, a monkey's would be the size of an envelope, a chimpanzee's the size of an A4 sheet of paper, and a human's the size of four A4 sheets. The relative sizes of cortical areas that are not dedicated to specific sensory functions, such as sight, hearing, and smell, increase from animals such as rats through to humans. The fact that the neocortex has been evolving to such a high level in so short a time implies that it must have been subject to very strong selection pressures. It also suggests that the mechanisms that generate the neocortex of the primates cannot be too different from those that generate the cortex of even the simplest of vertebrates; it is inconceivable that in such a relatively short space

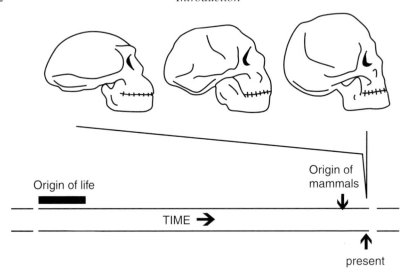

FIG. 1.1. The evolution of man. The three skulls are of *Homo erectus (left)*, *Homo sapiens neanderthalensis (centre)*, and *Homo sapiens sapiens (right)*. *Homo erectus* ranged across Africa into Eurasia from about 1.5 million to 300 000 years ago; *Homo sapiens* species came into existence about 300 000 years ago. The enlargement of the brain from *Homo erectus* to *Homo sapiens* is indicated by the increased size of the skull. It is estimated that *Homo erectus* had a brain volume of 775–1100 cm^3, whereas that of *Homo sapiens* species is put at 1200–1600 cm^3 (by comparison, chimpanzees have brains of 280–450 cm^3 and gorillas have brains of 350–750 cm^3). The time-line drawn below (approximately to scale) indicates the relative times of key events in evolution and illustrates how rapidly *Homo sapiens* has evolved.

of evolutionary time, entirely different developmental strategies were evolved for each different species.

During evolution there has been an enormous increase in the number of cells involved in cortical development. Considering the increase in brain volume and assuming that the brain cells of earliest man were as densely packed as those in the brain of modern man, it has been estimated that about nine billion cells were added to the brain during human evolution. That increase resulted in a doubling of brain size to its present content of approximately 15 billion cells (Smith, 1984). Probably most of these new cells would have been added to the cerebral cortex. Expressed in this way, this seems like a huge increase but it must be remembered that only one extra doubling of a population of cells is required to produce twice as many cells.

Cellular development is controlled both internally, by intracellular processes determined largely by the genes expressed in that cell, and by extracellular signals. Whereas the development of cells in some regions of the nervous system appears to be tightly regulated at the genetic level, developing neocortical cells may have more flexibility and their control may rely heavily on cell–cell signalling.

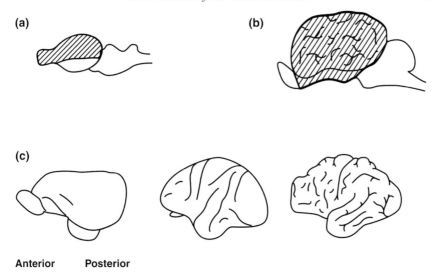

(a)

(b)

(c)

Anterior   **Posterior**

FIG. 1.2. The evolution of the cortex. (a) A primitive tetrapod. The cortical regions (hatched) make a relatively small contribution to total brain weight and contain no neocortex. (b) An advanced mammal. The neocortex, with its distinguishing cell types, cellular organization, and functions, dominates the brain and makes a relatively large contribution to total brain weight. (c) The disproportionate increase in the size of the neocortex in mammalian evolution is achieved by the extreme folding of the cortical surface. These drawings show the cortices of a tree shrew (*left*), monkey (*centre*), and human (*right*). The brains are not drawn to the same scale.

As the number of neocortical cells increased, it is most likely that each retained an essentially unaltered, and presumably relatively simple, intrinsic developmental programme that, when operated on and supplemented by extracellular signals, guided the cell to a complex and useful phenotype. There are many similarities between the development of the neocortex of the most widely divergent mammals, and neocortical cells have a profound ability to execute a flexible programme that enables them to alter the course of their development in the face of altered extracellular cues. It is unlikely that there would have been time for the cortex to have evolved to the extent that it has if a blueprint encoded at the genetic level required extensive modification as more and more cells were added. These considerations indicate that, in response to an ever-increasing population of neocortical cells, modifications to cortical development during evolution are likely to have involved quantitative and/or qualitative changes in extracellular signalling rather than numerous changes at the genetic level. Cell–cell signalling may play a particularly important role in the development of cortical cells, perhaps more than in other regions of the nervous system that have changed to relatively lesser degrees in evolution. It is worth noting that mammals provide their progeny, both pre- and postnatally, with an environment that is relatively stable and stereotyped, allowing their growing offspring to rely on the provision of appropriate environmental signals to complete the development of the neocortex.

None of the above is intended to give the impression that there have been no changes at a genetic level during cortical evolution. Despite the tremendous similarities in the processes and, presumably, the mechanisms of neocortical development in the most widely divergent vertebrate species, there are also clear examples of significant differences. For example, the primate has evolved an elaborate cortical system for the detection of colour whereas non-primate species have not; the afferents from the lateral geniculate nucleus (LGN) in the thalamus terminate mainly in the primary visual cortex (striate cortex or V1) of primates and rodents, whereas in carnivores such as the cat they innervate both striate and extrastriate visual cortex (Stone, 1983). It is quite possible that the evolution of such differences has been the result of modifications to the genes whose expression underlie neocortical development. Indeed, some genetic changes may have been crucial for allowing the emergence of new neocortices with an increased potential to interact with their environment.

2   SCOPE

We seek to explain what is known about the fundamental mechanisms that underlie the development of the neocortex of mammals. We shall draw on supporting evidence from other species, particularly other vertebrates. Much of our discussion will be targeted at *visual* cortical development as this system provides an excellent model for more general problems of development and it has been the most extensively studied. In the developing cerebral cortex, the fate of each cell at any given time of development is determined by a complex set of signals derived from its own genes and from extracellular sources, both inside and outside the growing organism. Clearly, many of the processes that occur in cortical development are common to many other developing systems (for example, the control of the cell cycle or the mechanisms of axonal extension). The thread of the book follows the sequence of cortical development from the time at which the forebrain develops from the neural plate up until the cortex reaches its adult form.

The book has three aspects to it which distinguish it from most other texts on the development of the neocortex.

Focus and range of systems covered. In interpreting neocortical development we use supporting evidence from other systems and species.

Levels of description. Many classic texts of developmental biology concentrate on the development of the size and shape of cells and their processes, their lineage, and the molecular basis for the interactions between cells observed during development. Many more modern texts are concerned with how specific genes are expressed in the developing nervous system. In our text an account of the development of the biology of cortical cells and the morphology of the structures that they form is interwoven with a detailed account of their biochemistry and the genetic origin of the factors that are thought to control key developmental processes.

Experiments and models. Whilst the primary account of the development of the neocortex necessarily is of the results of experimental neuroscience, where appropriate the results are interpreted on the basis of the various formal models that have been proposed.

The design of formal models to test hypotheses relating to specific biological questions is an activity that is now common to many areas of biology, particularly developmental biology and neurobiology. The type of model that we consider is formulated as a set of equations intended to represent the actions of the cellular or subcellular elements and their interactions in the biological system under consideration. Solution of the equations, either analytically or by computer simulation, specifies how, according to the model, the systems under consideration will behave under the given conditions. Here we consider models of the programme that the developing system undergoes.

The construction of formal models represents the most extreme version of the activity that people indulge in when they 'develop an idea for how a system works'. Using a well-constructed model has the advantages that the designer is forced to make a logically consistent hypothesis and the predictions from the model will be clear and reproducible by others; often the consequences drawn from hypotheses involving a large number of interacting elements (such as nerve cells) can only be found by constructing a formal model. The disadvantages are that the assumptions on which the model is based may be questionable, or the model may be too simple, or the conclusions drawn from the model may be untestable. The first of these disadvantages is often encountered in models formulated in developmental neurobiology. In many cases, to account for phenomena at the level of the cell, for example, strong assumptions about the underlying biochemical processes may have to be made which intuitively might be plausible but in fact are unjustified. This type of modelling activity, called computational neuroscience, has existed since at least the 1920s (Rashevsky, 1938; McCulloch and Pitts, 1943) but only recently has it been accepted as one of the ways to attack neurobiological problems (Sejnowski *et al.*, 1988). The current interest may be because modellers now tend to analyse specific systems rather than constructing general theories of brain; or that the models are more sophisticated, which is a consequence of the increased power of current computers that enables more realistic models to be simulated; or that it is difficult to work out how arrays of neurons might interact without recourse to mathematical and simulation studies. The modelling work described here should be distinguished from modelling of a purely *mathematical* nature where it is attempted to describe in mathematical form how the key measurable attributes of the system depend on other parameters but without requiring the proposed mathematical relationships to have any interpretation in the underlying biology.

The functioning of the nervous system depends critically on the roles adopted by the specific cells and their relationships with other cells. The basic question addressed in all modelling enterprises in developmental neurobiology focuses on how the individual members of a set of cells acquire differences one from another that enable them (i) early in development to adopt different developmental paths and differentiate into different structures; (ii) later in development, to make different patterns of connections. Both cases can be said to involve pattern formation. As we shall see, similar theoretical concepts have been used in both cases although they involve different types of pattern: in the first case the pattern is a property of the cells themselves and in the second case the pattern is in the *relation* between nerve cells.

In both cases, most models concentrate on the possible source of the information that enables different cells to act differently (Is it acquired from the genes or from the environment; from the presynaptic cell or the postsynaptic cell?) and how this information is signalled to the cells (By molecular or by electrical signalling; diffusion or active transport?). Over the course of this book we shall see how the same basic concepts of information processing constantly recur. Although in many models the spatial and temporal aspects of the signalling of information are considered, so far there have been few models that incorporate the physical constraints of the real neurobiological system under investigation.

Usually models are constructed in one of two ways. *Top-down* modelling is concerned with constructing a model system containing the machinery that enables it to have specific properties (such as an ordered map of connections between two sheets of cells); *bottom-up* modelling is concerned with investigating what properties of the model system arise from the known, or assumed, interactions between its elements.

3 FUTURE CHALLENGES

Our knowledge of biological processes is necessarily constrained by existing technologies. If this book had been written 10–15 years ago, the bulk of it would have concerned work using electrophysiological and neuroanatomical methods to study the development of receptive field properties and the emergence of cortical maps of the sensory periphery. In terms of mechanisms driving the developmental changes, there would have been a proportionately greater emphasis on the role of neural activity in the formation of ordered patterns of connections. However, since then there have been massive advances in molecular biological technologies and they have been applied extensively to the study of cortical development in the past few years. As a result, our understanding of the genetic control of cortical development is increasing rapidly, as reflected by the prominence given to this aspect of cortical development in our early chapters.

At the other end of the spectrum of development, there remains a huge gap in our understanding of the mechanisms that generate the functional properties of the cerebral cortex (Chapter 7). The cortex is immensely complex, containing vast numbers of cells connected by even larger numbers of synapses. The functional properties of individual cortical cells, groups of cortical cells, or all cortical cells together is not merely a product of which cells are connected to which other cells, but is also dependent on the functional properties of the synapses that connect them. There is currently no way to observe all these connections and to measure their individual functional properties as they develop. As our early chapters will show, it is quite possible to make statements about general mechanisms of cortical development, such as those that guide connections to an appropriate multicellular region, or those that refine cortical connections. But at present there is no prospect of being able to discover what controls the development of specific patterns of connections on and between individual cortical cells and how the functional properties of each synapse are determined. Therefore, a profound and detailed understanding of the mechanisms that generate the fine details of a biological circuitry with the functional capacity of the cerebral cortex remains an enormous challenge for the future.

4   UNDERSTANDING DISEASE THROUGH UNDERSTANDING DEVELOPMENT

Understanding the mechanisms of cortical development will have great impact on our ability to comprehend and treat neurological disease. Disease of the nervous system affects most people at some stage of their life. Some disorders are known to result from genetic defects. An example is the human condition periventricular nodular heterotopia, which is characterized by an abnormality of cortical migration (Gleeson and Walsh, 1997). Others disorders are caused by injury to the brain, perhaps through hypoxia, infection or exposure to other environmental agents such as alcohol or drugs of abuse, particularly during gestation (Evrard *et al.*, 1997). Then there are neoplastic and degenerative diseases, whose aetiologies have features in common with the mechanisms that regulate the normal development of cells and connections. For example, the processes that control cell proliferation and/or cell death become disrupted in cancer. The symptoms of such diseases are associated with recognized gross morphological or histological abnormalities in the nervous system; descriptions of the symptoms and pathological changes in these conditions are outside the scope of this book, and we refer the reader to standard textbooks of pathology or reviews of recent work, such as those by Roberts *et al.* (1995), Evrard *et al.* (1997), Gleeson and Walsh (1997) and Galaburda (1997). There are some diseases of the brain whose aetiology and pathology remain controversial. These include psychiatric disorders whose primary symptoms are abnormal behaviour and which have been described as 'functional' or 'non-organic' conditions, implying that they cannot be explained by defects in the structure and biochemistry of the brain. While it is certainly true that we are a long way from having a clear understanding of the neural basis of normal and abnormal behaviours, it is increasingly accepted that normal and abnormal mental processes and behaviours are caused by physical events that occur in the nervous system. Linked with this is the issue of the nature of consciousness. In this book we do not discuss it, since conscious awareness is inferred from the behaviour of an individual but is not directly observable and is therefore not accessible to experimentation. In all other respects, the brain can be viewed as a highly complex machine and the concept that higher mental processes have an origin outwith the neural circuitry of the brain is becoming less credible.

This is illustrated well by changing views on the relatively common illness, schizophrenia. This condition is characterized by disorders of thought and emotion, a lack of motivation, hallucinations, delusions, and disturbances of expression and movement. Intellectual capacity is often undiminished. The estimated risk of schizophrenia at some time in life is 0.5–1.0%, it is more common in males than females, and most cases begin between the ages of 15 and 45. Schizophrenia has been recognized for over 100 years but there has been debate over its aetiology. For example, some workers have suggested that it is not a disease but rather a response to environmental factors such as emotional pressure from family and society. Such debates have been settled in favour of its being a disease. Recent techniques for *in vivo* brain imaging have shown neuropathological changes associated with chronic schizophrenia, such as ventricular enlargement and a reduction in cortical grey matter (Suddath *et al.*, 1990), and have provided clear evidence of the biological nature of schizophrenia.

In recent years, the hypothesis that schizophrenia is a developmental disorder rather than a degenerative one has gained support (Jones, 1995; Roberts *et al.*, 1995; Ross and Pearlson, 1996; Raedler *et al.*, 1998). A genetic component has been postulated on the basis of twin, adoption, and family studies (Kidd, 1997; Murphy *et al.*, 1996; Karayiorgou and Gogos, 1997). A variety of observations have pointed to there being a developmental neuropathology underlying this condition. These have included reports of abnormal lamination in the entorhinal cortex and abnormal distributions of white matter neurons in the frontal lobes, observations that suggest abnormalities of cell migration and/or cell death during development (Raedler *et al.*, 1998; Jones, 1995; Akbarian *et al.*, 1996b). Changes in the numbers of GABA receptors on cortical neurons and of the expression of glutamatergic NMDA receptors in the prefrontal cortex have been reported (Benes *et al.*, 1996; Akbarian *et al.*, 1996a). Perturbation of proteins involved in synaptogenesis has been found in the cortex, suggesting defects in synaptic organization and function (Perrone-Bizzozero *et al.*, 1996; Glantz and Lewis, 1997; Gabriel *et al.*, 1997). The evidence for a developmental origin for schizophrenia is not yet conclusive, but it continues to accumulate and the case is becoming increasingly convincing.

In conclusion, neurological and psychiatric diseases include some of the most intractable problems for modern medicine. Many such diseases have a developmental origin and the example of schizophrenia indicates that such abnormalities may be more frequent than currently we appreciate. This example also illustrates how understanding the mechanisms of normal cerebral cortical development can suggest new ways to search for abnormalities associated with these types of disease.

2
Early development of the telencephalon

1 MAMMALIAN EMBRYOGENESIS AND EMERGENCE OF THE FOREBRAIN

Brain develops from embryonic ectoderm, one of the three germ layers of the embryo, the other two being endoderm and mesoderm. Figs. 2.1 and 2.2 summarize the main features of embryogenesis, the origin of ectoderm, and the emergence of brain. Detailed descriptions of this process and its interspecies variations can be found elsewhere. For example, Alberts *et al.* (1994) provides an excellent account of general principles; information in Valverde and Lichtman (1985) is particularly relevant to neural development; Kaufman (1992) offers an altas of specifically mouse embryogenesis. The following books contain considerable detail on the process of specifically forebrain development: Schambra and Silver (1992); Paxinos *et al.* (1991), and Paxinos and Watson (1982) provide atlases of the forebrain and its development in rodents; Bayer and Altman (1991) includes morphological data on early cortical formation. Much of our knowledge of early embryogenesis is derived from studies of amphibia, whose large eggs and embryos are relatively easy to observe and manipulate, and many of the main features are similar in mammals. However there are important differences. Many of these are due to the protective environment of the uterus and to the provision of nutrition by the placenta. Others are differences of geometry in otherwise homologous processes. The present overview relates to mammalian development, in particular the embryogenesis of the mouse. Among mammals, this species is more suitable than any other for

(a)

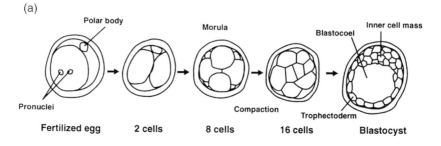

(b)

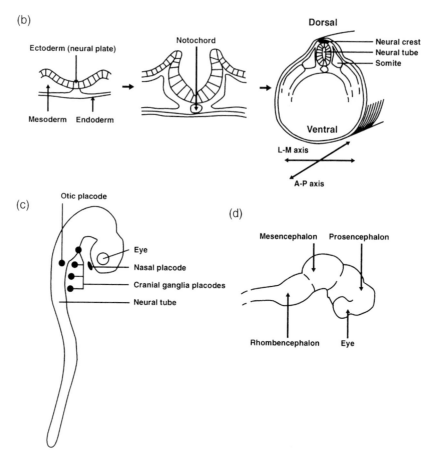

FIG.   2.1.   (a) Early development of the mouse embryo. The fertilized egg contains two haploid nuclei (the maternal and paternal pronuclei) and the polar bodies (the products of meiosis, which eventually degenerate). Subsequent mitoses generate the morula. The cells of the morula become compacted and, as they continue to divide, a fluid-filled cavity (the blastocoel) opens among them, forming the blastocyst. The embryo forms from the inner

genetic studies and for the analysis and experimental manipulation of gene expression in the living animal through transgenic techniques (described in Chapter 3).

The fertilized egg contains the maternal and paternal DNA in its haploid pronuclei (Fig. 2.1). The pronuclei fuse to form the diploid nucleus of the zygote, which divides to produce first the morula and then the blastocyst, which implants. Blastocyst formation involves cellular compaction (cells become more tightly cohesive and the surface of the morula becomes smoother) and the opening of a central fluid-filled cavity (the blastocoel). The blastocyst comprises the trophectoderm, which gives rise to the placenta and extraembryonic membranes (i.e. structures which are discarded at birth), and the inner cell mass, which contributes to extraembryonic structures and to the embryo proper (Fig. 2.1a). As described in Chapter 3, an understanding of these first developmental events, the adaptability of the morula, and the potential of cells in the morula and blastocyst have contributed crucially to our ability to study later events through genetic and transgenic techniques.

The blastocyst continues to develop by processes that include gastrulation and neurulation. Gastrulation leads to the generation of the three primary germ layers of the embryo, namely the endoderm, mesoderm, and ectoderm (Fig. 2.2). The endoderm (on the inside) forms the gut, associated organs (such as the salivary glands, liver, and pancreas), and the lungs. The mesoderm gives rise to two tissues in the embryo, the mesenchyme and the notochord. Mesenchyme is a loose meshwork of cells that forms cartilage, bone, and other connective tissue. The notochord is a rod of cells that runs anteroposteriorly and defines the central axis of the body (Fig. 2.1b). It plays a crucial role in the induction of overlying neural tissue and is the precursor of the vertebral column. The musculature, much of the urogenital system, and the vascular system are also derived from mesoderm. The ectoderm forms the outer epithelium of the body (epidermis) and the neural plate (Fig. 2.1b), from which the nervous system develops. Early in embryogenesis, the neural ectoderm (neuroepithelium) becomes separated from the surface ectoderm by a boundary zone that becomes progressively clearer in the region of the head and elsewhere

---

cell mass and the placenta forms from the trophectoderm. (b) Development of the neural tube. The diagrams show cross-sections through the dorsal ectoderm (neural plate), which folds to form the neural tube. Where the lateral edges of the neural plate fuse and separate from the surface ectoderm, the neural crest is formed (this is the origin of the peripheral nervous system). The somites and notochord derive from mesoderm. The body axes are indicated: L, lateral; M, medial; A, anterior; P, posterior. (c) Drawing of the neural tube, showing the positions of the placodes (thickenings of the surface ectoderm) that give rise to certain sensory cells and neurons. The otic placode forms the inner ear and associated neurons. The nasal placode forms olfactory neurons. The cranial placodes contribute to cranial sensory ganglia that innervate the head and neck. Note that the neurons of the eye originate from the neural tube (see d). (d) Major subdivisions of the brain of a mouse embryo at about mid-gestation. The prosencephalon is the forebrain, the mesencephalon is the midbrain, and the rhombencephalon is the hindbrain.

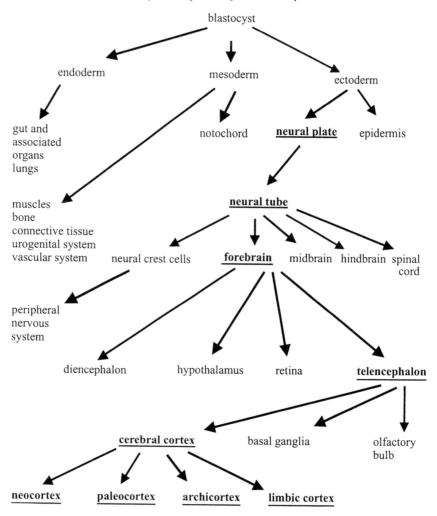

F I G . 2 . 2 . Flow diagram of the origin of the cerebral cortex.

along the embryonic axis. Although the endoderm, mesoderm, and ectoderm give rise to substantially different tissues in the mature animal, they do not develop independently. Interactions between them are essential for normal development (Ruiz i Altaba, 1994). In the early stages of embryogenesis, transplanting mesoderm to another site below the ectoderm can induce the formation of an ectopic neural tube (Wessells, 1977). More recent work has shown that the notochord can induce the development of regionally specific cell types in adjacent CNS (neural tube) through the secretion of diffusible morphogens (Chapter 3).

As illustrated in Fig. 2.1b, neural folds arise in the neural plate, appose, and later fuse to form the neural tube (a process called neurulation). As the process of fusion extends rostrally and caudally from its site of initiation, some cells break loose from the epithelium at its point of separation from the epidermis and migrate through the mesoderm. These are called neural crest cells. They give rise to the peripheral nervous system and, in the head, to cartilage, bone, and other connective tissues (elsewhere in the body these are mesodermal derivatives). The special sense organs for the detection of light, sound, and smell derive from the ectoderm. The retina forms from the neural tube, whereas the inner ear and its neurons, the olfactory neurons, and neurons that provide the rest of the sensory innervation of the head and neck arise from thickenings of the surface ectoderm called placodes (Fig. 2.1c). Eventually, the neural folds overlying the future forebrain fuse across the ventral midline to form the forebrain vesicle (the primary prosencephalic vesicle) with its two principle evaginations, the optic vesicles (future retinae and optic stalks). Figure 2.1d illustrates the three primary brain vesicles formed at the anterior end of the neural tube, namely the forebrain vesicle, the midbrain vesicle (mesencephalon), and the hindbrain vesicle (the rhombencephalon).

The development of the forebrain vesicle, which will eventually produce the forebrain (prosencephalon) of the adult, is illustrated in Fig. 2.3. The adult forebrain is extremely complex and detailed descriptions of its anatomy can be found elsewhere (we suggest Paxinos and Watson, 1982). However, its embryonic primordium is much simpler while containing major adult features from an early stage (from about mid-gestation in rodents). In broad terms, the forebrain of all but the youngest embryos can be divided on morphological and functional grounds into the diencephalon, hypothalamus, retinae, and telencephalon. These regions can be further subdivided as development progresses. For example, a major component of the mature diencephalon is a collection of anatomically discrete nuclei known collectively as the thalamus, through which sensory information from the periphery is relayed to the cerebral cortex (axonal connections between thalamus and cortex develop during the second half of gestation in rodents). The telencephalon, which derives from bilateral swellings of the primary prosencephalic vesicle (Fig. 2.3d), includes the cerebral cortex, basal ganglia (large groups of neurons lying under the cortical mantle, involved in the control of movement), and olfactory bulb. In higher mammals, the most prominent region of the cerebral cortex is the neocortex (phylogenetically its most recent component), which is surrounded by other phylogenetically older cortical regions known collectively as the paleocortex, archicortex, and limbic cortex, areas that include the hippocampus and olfactory cortices. In subsequent chapters, we examine what is known about the mechanisms that generate the major divisions of the forebrain, leading to the emergence of the cerebral cortex, and the processes by which the cortex forms axonal connections with subcortical structures.

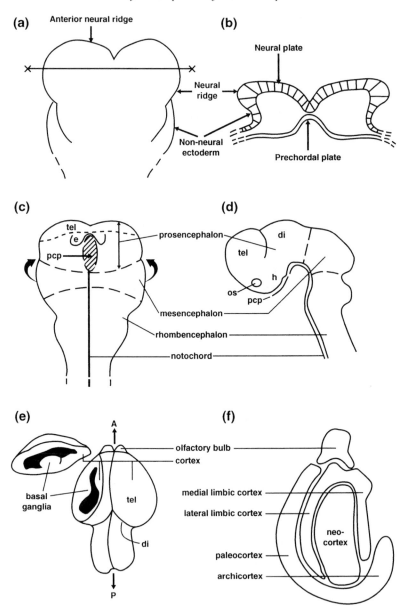

(a) Anterior neural ridge

(b) Neural plate

Neural ridge

Non-neural ectoderm

Prechordal plate

(c)

tel
e
pcp
prosencephalon
mesencephalon
rhombencephalon
notochord

(d)

di
tel
h
os
pcp

(e)

A
basal ganglia
tel
di
P

(f)

olfactory bulb
cortex
medial limbic cortex
lateral limbic cortex
neo-cortex
paleocortex
archicortex

FIG. 2.3. (a) Diagram of the anterior neural plate, seen from the dorsal aspect. The edge of the neural plate joins the non-neural ectoderm at the neural ridge. The section marked X–X is shown in (b). (b) Cross-section of the anterior neural plate at the level marked in (a). (b) Cross-section of the anterior neural plate at the level marked in (a). (c) Diagram of the anterior neural plate showing the origins of the major components of the brain. The neural plate rolls up as indicated by the filled arrows. (d) Appearance of

2 A FATE MAP OF THE ANTERIOR NEURAL PLATE

A fate map of a region of a developing organism shows what will become of each part of that region during subsequent development. It is also possible to follow the fate of individual cells, starting at any chosen point in development; we shall refer to this process as the analysis of cell lineage, and it is discussed further in Section 7. Later in this book we shall use the term map in a different context, to describe the spatially-ordered representation of one structure within another (for example, the representation of the surface of the retina on the visual cortex, as mediated by the axonal connections that form between them). There should be no confusion between the use of this word in these two contexts. By the time that axonal connections have developed between different regions of the forebrain, these regions have taken on adult-like appearances that makes their eventual fates relatively clear. By contrast, the fate-mapping of multicellular regions is a more useful exercise during very early development, when structures such as the neural tube have not yet assumed adult-like morphologies. It is crucial to note that a description of the fate of a region (or of an individual cell in the case of lineage studies) in normal development implies nothing about the degree to which it is irreversibly committed to that particular fate as opposed to other fates (as discussed later). This is equally true no matter how the fates of different regions or individual cells are worked out; the terms 'map', 'lineage', and 'fate' are used purely descriptively and carry no implications about mechanisms.

To draw a fate map, small groups of cells at specific points in a structure must be labelled so that they can be distinguished from the surrounding cells and followed during subsequent development. For example, molecules recognizable on the basis of fluorescence, radioactivity, or reactivity with a specific antibody may be injected at defined points. These techniques have the disadvantage that there is dilution of the label as cell division continues, limiting the period of time over which cell fate can be followed. An alternative approach which does not suffer from this problem is to take two closely related species whose cells are distinguishable from each other, graft tissue from a specific point in one species into the equivalent point in the other, and follow the fates of the grafted cells. Using such techniques, detailed fate maps of the neural plate have been obtained for the axolotl, *Xenopus*, zebrafish, and chick (Jacobson, 1959; Eagleson and Harris, 1990; Woo and Fraser, 1995; Rubenstein *et al.*, 1998). The available evidence indicates that the organization of

---

the forebrain of a mid-gestation mouse embryo, after folding of the neural plate to form the neural tube. (e) Appearance of the murine forebrain at around birth, seen from the dorsal aspect. The left cerebral hemisphere is cut open to show the position of the basal ganglia. A, anterior; P, posterior. (f) Diagram of the left cortex of an adult rodent, flattened and showing its major subdivisions. Abbreviations: di, diencephalon; e, eye; h, hypothalamus; os, optic stalk; pcp, prechordal plate; tel, telencephalon. (After Rubenstein and Beachy, 1998; Bayer and Altman, 1991).

(a)   **(b)**

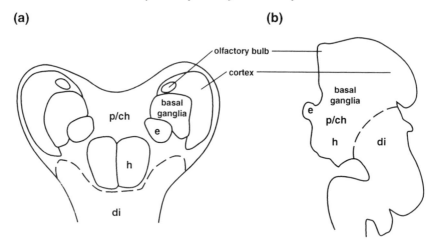

FIG. 2.4. (a) A fate map of the anterior neural plate. (b) Diagram of the embryonic brain showing the relative positions of the zones marked in (a). Abbreviations: di, diencephalon; e, eye; h, hypothalamus; p/ch, preoptic area and optic chiasm. (After Rubenstein *et al.*, 1998)

all vertebrate neural plates is highly conserved; this conservation probably extends to mammals, for which detailed fate maps are hard to obtain. Figure 2.4 shows a recently proposed fate map of the chick neural plate, supported by evidence from quail-into-chick grafts (Rubenstein *et al.*, 1998). Quail cells can be distinguished from chick cells using stains for a characteristic heterochromatic blob in their interphase nuclei (Le Douarin, 1982).

As can be seen in Fig. 2.4, the neural plate comprises a patchwork of regions that will give rise to the major forebrain structures. These primordial regions are laid out with the same topological relationships as their derivatives in the mature brain. Neither the cell movements of neurulation nor the disproportionate increase in the size of some of the neural plate primordia (e.g. the telencephalon and cerebral cortex) break their topological relationships, even though they change the three-dimensional structure of the forebrain so dramatically. At present, the fate maps of the anterior neural tube are rather coarse-grain; as technical improvements increase their resolution, it will be interesting to see the extent to which the subdivisions of the telencephalon and perhaps even of the cortex can be mapped on the neural plate.

3   THE DEVELOPING TELENCEPHALON

3.1   Anatomy

The principles of telencephalic development are similar in all species of mammal, although the timing varies. Corticogenesis is much faster in rodents than in carnivores and primates. Since much of our understanding of the mechanisms that regulate early forebrain development has come from studies of rodents, we shall continue to focus on embryogenesis in these species.

Figure 2.5 shows a series of sections through the developing telencephalon of the rodent embryo (for detailed atlases, refer to Bayer and Altman, 1991, Schambra and Silver, 1992 and Paxinos *et al.*, 1991). As the embryo enters the second half of gestation, the telencephalic vesicles appear as two dorsolateral expansions of the primary forebrain vesicle. These continue to enlarge, in the direction of the arrows in Fig. 2.5a (right). Over the following few days, the expansion of the telencephalic vesicles accelerates (Fig. 2.5b). They come to lie over the olfactory epithelium and their evaginated dorsolateral portions are now recognizable as primitive cerebral cortex. As shown in Fig. 2.5b, there is also an evagination of the more medial prosencephalic wall (marked di) to form diencephalic structures such as the thalamus, which surrounds the third ventricle. The disproportionate enlargement of the telencephalic vesicles continues (Fig. 2.5c); by the time of birth, its dorsal regions containing the developing cerebral cortex have ballooned to cover the diencephalon, which becomes situated deep within the brain. During this period, axons grow between subcortical structures such as the thalamus and the cortex (Fig. 2.5c); (De Carlos and O'Leary, 1992; Yuasa *et al.*, 1994; Molnar, 1998). These axons funnel through the ventral part of the telencephalon, forming a massive bundle of axons called the internal capsule. Next to the internal capsule is the region of neuroepithelium that will form the basal ganglia, usually referred to in the embryo as the ganglionic eminence (Fig. 2.5b,c).

Thus, by the time of birth, the major components of the telencephalon, including its afferent and efferent connections, are identifiable although they are by no means completely developed. As discussed later, axonal connections between the periphery and central structures are also in place from an early stage, allowing neuronal activity to start playing a role in further development (Chapters 3 and 4). By this stage, the telencephalon can be divided into two main regions, one ventral the other dorsal. The development of these two regions is discussed in the next section and mechanisms that regulate their different fates will be discussed in Chapter 3.

3.2   Specification of telencephalic regional identity

So far in this chapter we have provided a description of some of the early cellular events that take place within structures such as the neural plate, neural tube, telencephalon, and cerebral cortex during normal development. A major goal of current research is to understand how the fates of early neurectodermal cells are controlled at each stage of their proliferation, migration, and differentiation. Many workers in this field seek to explain how cells are guided along their developmental pathways and through their various decision points at a molecular level. Some of what we already know about the molecular regulation of early forebrain and cortical development is discussed in Chapter 3. Before looking at the regulatory

(a)

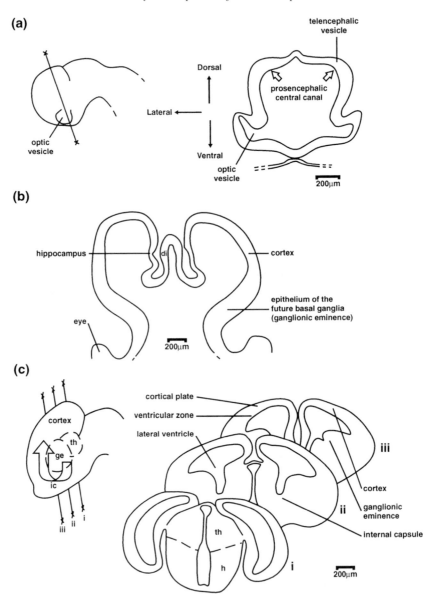

(b)

(c)

FIG. 2.5. (a) Section through the forebrain of a rodent embryo at around mid-gestation, cut at the level shown (X–X). Open arrows indicate the future growth of the telencephalic vesicles. (b) Section from a rodent embryo at a similar level to that in (a) but about two days later. The telencephalic vesicles have ballooned dorsally and laterally and are starting to cover the developing diencephalon (di). (c) Sections from a rodent embryo approaching birth, cut at three levels (i, ii, iii). The curved arrow shows the course taken by thalamocortical axons. These axons run from the thalamus (th) and penetrate the ganglionic eminence (ge) to form the internal capsule (ic). Abbreviation: h, hypothalamus. (After Bayer and Altman, 1991)

roles of specific molecules, we need to consider experiments designed to test the commitment of cells to the fates that they normally follow.

It is useful to distinguish between several processes in the commitment of cells to their particular fates. These are specification, determination, and potency.

1. If a cell or tissue is specified to become a particular cell type or structure, that means that it will develop autonomously into that structure during normal development, even if isolated from the rest of the embryo. Thus, a specified tissue is one that has some degree of information as to its fate and some degree of commitment to that fate. If perturbed it may still alter its fate; in other words, its commitment is reversible.

2. A cell or region that is determined differs from a specified one in that its commitment is irreversible, even if its environment is altered.

3. The potency of a cell or tissue is the total of all the fates that it can adopt if put into the appropriate environment. A pluripotent cell or tissue can develop into more than one type of cell or tissue; a totipotent cell or tissue can develop into any type of cell or tissue in the embryo.

During development of the telencephalon, a prominent anatomical boundary forms between its two main regions, the dorsal telencephalon (future cortex) and the ventral telencephalon (ganglionic eminence) (Fig. 2.4). Molecular analyses have shown that this is also a boundary in the expression domains of some regulatory genes such as Emx-1, Emx-2, and Pax-6, that are expressed in dorsal telencephalon, and Dlx genes, that are expressed in ventral telencephalon. As discussed further in this chapter, such genes may contribute to the specification of these two major anatomical regions of the telencephalon; but do the dorsal and ventral regions of the telencephalon develop independently?

One way to examine this issue is by studying the degree to which cells intermix between these two regions during their early development. Can these two regions be considered separate compartments, as defined in *Drosophila* embryology (Fishell, 1997)? This term was originally used to describe a multicellular region within which the progeny of every cell remain confined. Its use began in studies of the development of clones of cells in the imaginal discs of *Drosophila*. The anterior and posterior parts of the imaginal disc are compartments separated by a boundary at which there is no obvious barrier to cell mixing but which anterior and posterior clones do not normally cross (Garcia Bellido *et al.*, 1979). Further studies of these two compartments revealed that the regulatory gene *engrailed* is normally expressed in the posterior compartment but not in the anterior compartment but that if the expression of *engrailed* is disrupted, posterior clones can cross the boundary between the two regions. In this case, therefore, the evidence is that a difference in the expression of a regulatory gene restricts posterior and anterior cells to their own compartments. While it is true that different compartments may express different regulatory genes (which may confer on the cells in each compartment differences that prevent them intermingling), the converse is not necessarily the case: i.e. two regions are not necessarily different compartments just because they express different regulatory genes. Although there is evidence that cells in dorsal and ventral telencephalic regions aggregate preferentially with cells of their own type *in vitro* and that there may be less movement of cells across the border between ventral and dorsal telencephalic regions than within each region (Gotz *et al.*, 1996; Fishell, 1997), there is other evidence showing tangential migration of neurons (see below) across this border (Anderson *et al.*, 1997; De Carlos *et al.*, 1996). Probably it is unwise to consider the ventral and dorsal telencephalic regions as separate compartments.

Given that cells intermix between the dorsal and ventral telencephalon, another question concerns the degree to which precursor cells in these regions are committed to their different fates during embryogenesis. How can we learn what degree of commitment a telencephalic cell possesses at any given stage of its development? One approach that has been adopted is to challenge the cell by altering its environment and then examining whether this alters its fate. This is a useful approach, although it has the major limitation that it is not possible to alter a cell's environment in all possible ways and it is not possible to examine every aspects of the cell's fate. These limitations are sometimes ignored and this leads to inappropriate generalizations about a cell's commitment to the developmental path that it follows. It is possible to decide when a cell is not irreversibly committed (i.e. not determined) to a particular fate, meaning that its fate can be altered by challenging its development, for example by transplanting it to a new site. But it is not possible to conclude that a cell **is** irreversibly committed, in an absolute sense, only that it **remains** committed **under the given experimental condition**. To avoid reaching wrong conclusions, it is as well to adopt a strict terminology in the interpretation of experiments that address the issue of cell commitment.

In a recent series of experiments, from several laboratories, ventral telencephalic cells were dissociated and injected into the cerebral ventricles, offering them the potential to integrate not only into ventral telencephalic regions but also at other sites (Fishell, 1995; Campbell *et al.*, 1995; Brustle *et al.*, 1995). The overall conclusion from these studies was that ventral telencephalic cells are able to integrate and differentiate appropriately, in terms of their morphology, gene expression, and axonal connections, in other telencephalic regions. There were some differences between the details of the results of the different experiments, that probably resulted from differences in the ages of the transplanted cells and the methods used to prepare them (Fishell, 1997), but they all indicate that the regional fates of telencephalic cells are not determined (i.e. they are not irreversibly specified) during forebrain neurogenesis. Thus, it is likely that the phenotypes of embryonic telencephalic cells are determined by instructions not only from within the cells themselves but also from their environment. It is likely that each cell's internal instructions are influenced by environmental cues in that cell's history and that the potential of these cells to adopt a variety of fates is reduced as development advances. While there are clear differences between the dorsal and ventral regions of the telencephalon in terms of cell types, tissue morphology, gene expression, and so on, the origins of the instructions that confer these differences remain unknown.

4 ANATOMY OF THE DEVELOPING NEOCORTEX

As we have seen, the cerebral neocortex is the most prominent region to emerge from the dorsal telencephalon of the mammalian forebrain. In the adult, the neocortex has six principal layers, numbered 1 (most superficial) to 6. In some higher species, particularly primates, these are subdivided. The cortical layers have different appearances (due to their different complements of neuronal subtypes), different patterns of afferent and efferent axonal connections, and express different sets of genes. They are formed from the neuroepithelium of the dorsal telencephalon.

At the stage when the telencephalic vesicles bulge from the prosencephalon, they comprise only germinal neuroepithelium and present a relatively homogeneous appearance throughout their depth, with mitotic spindles of dividing cells visible close to the ventricular surface (Sauer, 1935; Uylings *et al.*, 1990; Bayer and Altman, 1991). Subsequent development involves the production of at least three broad classes of cell by division in the neuroepithelium: (i) postmitotic neurons (that will not redivide during the animal's lifetime); (ii) glial cells (that support the development and function of neurons); and (iii) new progenitor cells (that redivide to produce neurons and/or glia). In most species of mammal most postmitotic neurons are generated (or 'born', in the commonly used parlance of this field of research) prenatally. A newborn postmitotic neuron is initially referred to as a neuronal precursor cell, since it must undergo migration and differentiation before becoming a mature neuron. The major phase of gliogenesis occurs after neurogenesis is complete and continues postnatally. The large pools of progenitor cells of the developing cortex disappear postnatally, although there is evidence that some progenitors retain the ability to divide even in the adult and may therefore be classified as true stem cells which have been defined as retaining the ability to divide throughout the lifetime of an organism. Although most cortical progenitors are not stem cells by this definition they are sometimes described as such on the basis that they divide for a prolonged period (Lillien, 1998).

The sequence of events that leads to the production of the six-layered cerebral cortex from the neuroepithelium of the dorsal telencephalon is summarized in Fig. 2.6. Throughout corticogenesis, there are temporal gradients of maturation with anterior (sometimes termed rostral) and ventral regions developing ahead of posterior (sometimes termed caudal) and dorsal regions; in rodents, the less advanced regions lag behind the more advanced regions by one or two days-worth of development (the dorsoventral gradient is greater than the anteroposterior gradient). The first step in lamination of the dorsal telencephalic wall is its division into an inner layer of proliferating cells, called the ventricular zone (Boulder Committee, 1970), and an outer layer known as the primordial plexiform layer or the preplate (Fig. 2.6) (Marin-Padilla, 1971; Smart, 1983). The preplate contains prospective Cajal–Retzius cells, which have long tangential (i.e. parallel to the surface of the cortex) processes, as well as other polymorphous cells. This structure, proposed to be the mammalian homologue of a phylogenetically ancient (reptilian) cortex, may constitute a morphogenetic framework within which the main layers of the mature mammalian cortex develop (Marin-Padilla, 1971, 1978; Bayer and Altman, 1991). Cajal–Retzius cells are born in the ventricular zone early in cortical neurogenesis (Raedler and Raedler, 1978) and begin to differentiate before other cortical layers have begun to form (Cajal, 1911; Uylings *et al.*, 1990; Frotscher and Soriano, 1998).

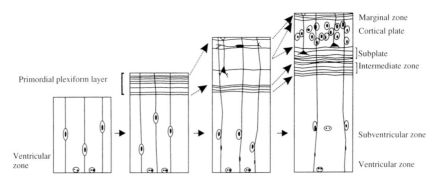

FIG.   2.6. Stratification of the cerebral wall. Cortical development begins with the appearance of a population of cells alongside the lateral ventricle, known as the ventricular zone (VZ). This population of cells gives rise to most of the neurons and glial cells of the cerebral cortex. Once generated, neurons migrate towards the pial surface and complete their differentiation in the cortical plate, which is the forerunner of the mature cerebral cortex. Both the generation and migration of neurons occurs over an extended period. Neurons for the deeper layers of the cortex are generated and then migrate away from the VZ earlier than the neurons destined for progressively more superficial layers. Following the cessation of neuronal production there is a massive production of astrocytes and oligodendrocytes, which continues postnatally. Two distinct proliferative populations arise from the original proliferative population which are referred to as the pseudostratified ventricular epithelium (PVE) and the secondary proliferative population (SPP). These two cell types differ in their distributions within the cell wall and also in their proliferative behaviour.

Cerebral stratification in the mouse. Neurogenesis in the mouse neocortex occurs from embryonic day 12–17 (E12–E17) (Gillies and Price, 1993a), whereas gliogenesis occurs after this, mostly postnatally. The PVE lies immediately adjacent to the ventricle and is present from the outset of evagination of the cerebral hemispheres. This population gives rise to the majority of neurons within the neocortex, but is also a proliferative zone for the radial glial cells of the astroglial lineage.

Apart from the radial glial cells the first born neocortical cells normally form two layers, one above and one below the developing cortical plate, known as the marginal zone and the subplate. This has been studied by injecting bromodeoxyuridine into pregnant animals on E11 and looking at this distribution of labelled cells at various time points post-injection. By studying the distribution of cells labelled on E11 and E13 it appears that the majority of these cells form the subplate, with slightly less that are destined for the marginal zone. Shortly after birth these cells appear to have disappeared and it is thought that they die (Price *et al.*, 1997). On E13–E14, the cerebral wall is bilaminar consisting primarily of the VZ and overlying primitive plexiform layer comprising approximately 70% and 30% of the total width of the cerebral wall respectively. This increase in width of the VZ is due to cells of the PVE dividing rapidly to increase the size of the population of progenitors.

As the cortex thickens, two additional layers appear above the ventricular zone, namely the intermediate zone and the cortical plate (Fig. 2.6). The intermediate zone, immediately overlying the ventricular zone, contains a lower density of non-mitotic cells; the cortical plate, lying superficial to the intermediate zone in the midst of the preplate, is composed of densely-packed cells. The intermediate zone will eventually contain the major afferent and efferent axonal tracts of the cerebral cortex (future white matter) and the expanding cortical plate will transform into layers 2–6 of the cerebral cortex. The formation of the cortical plate splits the preplate into superficial and deep components, called the marginal zone and sub-plate respectively (Fig. 2.6). The marginal zone will eventually form layer 1 of the adult cortex. The subplate is a transient structure containing highly differentiated neurons (Allendoerfer and Shatz, 1994), at least many of which are fated to die postnatally (this is discussed further below).

As the cortical plate emerges, another layer becomes visible between the ventricular and intermediate zones, the subventricular zone (Fig. 2.6). This cell-dense zone contains dividing cells and is a secondary germinal layer set up by cells produced in the ventricular zone. Initially, it is thinner than the ventricular zone

---

At E14 mitosis is restricted to the lining of the ventricular surface. However, mitoses at a distance from the ventricular edge, signalling the emergence of the SPP, are initially recognized on E13 at the outer margin of the VZ. (The SPP arises from the PVE, but tends to have a more diffuse and widespread distribution extending from the interface of the VZ and subventricular zone or SVZ, outward across the whole width of the intermediate zone.) When the SPP first emerges at the outer margin of the VZ it consists only of 11% of the total proliferative population. At E14–E16 the proliferative population of the cerebral wall is therefore constituted of cells of the SPP and PVE. Over the next 24 hours full stratification of the cerebral wall emerges. At E15 the VZ has reached its maximum thickness and then declines to approximately 50% of its maximum value by the end of E16. In the E15–E16 interval there is a dramatic change in the relative abundance of cells of the PVE and SPP. The number of SPP cells increases more than twice, contributing to 35% of the total proliferative population of the cerebral wall (a 300% increase over 48 hours), whilst that of the PVE is reduced by nearly 40%. In contrast to the reduction in width of the VZ and corresponding dramatic reduction in cell numbers in the PVE, the rest of the cortical strata (molecular layer, cortical plate, intermediate zone and SVZ) increase in width through E16. Although the subplate is still present at this point it starts to decrease in width until it has completely disappeared shortly after. Between E16 and E18 a similar pattern is observed. By E17 the PVE ceases to exist while the proliferative activity of the SPP continues postnatally and eventually becomes confined to the subependymal layer. Although the SPP is still proliferatively active, the SVZ reduces dramatically in width at a similar time to the disappearance of the subplate. These proliferating cells hence tend to be located in the overlying intermediate zone/white matter and the single cell layer of ependymal cells. This ependymal layer is present in adulthood and is thought to contain a population of neural stem cells. Differences in the properties and proliferative behaviours of the SPP and PVE reflect upon the two distinct histogenic roles of the two populations. The PVE is the source of neurons whereas the SPP is the source of glial cell types (not radial glial).

By E18/E19 the thickness of the overlying intermediate zone/white matter and developing cortical plate are at their maximum widths, with all neuronal cells having exited the cell cycle and migrated to their final laminar distribution within the developing cortex.

but it gradually enlarges. Late in gestation, by which stage the ventricular zone is disappearing, it is considerably thicker than the ventricular zone (Fig. 2.7) (Bayer and Altman, 1991). Its borders with the ventricular zone and the intermediate zone are not always easy to define, particularly late in embryogenesis. Its appearance is different from that of the ventricular zone: the radial rows of cell bodies seen in the ventricular zone are lost in the subventricular zone. The intermediate zone has been defined by the absence of mitotic cells or by the presence of tangential fibres, but the exact position of its border with the subventricular zone varies with the method used (Uylings *et al.*, 1990). Figure 2.7 summarizes the development of the cortical wall, the disappearance of some of its transient layers, and the main products of cell division at each stage.

5 CELL PROLIFERATION AND MIGRATION IN NEOCORTICAL DEVELOPMENT

The cellular processes that underlie the anatomical changes described in the preceding section have been well studied in a wide range of species over the past several decades. Essentially, these processes involve the generation of neurons at or near to the ventricular side of the cortical wall and their subsequent migration towards the pial surface, where they differentiate (Angevine and Sidman, 1961; Rakic, 1974, 1988, 1997; Lund and Mustari, 1977; Smart and Smart, 1982; Luskin and Shatz, 1985a,b; Shatz and Luskin, 1986; Jackson *et al.*, 1989; Gillies and Price, 1993a; Caviness *et al.*, 1995).

Both the processes of cortical cell proliferation and migration can be studied by labelling DNA during its replication. Tritiated thymidine, and the now commonly used thymidine analogue bromodeoxyuridine (BrdU), are small chemicals readily taken up by cells and incorporated into newly synthesized DNA. Since they are cleared from the circulatory system within hours of being injected into an animal, they can be used to label selectively those cells undergoing cell division at the time of administration. Provided the labelled cells do not undergo numerous redivisions before the tissue is examined, which would dilute the tritiated thymidine or bromodeoxyuridine in the DNA, they can be identified in histological sections. This condition is met for newly generated neurons. These cells do not redivide and can be labelled during neurogenesis in the embryo and identified at any later age, right through adulthood, by autoradiography in the case of tritiated thymidine and with an antibody in the case of bromodeoxyuridine.

5.1 Proliferation

The cell cycles of eukaryotic cells can be divided into four successive phases (Fig. 2.8a). These are (i) M phase (M stands for mitosis), during which the nucleus and cytoplasm divide, (ii) G1 phase (G stands for gap), between the end of M phase and the onset of DNA synthesis, (iii) S phase (S stands for synthesis), during which

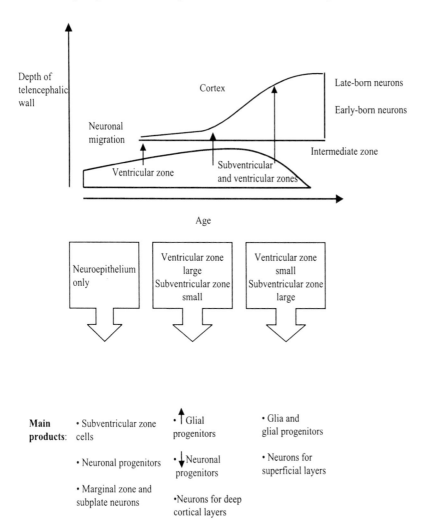

F I G .   2 . 7 .   Diagram illustrating the changes in the relative thicknesses of the proliferative zones (the ventricular and subventricular zones) and the cortex (cortical plate, marginal
zone, and subplate) in the dorsal telencephalic wall during embryogenesis and very early
postnatal life. Initially, at around mid-gestation, the telencephalic wall comprises mostly
proliferating cells. These cells form the primordial plexiform layer (which is later split to
form the marginal zone and subplate) and contribute to the subventricular zone. Later on,
neurons start to migrate to form the cortex (deep layers first, superficial layers later). As
embryonic development continues, the ventricular zone shrinks and the subventricular zone
becomes the larger component of the proliferative zone. Most glial cells are produced after
neurogenesis is finished. Around birth and in the early postnatal period, the proliferative
zone disappears. (After Caviness *et al.*, 1997; Bayer and Altman, 1991)

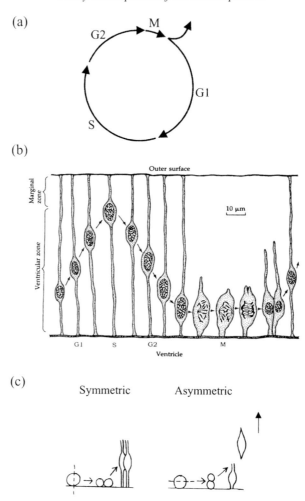

FIG.   2.8.   (a) The four phases of the cell cycle. (b) Diagram of a section through the early telencephalic wall, showing the movement of the nuclei of the progenitor cells (called interkinetic movement) during the four phases of the cell cycle. Cells divide at the ventricular edge but undergo S phase away from it. (c) Diagrams showing how progenitors may divide symmetrically, to generate two new progenitors, or asymmetrically, to generate one new progenitor and a neuronal precursor which migrates away towards the pial surface.

DNA in the nucleus is replicated, and (iv) G2 phase, between the end of S phase and the next M phase. The length of the cell cycle varies enormously, depending on the cell type and the stage of development. Most of the variation is in the length of the G1 phase. Some cells, such as neurons, become arrested in G1 phase in a quiescent state known at G0. The lengths of the different phases of the cell cycle can be measured by administering substances such as tritiated thymidine and/or bromodeoxyuridine, that are incorporated into newly synthesized DNA. When these substances are given as a single pulse (which lasts for up to several hours if it is from an injection into an animal) to a population of cells that is growing steadily and in which all the cells are proliferating at similar rates, the proportion of cells that are labelled will reflect the overall length of their cell cycles relative to the length of their S phases. High proportions of labelled cells indicate that their S phases occupy a large portion of their cell cycles (as it turns out, S phase varies less in duration than other phases, and so this outcome is most likely to be because the cells are proliferating rapidly, i.e. their overall cell cycle times are short); low proportions of labelled cells indicate the opposite. This approach can be extended: by varying the time between the administration of the tritiated thymidine or bromodeoxyuridine and the counting of the labelled cells, by successive administrations to give a variable length of pulse, or by administering first one type of label and later the other, the lengths of the four phases of the cell cycle can be deduced.

Many studies have used these methods to characterize the proliferative process in the developing cortex throughout neurogenesis (Waechter and Jaensch, 1972; Schultze and Korr, 1981; Schmahl, 1983; Takahashi *et al.*, 1992a,b, 1993, 1994, 1995a, 1996; Miller and Kuhn, 1995). These studies have shown that the overall length of the cell cycle increases progressively throughout cortical neurogenesis, becoming nearly twice as long at the end of this period as at the beginning. As in other cell types elsewhere in the body, this is due to the lengthening of the G1 phase; neither S phase nor G2 and M phases vary systematically during neurogenesis.

During the cell cycle, ventricular cell nuclei move intracellularly. In S phase (DNA replication; Fig. 2.8a) the nuclei are away from the lumenal surface of the ventricular zone, and in G2 they move to the ventricular surface to undergo mitosis (Fig. 2.8b) (Sidman *et al.*, 1959; Fujita, 1964). It has been assumed for some time, supported by recent evidence from Chenn and McConnell (1995), that there are two types of cell division in the ventricular zone, symmetric and asymmetric (Fig. 2.8c) (Mione *et al.*, 1997). Symmetric division by vertical cleavage may generate daughters that both become stem cells. Asymmetric division by horizontal cleavage may generate one daughter that migrates to the cortical plate and one that remains as a stem cell in the ventricular zone. Thus it is suggested that symmetric divisions may be more common early in corticogenesis, when the pool of stem cells is expanding, and asymmetric divisions may be more common later in corticogenesis, when neuronal production is greater. These observations suggest a relationship between the rates and the types of division in the ventricular zone and they raise two intriguing possibilities: whatever regulates the proliferation rate may also regulate cleavage type, ensuring that it is appropriate for the acquired rate; that the factors that regulate proliferation rate may do so by acting primarily on the type of cleavage. A major challenge for future research is to test these hypotheses.

Although this descriptive framework for early cortical neurogenesis is now well-established, numerous questions remain. One major issue concerns the way in which region-specific numbers of neurons, glia, and progenitor cells are regulated during development. Given that the telencephalon becomes relatively much larger than other forebrain regions, its net production of neurons and glia must outstrip that of the other areas. At a finer level, the net production of neurons and glia is likely to vary between regions of the telencephalon itself and within its subdivisions, including the cerebral cortex. The number of neurons and glia in a region of adult forebrain, telencephalon, or cortex will be the result of the number produced in that region plus the number that migrate into it, minus the number that die in that region and/or migrate away from it. As we shall see below, there is evidence that significant numbers of cells migrate between some regions of the developing forebrain and even between regions of the cortex itself (referred to as tangential migration), despite the predominance of the radial migratory pathway described below. With regards to cell death, recent evidence suggests that the removal of significant numbers of cells occurs from a very early time, beginning during cortical neurogenesis itself and continuing into postnatal life (Finlay and Slattery, 1983; Finlay and Pallas, 1989; Blaschke *et al.*, 1996). The mechanisms that may regulate cell death in the developing cortex are discussed in Chapter 6. Although differential rates of cell death may contribute to the development of cortical regions with different histological appearances (or cytoarchitectonics), it is not yet clear to what extent they contribute to the overall differences in cell numbers between different regions of the forebrain and cortex. With regards to the initial proliferation of cells in the different regions of the anterior CNS, recent work has shown that different regions of the forebrain and cortex have different proliferative rates (Warren and Price, 1997; Dehay *et al.*, 1993). At the level of the major subdivisions of the forebrain (i.e. into the telencephalic and diencephalic vesicles), it is now recognized that some regulatory genes have region-specific patterns of expression at the anterior end of the neural plate and neural tube and can control region-specific proliferative rates (Xuan *et al.*, 1995; Warren and Price, 1997). Secreted growth factors, many of which may play multiple roles throughout forebrain and cortical development, may also be important in regulating proliferative rates. Regulatory genes and secreted factors that may control the emergence of forebrain regions each with specific characteristics, including specific numbers of cells, are discussed in Chapter 3.

At the level of the cerebral cortex, mechanisms must be in place to regulate temporal changes in neuronal and glial proliferation. Cortical neurogenesis begins relatively slowly but later accelerates until, near the end of embryogenesis, neurogenesis gives way to gliogenesis (Caviness *et al.*, 1995). In addition, the rates of cortical neurogenesis may be regulated spatially. For example, Dehay *et al.* (1993) have shown that proliferative rates vary between different regions of the ventricular zone in primates. How region-specific rates of production of cortical neurons, and perhaps later glial cells, are regulated remains mysterious. Recent *in vitro* experiments have suggested that diffusible factors released by the thalamus can influence the parameters of the cell cycle of cortical progenitors (Kennedy and Dehay, 1997). *In vivo*, such factors may be provided to the developing cortex by thalamocortical afferents, with differences between proliferation rates in different areas being related to the presence, absence, or differences in the nature of these afferents (Kennedy and Dehay, 1997).

5.2   Cell migration

The suggestion that neurons migrate was first made over a hundred years ago, but experimental evidence had to wait for the development of electron microscopy and tritiated thymidine autoradiography in the latter part of this century. As a result of the use of these techniques, the principle that neurons migrate during cortical neurogenesis is now well established. As discussed below, there is still considerable ambiguity regarding the processes of cortical gliogenesis. This topic has received less attention probably in part because many glial cells continue to divide as an animal ages, making them harder to study with DNA labelling methods.

Early in the ultrastructural analysis of cortical neurogenesis, it was realized that postmitotic neuronal precursors generated in the proliferative region of the neuroepithelium migrate through the intermediate zone (future white matter) in close apposition to the elongated shafts of glial cells that span the cortical wall, termed radial glial cells (Fig. 2.9). Radial glial cells are formed early in cortical neurogenesis. They persist throughout the period of neuronal migration, during which time they stop dividing temporarily and guide and support the migration of at least a large proportion of cortical neuronal precursors (Schmechel and Rakic, 1979). As shown in Fig. 2.9b, migrating neurons contact the processes of other cell types as they traverse the intermediate zone, but they appear to have a preferential adhesion to radial glial processes (Rakic *et al.*, 1994; Rakic, 1997). The molecular mechanisms that may underlie this gliophilic migration are discussed in Chapter 3.

Neuronal precursors migrate in the order in which they are generated. The first-born neurons form a continuous population around the edge of the telencephalon (the preplate; Fig. 2.6). This population is later split tangentially by cells migrating to form the cortical plate. The earliest generated cells become distributed either superficial to the cortical plate in the marginal zone (future layer 1), where they form the earliest differentiating neurons (the Cajal–Retzius cells), or deep to the cortical plate in the subplate, a transient structure (discussed later) that may have considerable importance for the development of cortical circuitry (Luskin and Shatz, 1985b; Wahle and Meyer, 1987; Ghosh *et al.*, 1990; Wood *et al.*, 1992). Neuronal precursors that form the deep layers of the cortical plate itself are born earlier than those destined for superficial layers. As cells arrive in the cortical plate they assume progressively more superficial positions. Thus, the main cortical layers are normally laid down from inside to outside and, as has been known since the early 1900s, differentiation follows the same sequence (Cajal, 1911). These events are illustrated using our own data on mouse development in Fig. 2.10 (Gillies and Price, 1993a). Although the timing of layer formation differs enormously between species, lasting from several days in rodents to many weeks in primates, the pattern of development shown in Fig. 2.10 is the same.

(a)

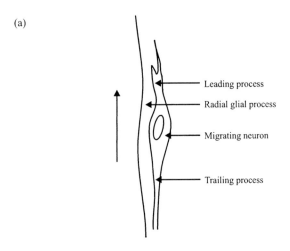

- Leading process
- Radial glial process
- Migrating neuron
- Trailing process

(b)

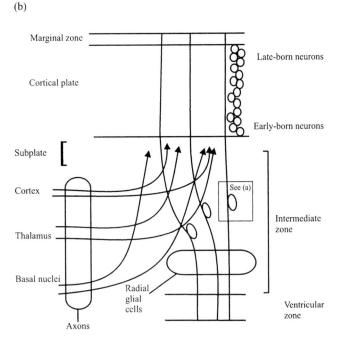

Marginal zone

Late-born neurons

Cortical plate

Early-born neurons

Subplate

See (a)

Cortex

Intermediate zone

Thalamus

Basal nuclei

Radial glial cells

Ventricular zone

Axons

F IG .   2 . 9 . (a) Diagram of a migrating cortical neuronal precursor travelling along a radial glial fibre, in the direction of the arrow. (b) Illustrates the major components of the environment through which cortical neuronal precursors migrate. As migration proceeds, axons are arriving in the developing cortex from other cortical areas (callosal and ipsilateral corticocortical axons) and from subcortical structures (such as the thalamus and basal nuclei). (After Rakic, 1997)

(a)

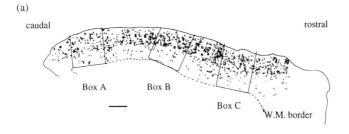

(b)

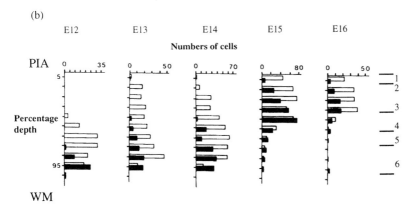

FIG. 2.10. (a) Camera lucida drawing of a parasagittal section through the left cerebral cortex of a normal mature mouse that had been injected with bromodeoxyuridine on
embryonic day 15. The positions of all labelled cells are marked by dots. Three areas of
the cortex were selected for analysis (Boxes A, B, and C). WM, white matter; scale bar,
0.5 mm. (b) Quantitative analysis of results shown in (a). Histograms of numbers of bromodeoxyuridine labelled cells (filled bars, densely labelled, born on embryonic day 15;
open bars, lightly labelled, many are born later than embryonic day 15) against depth, as
a percentage of the distance from the pial surface to the grey matter/white matter (WM)
border. Data are from Box A in mice that had been injected on embryonic days (E) 12, 13,
14, 15, 16. Positions of cortical layers are indicated on the *right*. Note that the deep layers
are created before the superficial layers. (Gillies and Price, 1993a)

Another issue that has attracted attention in recent years concerns the significance of the cortical precursors that do not follow a strictly radial pathway but
become dispersed in a tangential direction (Hatten, 1993; Rakic, 1995). O'Rourke
et al. (1992) studied the migration of cells through the intermediate zone in cultured explants of the developing telencephalon of ferrets. They observed that,
although the majority followed the direction of the radial glia, a significant proportion migrated orthogonal to the radial glia. This *in vitro* finding is supported
by *in vivo* evidence that many migrating neurons are oriented non-radially and

that neurons may use substrates other than glial cells (e.g. axons) in novel ways to migrate tangentially (Valverde *et al.*, 1989; O'Rourke *et al.*, 1995). Further studies have shown tangentially oriented postmitotic neurons in the ventricular and sub-ventricular zones and have demonstrated that these cells can migrate long distances within these regions (O'Rourke *et al.*, 1997; Menezes and Luskin, 1994). These results indicate that a model of corticogenesis based entirely on radial migration, as illustrated in Fig. 2.9, needs modification, although it is important to bear in mind that the proportions of cells that deviate from the radial pathway may vary from species to species. In addition to these reports of the tangential movements of postmitotic neuronal precursors in the intermediate and proliferative zones, there is evidence that progenitor cells (cells that will undergo division to generate postmi-totic cells) also move tangentially within the ventricular zone (Fishell *et al.*, 1993; Reid *et al.*, 1995). Part of this evidence comes from studies using retroviruses to examine lineally related cells (discussed in Section 7). As yet, it is not clear what cellular and molecular processes and substrates guide these tangential migrations. It is possible that the cells that follow them have distinct fates in the mature cortex (Anderson *et al.*, 1997).

In addition to tangential migration within the cortex, there is good evidence for the movement of neuronal precursors over long distances between forebrain structures, including the olfactory bulb, the lateral ganglionic eminence (Figs 2.4 and 2.5), and the cerebral cortex. For example, interneurons of the olfactory bulb originate in the telencephalic subventricular zone. Their migration is not guided by glial cells or axonal processes, but rather the cells move over one another in a process described as chain migration (Wichterle *et al.*, 1997; Lois *et al.*, 1996). This process, which is dependent on N-CAM (neural cell adhesion molecule) and which persists into adulthood, is a further illustration of the fact that neurons use multiple strategies to migrate in the forebrain. It seems very likely that several recognized or as yet unknown methods may be used by migrating neuronal precursors even within a single structure such as the cerebral cortex, perhaps with different forms of migration predominating at particular times in development.

Other tangential migrations of neurons into the cerebral cortex include the move-ment of precursors from the subventricular zone in and around the olfactory bulb into the marginal zone, over the entire cortex, and the tangential migration of cells from the lateral ganglionic eminence into the marginal and intermediate zones of the cortex. The former migration is thought to contribute neurons called subpial granule cells that, together with the Cajal–Retzius cells (see above), comprise the major cell types in the marginal zone (Gadisseux *et al.*, 1992). The latter migration is thought to contribute a substantial number of GABAergic interneurons to the cortex (De Carlos *et al.*, 1996; Anderson *et al.*, 1997) and is dependent on the expression of the regulatory genes Dlx1 and 2 (see Chapter 3) (Anderson *et al.*, 1997). The results of these studies of tangential cell migrations indicate that the cerebral cortex is not generated exclusively by the progenitor cells within it, but that it receives a major contribution of cells from adjacent anatomically distinct regions.

6 THE SWITCH FROM NEUROGENESIS TO GLIOGENESIS

Although many studies of the development of the CNS focus on the formation of neurons, there are about ten times as many glial cells as neurons in the mature brain. It is widely accepted that the main role of glial cells is to support the development and function of neurons, although it is likely that we do not yet know their full repertoire of activities. The specialized function of radial glial cells in guiding migration, described above, is a good example of how glia act in development. In the adult CNS, the best understood glial cells are the oligodendrocytes, which wrap themselves around the axons to provide their insulating myelin sheaths. These sheaths are essential for neurons to transmit action potentials at an appropriate speed (in the peripheral nervous system, myelin sheaths are provided by Schwann cells). Apart from oligodendocytes, the CNS contains astrocytes, ependymal cells, and microglia (Fig. 2.11). Astrocytes are plentiful, but their functions are less clear than those of oligodendrocytes. They have many processes radiating from the cell body. These may end on the surfaces of neurons, on the external surface of the CNS or on endothelial cells of blood vessels in the CNS (where they contribute to the blood–brain barrier, which regulates the passage of molecules into the brain and hence controls the environment of its neurons). Ependymal cells line the central cavity of the CNS, the central canal of the spinal cord and the ventricles of the forebrain, formed after neural tube closure, and may help to regulate the chemical composition of both the CNS and the fluid which bathes it and fills its central cavity (the cerebrospinal fluid). Microglia are the equivalent of the macrophages found elsewhere in the body. These cell types have the capacity to ingest large particles, such as micro-organisms and cellular debris, in a process called phagocytosis. They originate from haemopoietic (blood-forming) tissue.

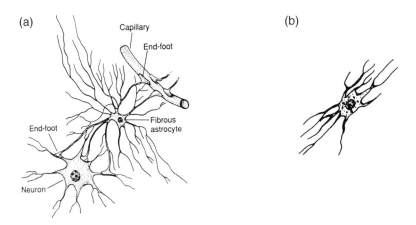

FIG. 2.11. Drawings of two of the four types of glial cell found in the cerebral cortex. (a) Astrocyte. (b) Oligodendrocyte. (After Kandel *et al.*, 1991)

With the exception of microglia, the glial cells of the CNS share a common embryonic origin with the neurons. As neurectodermal cells divide, migrate, and differentiate, at some point each must follow a specific developmental pathway leading to the differentiation of it or its descendants into one of the numerous glial or neuronal cell types in the mature CNS. The complexity of the developing CNS, in terms of such factors as the numbers of cells that it contains, their ability to migrate from region to region, and its heterogeneity, makes an analysis of the developmental pathways open to and taken by individual cells in the CNS a daunting task even in discrete anatomical regions such as the cortex. Experiments which attempt to trace the lineage of cells in the CNS (i.e. their lines of descent) have shed some light on this issue and are described in the following section. Other experiments have studied the routes by which populations of neurons and glia develop, for example by labelling cohorts of cells born on a particular day with tritiated thymidine or bromodeoxyuridine and following their fates. This approach is described above for neurogenesis; its application to the study of gliogenesis is more complicated. First, many glial cells have the potential to redivide throughout an organism's life (which means they may lose markers incorporated into their DNA) and, secondly, the approach requires the experimenter to recognize if cells carrying a DNA marker are glial. This would be best achieved with the use of glial-specific molecular markers, but as yet there are relatively few that are suitable (Cameron and Rakic, 1991).

Despite these problems, several conclusions have been reached concerning the development of populations of glial cells in the cortex. It is well accepted that, although some glial cells appear early in cortical development, the vast majority are generated after neurogenesis is complete. In general, therefore, there is a switch from the production of predominantly neurons to the production of glia. This occurs during late gestation in many species. At around this time, once neuronal migration is complete, the early generated radial glial cells transform into astrocytes (Schmechel and Rakic, 1979; Levitt and Rakic, 1980; Pixley and De Vellis, 1984; Benjelloum Toumi *et al.*, 1985; Misson *et al.*, 1988, 1991; Voigt, 1989; Takahashi *et al.*, 1990; Culican *et al.*, 1990; Cameron and Rakic, 1991; Goldman and Vaysse, 1991). Proliferation of cells near to the ventricular surface of the cortical wall gives rise to both cortical neurons and cortical glia although, as for cortical neurons, it is possible that some cortical glia migrate into the cortex having arisen from progenitors in adjacent structures. During neurogenesis, some of the cells born in the proliferative zone of the cortical wall do not migrate into the cortical plate but form a secondary proliferative population in the subventricular zone (Fig. 2.6; Bayer and Altman, 1991; Takahashi *et al.*, 1992a, 1995b). The nuclei of these cells do not undergo interkinetic movement as they progress through the stages of the cell cycle (an event seen during neurogenesis, Fig. 2.8). This secondary proliferative population is thought to be a major source of cortical glial cells, contributing both astrocytes (additional to those formed by the transformation of radial glia) and oligodendrocytes (Gressens *et al.* 1992; our unpublished observations).

7 CELL LINEAGE

To consider the possible mechanisms generating the cortex, we must have a reasonably detailed description of how the cells of the cortex behave during its development. Ideally, we would start with a complete description of the routes by which the different cell types are generated, i.e. their lineages. In the embryos of simple invertebrates whose development is discernably invariant from individual to individual, it is relatively straightforward to trace normal cell lineages. In these species, such observational studies, which require little more than a good microscope, were begun over a hundred years ago (Whitman, 1878, 1887), and have formed the basis for subsequent experimental manipulations aimed at elucidating the mechanisms that determine each cell's fate (Weisblat *et al.*, 1978; Weisblat and Shankland, 1985). In theory, similar processes of observation and experiment can be applied to the developing cortex; in practice, the complexity and inaccessibility of this tissue means that even to observe the behaviour of its cells requires the application of complex techniques that often carry with them problems of interpretation. Even when the techniques have been developed, the invariance of cell lineage seen in invertebrates may not be present. Thus, much of the work on the development of the cortex has been descriptive, and inevitably the distinction between observation and experiment is blurred.

The lineage of a cell is a description of its ancestry; from another point of view, precursor cells produce mature cells via a line of descent or lineage. For simpler organisms such as the leech, it is useful to ask questions about the lineal relationships of *individual* cells in the adult organism (Weisblat *et al.*, 1978; Weisblat and Shankland, 1985), but in the cerebral cortex such considerations can only concern different cell types. There is an immense range of neuronal and glial phenotypes in the mature cerebral cortex; cortical cells with similar functional or morphological properties can be placed in groups whose sizes and number depend on the criteria used to define them. Clearly, all the different cortical cells have a common origin and all derive from neurectodermal cells. It would be of great interest to know whether, at particular developmental stages, cortical precursors give rise to only one class of cell, or to a specific set of classes. The discovery of stereotyped lineages would allow us to ask more useful questions about the mechanisms controlling the development of certain classes of cell, as is possible for individual cells in simpler organisms. However, the experiments required to study cell lineages in the cerebral cortex are far from straightforward. Apart from the problems of categorizing different cells in the mature cortex, there are the major problems that the pool of precursors in the ventricular zone appears relatively homogeneous and is inaccessible. Different types of precursor cannot be individually identified, as they can be in invertebrates, and so their lineages cannot be studied directly. But, despite these and other more technical problems, methods have been devised that have led to some tentative conclusions about the lineages of very broad classes of cortical cell, namely pyramidal, non-pyramidal, and glial cells of ectodermal origin (i.e. excluding blood-derived microglia, see Section 2.6). It is encouraging that these conclusions are to some extent similar to those for lineages in the retina, that have been deduced with methods that can not be applied to the cortex (Turner and Cepko, 1987; Holt *et al.*, 1988; Wetts and Fraser, 1988). While the mature retina and cerebral cortex have obvious structural and functional differences, they both arise from the prosencephalon and the preservation of some developmental mechanisms might be expected. However, it is important to appreciate that conclusions from work on cell lineage in the cerebral cortex remain controversial, and consensus on some issues may take several more years of detailed experimentation. In addition, recent data has led to the astonishing conclusion that up to 70% of cortical cells may die during development (Blaschke *et al.*, 1996), and this has implications for studies of both cerebral cell proliferation and lineage. The possibility that massive cell death might eliminate entire branches of lineage trees before clonally related cells are examined implies that current data may severely underestimate clonal sizes.

Most conventional lineage tracers are enzymes (such as horseradish peroxidase) or fluorescent molecules (such as lysinated rhodamine dextran) that are injected intracellularly and are carried over into the progeny of a cell as it divides. One important limitation with such methods is that, after many cell divisions the injected substance will become very dilute and may no longer be detectable. The study of cell lineages in the cerebral cortex has become possible through the use of retroviral markers, where there is no such dilution. The life cycle of a retrovirus includes the incorporation of its genome into that of the infected cell (Varmus, 1988) (Fig. 2.12). A wild-type retrovirus normally directs the cell it has infected to produce new retroviral particles that can then infect other cells. By manipulating the genome of the retrovirus it is possible to prevent the creation of new particles in an infected cell. It is also possible to introduce into the viruses genes that code for molecules that are detectable by histochemistry. One example is the lacZ gene that codes for β-galactosidase, a bacterial enzyme that acts on 5-bromo-4-chloro-3-indolyl-β-D-galactopyranoside (X-gal) to produce a blue colour in the cell. More recently, alkaline phosphatase has been used as a histochemical marker (Reid *et al.*, 1995). This has the advantage of producing an intense staining of the cells and their processes, allowing a finer level of analysis of their morphologies. When an engineered retrovirus infects a cell, its genome should be incorporated into that of the host cell and be passed on to all its progeny, without being transferred to cells that are not clonally related. Clearly, then, genetically engineered retroviruses have the potential to be very powerful lineage tracers. Engineered retroviruses do not need to be injected intracellularly, a procedure that would be very difficult in the ventricular zone. Instead, the viruses can be injected into the ventricular space of the cerebral vesicles in a concentration that is calculated to produce only a small number of infections per fetus. Thus, when the cortex is studied at a later stage, only a small number of labelled cells should be found.

In the first studies that used these methods, it was assumed that if labelled cells were clustered together they were clonally related. This was a problem as the extent and direction of movement of neurons was unknown. On the hypothesis

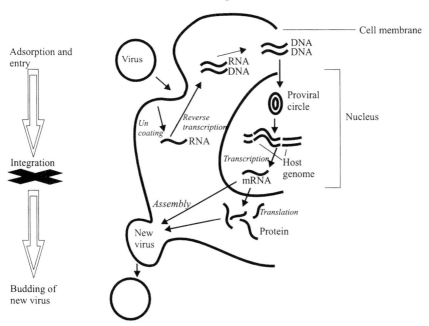

F I G .   2 . 12 . Life cycle of a wild-type retrovirus. Retroviruses enter the host cell through an interaction at the host cell surface. The viral genome is in the form of RNA and this is reverse transcribed into DNA. The DNA enters the nucleus in a double-stranded circular or linear form and is integrated into the host genome. A wild-type replication competent virus makes more virus by expressing viral structural genes. Viruses used for lineage tracing do not include the genes for production of new retroviral particles, blocking the second half of the process (✖).

that cortical neurons migrate on radial glial fibres from the ventricular zone to the cortical plate (Rakic, 1972, 1988), it was reasonable to assume that sequentially generated daughter cells from one neuroepithelial stem cell might move radially along the same or adjacent glial cells and so end up very close together in the cortex. Rakic (1988) postulated that this process leads to the production of ontogenetic columns, in which the daughter cells of each stem cell lie above each other in the radial direction with the younger cells being progressively more superficial. However, other evidence has suggested that there is considerable lateral spread of cells migrating from the ventricular zone to the cortical plate. Although early retroviral studies of lineage in the developing neocortex indicated that a clone of cells descended from a single progenitor can spread laterally by up to 0.5 mm (Luskin *et al.*, 1988; Price and Thurlow, 1988; Walsh and Cepko, 1988; Austin and Cepko, 1990), subsequent work has shown that clones can spread tangentially over much wider distances.

The most recent work on cortical lineages has avoided this problem by using libraries of retroviral vectors carrying a large number of DNA tags, each of which can be distinguished by the polymerase chain reaction (PCR) (Reid *et al.*, 1995). Essentially, the method involves the injection of a library of such vectors. After development is complete and retrovirally labelled cells have been detected, each labelled cell is dissected from the tissue and analysed by polymerase chain reaction. As there are relatively few infections after injection, and a large number of different tags, there is an insignificantly small probability that labelled cells carrying the same tags are derived from more than one infection. Using this method, Reid *et al.* (1995) have shown that, as previous studies had hinted, many clones are very widely dispersed throughout the cortex. Indeed, they found some clones that spanned both neocortical and non-neocortical areas, such as hippocampus, piriform cortex, and perirhinal cortex (providing further evidence that different telencephalic regions are not separated from each other by lineage-restriction boundaries and would not be considered as compartments; see Section 3.2).

Reid *et al.* (1995) found that clonally related cells were distributed in clusters which were not randomly distributed (each of which would correspond to the clusters analysed in earlier studies). They suggested that these clusters are generated by the tangential movement of precursor cells through the ventricular zone (Fig. 2.13). Such a hypothesis is in good agreement with previous reports of cell movement in the ventricular zone *in vitro* (Fishell *et al.*, 1993). Moreover, these findings imply that migratory multipotential progenitors divide to produce non-migratory precursors that then divide several times to generate clusters of neurons. This hypothesis is in agreement with data from the use of retroviral tracers in primates (Kornack and Rakic, 1995), and with *in vitro* evidence that, early

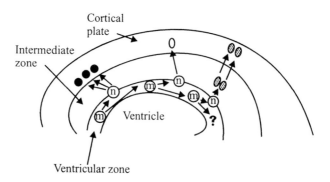

FIG. 2.13. A model for cell lineage in the cortex based on the use of retroviral markers during cortical neurogenesis. In this model, migratory multipotential progenitors (m) divide at intervals. The migratory cell generates a non-migratory cell (n) and another migratory cell. Non-migratory cells may divide no further or they may divide one or more times and many of them or their progeny will migrate radially. Thus, the results of injecting retroviral markers will depend on the age at which the injection is made. Earlier injections would be expected to result in a greater proportion of large widespread clones; later injections would be expected to result in a greater proportion of smaller clones. (After Reid *et al.*, 1995)

in corticogenesis, multipotential progenitors predominate whereas later they are replaced by multiple populations of more highly specified precursors (Williams and Price, 1995).

Numerous retroviral studies that predated the introduction of libraries of vectors and that relied on the analysis of clones based on the proximity of labelled cells provided evidence for the existence of many progenitors that generate similar neuronal or glial cell types (Parnavalas *et al.*, 1991; Grove *et al.*, 1993; Luskin *et al.*, 1988, 1993; Mione *et al.*, 1994, 1997; Goldman and Vaysse, 1991). Parnavalas *et al.* (1991) and Mione *et al.* (1997) suggested that the ventricular zone contains progenitor cells that produce either pyramidal cells and/or astrocytes or non-pyramidal cells or glial cells. Other studies have shown that a smaller proportion of progenitors are multipotential and produce several cell types (Temple, 1989; Reynolds and Weiss, 1992; Davis and Temple, 1994; Price and Thurlow, 1988; Walsh and Cepko, 1988, 1992). Results from Luskin *et al.* (1988), Walsh and Cepko (1988) and Price and Thurlow (1988) have suggested that there are two cortical lineages, one generating grey matter astrocytes and the other generating pyramidal, non-pyramidal, and white matter glial cells (reviewed by Price 1991). The model of Reid *et al.* (1995) reconciles these studies, that previously appeared to conflict. In this model, migrating precursors would be multipotential and non-migrating precursors unipotential (Fig. 2.13).

Another important issue in the development of the cerebral cortex is whether the same precursor cells produce all the cortical laminae. The use of chimeric mice and retroviral lineage markers have led to the suggestion that separate precursors produce deep and superficial layer neurons during normal cortical development (Price and Thurlow, 1988; Fishell *et al.*, 1990; Crandall and Herrup, 1990; van der Kooy *et al.*, 1992). However, other studies using retroviral lineage tracers have indicated that clones can cover all cortical plate layers from 2 to 6 (Luskin *et al.*, 1988). It is not clear what proportion of precursors generate clones that contribute to all cortical layers. If the proportion is low, and the superficial layers are generated from a different pool of precursors, then a site for these precursors (that become active later in cortical formation) must be found outside the ventricular zone. There are no quiescent cells in the ventricular zone throughout cortical neurogenesis; on each day all cells divide and can be labelled with [^{3}H]thymidine infusions lasting for up to about 14 h (Waechter and Jaensch, 1972). It has been suggested that the neurons in the superficial cortical layers are generated in the subventricular zone, the region immediately adjacent to the ventricular zone, since this zone expands as the superficial layers are forming whereas the ventricular zone shrinks (Smart and Smart, 1982). However, what seems more likely is that the subventricular zone is the source of cortical glial cells (Bayer and Altman, 1991; Takahashi *et al.*, 1992a, 1995b).

Retroviral techniques have provided considerable insight into the ways in which cortical cells are formed, and have generated hypotheses concerning the times at which decisions about differentiation are made. Overall, the evidence from these studies taken together with the results of other work, including *in vitro* evidence (Gadisseux *et al.*, 1989; Voigt, 1989; Temple, 1989; Guthrie, 1992), suggests that there are two main lineages in the cerebral cortex: one generates astrocytes and radial glial cells, which later become astrocytes (Gadisseux *et al.*, 1989), the other generates both main types of neuron and white matter glia. Recent *in vitro* studies have suggested that, during cortical neurogenesis, the proliferative zones of the cerebral cortex containing intrinsically different progenitors that vary in the numbers of neurons that they can generate (Qian *et al.*, 1998).

In conclusion, the present position on the dynamics of cortex formation is that the vast majority of neurons in the cortex are produced in the ventricular zone, and that most neuronal progenitors produce a clone of cells destined to contribute to most cortical layers. The ventricular zone is heterogeneous, comprising cells with intrinsically different developmental programs. The potency of cortical progenitors may vary with time. At least some are multipotent, generating pyramidal, non-pyramidal, and glial cells. Whether others produce a narrower range of cell types because their potency is restricted or because they receive different signals is not clear. Cortical glial cells are produced mainly in the subventricular zone.

8   HOW ARE THE FATES OF CORTICAL CELLS DETERMINED?

8.1   Cells that persist. I. Laminar fates

In a series of elegant experiments, McConnell and her co-workers showed that neocortical cells are instructed, by as yet unidentified environmental cues, to migrate to specific neocortical laminae as they are being born in the ventricular zone (McConnell, 1988; McConnell *et al.*, 1989; McConnell, 1991; McConnell and Kaznowski, 1991). This conclusion was based on results from heterochronic transplants in which dividing ventricular zone cells from one animal (in which deep layers were being born) were labelled in S phase. After various periods of time they were moved to the ventricular zone of animals of a different age (in which superficial layers were being born). Provided the cells were allowed to go beyond S phase before transplantation, they migrated to laminar positions appropriate for their birthdate in the donor rather than to positions adopted by their new neighbours in the host ventricular zone (i.e. they had already been instructed in the donor). When transplantation was done earlier, they took on the fates of their new neighbours in the host (i.e. they were multipotent on removal and were instructed by cues in the host). The extent to which these cells differentiate in a manner appropriate for their birthdate or for their eventual neocortical position is not yet clear. Current work is focusing on the search for specific molecular markers of cells in each cortical layer in normal brain so that this question can be addressed for a broader range of indicators of differentiation. At present, it is known that cells transplanted in G2 that migrate to layers specific for their birthday form axonal projections appropriate to those layers (McConnell, 1995).

More recent transplantation studies have indicated that, in the ventricular zone of older embryos, in which superficial layers are being generated, the potential of precursors is restricted. The evidence for this comes from the observation that these late-born cells appear to lose the potential to respond to altered environmental cues following heterochronic transplantation (Frantz and McConnell, 1996). However, other perturbations may be able to alter the laminar fates of the late-born cells, indicating that the restriction in the potential of late-born cells to respond to transplantation may not extend to other forms of manipulation. In these experiments, the fates of specific sets of cortical precursors were studied in mice in which earlier generated groups of cortical progenitors destined for deep layers had been destroyed with the antimitotic agent methylazoxymethanol acetate (MAM Ac) (Gillies and Price, 1993a). In the lesioned mice, many precursors that would normally have adopted fates in the superficial layers contributed to deep layers. The conclusion was that the developing telencephalon can compensate for the earlier destruction of specific precursors by altering the fates of neurons born later, perhaps as a result of feedback of cues from the remaining earlier born cells. This is a good illustration of the principle, discussed in Section 3.2, that a cell's commitment to a particular fate needs to be defined in terms of specific experimental manipulations. The task ahead is to understand why different manipulations either do or do not alter cell fate.

Based on studies with MAM Ac and the transplant work from McConnell's laboratory, it has been suggested that the determination of the fate of cells destined for the cortical plate involves the feedback of molecular cues from previously generated precursors/differentiated cells. These signals may come from earlier born cells that are either still in the ventricular zone (prior to their migration) or in the cortical plate/subplate (after their migration). It may be transmitted in various ways. For example, if the signal originates in the developing cortical plate or subplate, it may travel *via* corticofugal axons, that are known to extend along the edge of the ventricular zone from an early age (McConnell and Kaznowski, 1991). Alternatively, a signalling molecule (or molecules) may diffuse through the extracellular space from earlier generated cells in the ventricular zone or immediately overlying cortical plate. Another possibility is that membrane-bound factors on previously born cells still in the ventricular zone are detected by the newly-dividing cells. In recent work by Bohner *et al.* (1997), donor cells were cultured in various ways prior to transplantation to discover the nature of the interactions required for laminar fate cues. These experiments provided evidence that short-range signals induce progenitors to produce deep layer neurons. Such signals, be they axonally-transported, diffusable, or membrane bound, might change with age because, for example, different factors may be expressed at different times, or there may be a progressive change in the amount(s) of such factor(s).

8.2   Cells that persist. II: Areal fates

A question that has intrigued many developmental neurobiologists interested in corticogenesis is how its distinct areas emerge from the ventricular zone and early cortical plate. In the adult mammal, the cerebral cortex can be divided into areas that differ in their histological appearances. This is illustrated in Fig. 2.14, which shows the cytoarchitectonic fields of the human brain as defined almost a century ago by Brodmann (1909). These distinct fields were defined according to the relative thickness of cell and fibre layers and Brodmann was able to delineate sharp borders between neighbouring areas. This analysis of the human brain was

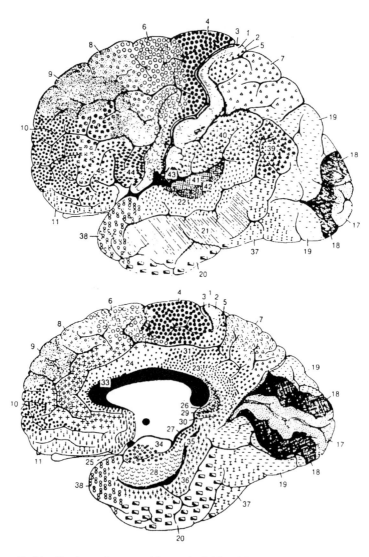

FIG. 2.14. Brodmann's cytoarchitectonic fields of the human brain marked on the left cerebral hemisphere, seen from the lateral (*top*) and medial (*bottom*) aspects. (After Brodmann, 1909)

extended to other species, showing that their cortices could also be subdivided into cytoarchitectonic fields, with equivalent fields occupying relatively similar positions. More recent studies have shown that areal differences in the patterns of cortical lamination seen by Brodmann either cause or accompany other differences. The proportions of different types of cortical neuron vary from area to area (Peters and Jones, 1984); for example, in primary sensory areas there is a relatively thick granular layer 4 containing stellate and/or small pyramidal cells (Fig. 2.15), whereas motor areas have a thicker layer 5 with large pyramidal neurons (Betz cells), many of which project to the spinal cord. The different areas of the cortex have different functional specializations that are dictated by the axonal connections that they receive and send to other parts of the nervous system; the issue of how these functional specializations map onto the cortex will be discussed in Chapter 5. Whereas morphological differences between different regions of the adult cortex are relatively obvious, the same is not the case for the early cortical plate, which has a homogeneous appearance. This led to the suggestion that areal differences in the cortex are induced by the afferent thalamocortical axons that innervate the cortex (Creutzfeldt, 1977). Indeed, there is now considerable evidence supporting a strong role for thalamic innervation in the development of many features of

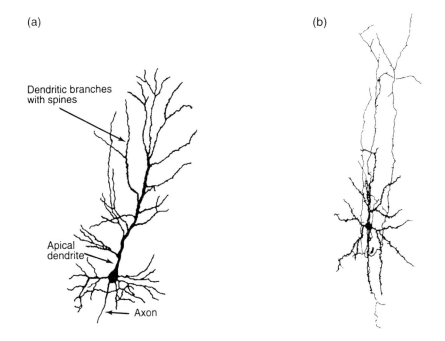

(a)   (b)

Dendritic branches
with spines

Apical
dendrite

← Axon

FIG.   2.15.   Drawings of two types of neuron found in the cerebral cortex. (a) Pyramidal cell. (b) Spiny stellate cell. (After Kandel *et al.*, 1991)

cortical organization, as discussed in Chapter 5 (Frost and Metin, 1985; Sur *et al.*, 1988; Rakic, 1976a, 1983; Schlagger and O'Leary, 1992; Shatz, 1996). However, there is also evidence that some area-specific differences are detectable before cortical innervation. Within the ventricular zone, there are regional differences in rates of proliferation (Dehay *et al.*, 1993; Kennedy and Dehay, 1997) that may account for differences in the numbers of neurons throughout the thickness of the mature cortical wall in different cortical areas (Rakic, 1976b). The abolition of the activity of cortical afferents does not prevent the development in the cortex of characteristic region-specific distributions of molecules, such as the enzyme cytochrome oxidase and neurotransmitter receptors, and of some elements of cortical functional architecture (Kuljis and Rakic, 1990; Rakic, 1995; Chapman *et al.*, 1996). Finally, there have been a number of reports of cortical area-specific gene expression that begins before or is independent of afferent innervation. Limbic system-associated protein (LAMP) is a cell-adhesion molecule expressed by neurons in prefrontal, perirhinal, entorhinal, and subicular cortex (Levitt, 1984; Zacco *et al.*, 1990). Latexin is a protein found in specifically the lateral part of the rodent cerebral cortex (Hatanaka *et al.*, 1994; Arimatsu *et al.*, 1999).

An unidentified gene (detected by the insertion of a reporter gene into the mouse genome in an enhancer-trap experiment) is expressed in the somatosensory cortex from before the time of afferent innervation (Cohen-Tannoudji *et al.*, 1994); the gene is still expressed if the developing somatosensory cortex is transplanted to an ectopic location but is not expressed by other regions of developing cortex even if they are transplanted to the somatosensory cortex. Other genes that regionalize the forebrain, telencephalon, and cortex are discussed in Chapter 3.

It is far from clear how cortical area-specific differentiation is achieved and our ignorance has fuelled a sometimes highly polarized debate on this matter. Some workers have emphasized the hypothesis that areal differences are imposed on the cortex by its afferents; others have stressed that specification of cortical areas may begin before innervation, an idea that has been termed the 'protomap hypothesis' (Rakic, 1988). The evidence described above indicates that cortical regionalization results from a cascade of events that builds on some degree of early regional specification within the embryonic ventricular zone. It is likely that a complex network of interactions between cortical neurons and their afferents elaborate and refine early regional differences in the ventricular zone and cortical plate. How regional specification within the ventricular zone arises in the first place, and details of the cascade of interactions that build on the early differences, are poorly understood. A further discussion of cortical regionalization and the influence of innervation is given in Chapter 5.

8.3 Cells that die

Paradoxically, many cells born during development are fated to die by a process called programmed cell death. The mechanisms that underlie this process are discussed in Chapter 6. Cell death shapes the development of the cortex; it refines cell numbers and connections and it leads to the disappearance of entire structures such as the subplate (Allendoerfer and Shatz, 1994; Price *et al.*, 1997). It even occurs in the proliferative zone of the embryonic cortex (Blaschke *et al.*, 1996; Thomaidou *et al.*, 1997).

Until recently, estimates of the rates of cell death in the proliferative zone, based on histological or electron microscopic studies, were put at only a few per cent of cells (Saunders, 1966). However, the development of extremely sensitive methods for the detection of cells that are beginning to die by programmed cell death has led to a recent upwards revision of these values (Blaschke *et al.*, 1996, 1998; Thomaidou *et al.*, 1997). Cells undergoing programmed cell death show fragmentation of their DNA (Chapter 6), and these breaks can be detected by DNA end-labelling long before cells show overt signs of death. It is not clear how much time elapses after DNA breaks appear before the cells die and their debris is cleared away. This makes it hard to deduce the percentage of cells that are removed by cell death from the cortical proliferative zone during neurogenesis using this method. Nevertheless, on average about 50% of proliferative cells show DNA breaks, with as many as 70% showing breaks on some gestational days (Blaschke *et al.*, 1996, 1998). This suggests that earlier studies may have underestimated the significance of this process.

With regards to cortical connections, studies by Rakic and his colleagues (Williams and Rakic, 1988) have shown that, in primates, there is a period of cell death in the thalamus (in its lateral geniculate nucleus, LGN, which projects to the visual cortex) before birth, about halfway through gestation. This period of cell death occurs well before the segregation of geniculocortical afferents to form ocular dominance columns. In rodents, the timing of cell death in the LGN is not so precisely worked out, although it appears to occur during the first few weeks after birth (Finlay and Pallas, 1989). One reason for this difference may be that rodents are born relatively immature. In these animals the period of cell death may overlap with the period of connectional refinement. Despite the apparent segregation of these phases in the primate, there is the possibility that similar molecular processes, and perhaps the same molecules, are involved in both. Certainly, *in vitro* experiments indicate that the ability of cells to survive and to elaborate neural processes are very closely related. This will be reconsidered in Chapter 6.

Many studies of cell death in the cortex itself have focused on the subplate. This is an unusual structure that has attracted much attention in recent years. Unlike the overlying cortical plate, current evidence indicates that many of its cells are fated to die after playing a crucial role in guiding thalamocortical, and possibly other long-range cortical projections, to their appropriate targets (Ghosh *et al.*, 1990; Ghosh and Shatz, 1992a; Allendorfer and Shatz, 1994). This structure is very much larger and more highly developed in phylogenetically more advanced species (Allendoerfer and Shatz, 1994), although it can be identified even in rodents (Bayer and Altman, 1990; Wood *et al.*, 1992; Price *et al.*, 1997). It is born and differentiates early, forming a rich network of connections with both cortical and subcortical structures (described below). As the cortex matures, the subplate largely disappears leaving only a few interstitial cells in the white matter below the cortex (Shering and Lowenstein, 1994). It has been suggested that cells of the marginal zone and the subplate form a morphogenetic framework in which the cortical plate develops.

The subplate also seems important for the later refinement of cortical afferents (Ghosh and Shatz, 1992b). The size of the subplate is species-dependent: larger subplates are found in larger brains, and in rodents the subplate is relatively small (Wood *et al.*, 1992; Allendoerfer and Shatz, 1994). The proportion of subplate cells that die during development may also be species-dependent. In the cat, almost all subplate cells die by four months postnatally (Allendoerfer and Shatz, 1994); in the hamster, although most subplate cells die, a significant proportion may persist into adulthood (Woo *et al.*, 1991). Controversial results have been obtained for the rat: several studies have indicated that developmentally regulated subplate cell death probably does occur in this species (reviewed by Allendoerfer and Shatz, 1994), although findings by Valverde *et al.* (1995a) in rodent have suggested that, at least from birth on, there is little neuronal death in the subplate. In mouse, there is much evidence that most subplate cells die and that this death may begin prenatally (Price *et al.*, 1997; Wood *et al.*, 1992; Gillies and Price, 1993b). What determines the death or survival of subplate cells *in vivo* is unclear. Certainly, the time of their death cannot rely on a cell-autonomous endogenously-timed death program, since the timing of subplate death can be readily manipulated both *in vitro* and *in vivo*. For example, subplate death occurs more rapidly in cortical slices cultured alone than it does *in vivo* (Wood *et al.*, 1992; Gillies and Price, 1993b), but this can be prevented by co-culture with the thalamus (Price and Lotto, 1996). Furthermore *in vivo* lesions of the thalamocortical pathway can alter the time at which subplate cells die (Molnar *et al.*, 1991). Finally, one can alter the timing of subplate death *in vitro* by altering the culture conditions (i.e. by adding thalamic tissue; serum-supplemented medium will also keep subplate cells alive) (Hohn *et al.*, 1993). These experiments suggest that a change in the trophic support that subplate cells receive from subcortical structures, such as the thalamus (Price and Lotto, 1996), may contribute to a change in their viability *in vivo*.

One possibility is that, *in vivo*, subplate neurons obtain thalamic factors by the well-established mechanism of retrograde transport along their axons (Korsching, 1993). However, recent observations mitigate against this possibility. Although some subplate axons may project to or through the internal capsule (De Carlos and O'Leary, 1992), and might even pioneer this pathway for subsequent layer 5 and layer 6 fibers (McConnell *et al.*, 1989), few subplate axons actually innervate nuclei within the dorsal thalamus itself (Clasca *et al.*, 1994, 1995; Molnar, 1994; Molnar and Blakemore, 1995a). If the thalamus is not a major target, most subplate neurons would probably not acquire thalamic factors retrogradely. On the other hand, it is well-documented that thalamic axons invade the subplate (Ghosh and Shatz,

1992a). Thus it is possible that thalamic factors are transported anterogradely along thalamocortical axons into the subplate. There is a precedent for the anterograde transport of trophic factors within the visual system, from the retina to the tectum (Catsicas *et al.*, 1992). With this in mind, Price and Lotto (1996) proposed the following sequence of events.

At around E16 to E17 in rodents, thalamocortical axons reach the subplate (Catalano *et al.*, 1991) where they may 'wait', the duration of the period being species-dependent (Allendoerfer and Shatz, 1994), and form transient synaptic contacts (Friauf *et al.*, 1990; Hermann *et al.*, 1994). During the waiting period, thalamic factors transported into the subplate may maintain its viability. However, once thalamic axons leave the subplate to innervate the overlying cortical plate (around birth in rodents), perhaps due to the up-regulation of growth-promoting substances in the cortical plate (Bolz *et al.*, 1993; Tuttle *et al.*, 1995), they take with them their trophic support. Consistent with this hypothesis is the observation that the onset of subplate death in mice occurs after the subplate starts to clear of thalamic innervation (Wood *et al.*, 1992; Price *et al.*, 1997).

Other mechanisms may also contribute to the timing of subplate death *in vivo*, but they seem less satisfactory as complete explanations. For example, the innervation of subplate cells (rather than the withdrawal of innervation) may push them towards death, possibly by exposing them to large amounts of glutamate, which is known to be toxic at high concentrations (Lipton and Kater, 1989). This theory would demand an explanation of why subplate cells should be more sensitive to the effects of innervation than the cortical plate, which is clearly not killed by innervation. A loss of trophic support from the thalamus might be one explanation. It seems unlikely that the thalamocortical contribution to the afferent innervation of subplate cells kills them since subplate death occurs after thalamocortical axons start to leave this region; this does not exclude the possibility that other afferent projections to the subplate play a role in triggering the death of these cells (e.g. those from other cortical areas, that develop later).

With regards to cell death in other cortical layers, Windrem and Finlay (1991) have shown that, by the end of the first postnatal week in the hamster, cell death is seen across all cortical layers *in vivo*, with a high incidence amongst cells destined for the superficial layers (i.e. E17-born cells). These authors also demonstrated that the neonatal lesions of the thalamus significantly increased cell death among postnatal cells destined to form the superficial layers, but not among postnatal cells destined for the other layers. At earlier embryonic stages, the viability of cortical plate neurons *in vitro*, including those of layers 6 and 4 that project to and receive innervation from the thalamus, appear to be unaffected by the presence or absence of a co-cultured thalamus (Price and Lotto, 1996). At this age, the survival of most cortical plate cells may be promoted by cortical factors; clearly, cortical cells that can survive without the thalamus at E19 may develop a dependency on the thalamus at later ages. Thus, depending on age, the thalamus may enhance the survival of cortical plate cells. In addition, influences from surrounding cortical areas may support cortical viability via corticocortical cells projecting between the superficial cortical layers (Haun and Cunningham, 1993; Price, 1995). These factors may act synergistically with thalamic influences. The next important task will be the identification of the molecules mediating these interactions.

3

Molecular regulation of early forebrain and cortical development

1 CONTRIBUTIONS FROM MOUSE DEVELOPMENTAL GENETICS

Over the past few decades, higher mammals with larger and more advanced brains, such as cats and primates, have been studied by many scientists interested in cortical development. Prominent examples are Nobel laureates David Hubel and Torsten Wiesel, who worked on cortical development and the effects of visual deprivation. Much of their work (as well as that of numerous researchers stimulated by their studies) was carried out on cats, described in Chapter 5. One reason for this tendency may be a desire to understand the development of the human brain and its perceptual and cognitive functions. Many features of the brains of higher mammals are poorly represented in other vertebrates, one clear example being colour vision. Furthermore, the techniques that are applied to the study of functional development of the brain, such as electrophysiological recording and behavioural tests (discussed in later chapters), may be extremely difficult in other animals. However, in recent years, the massive increase of research in mouse molecular genetics has begun to make significant contributions to our understanding of the molecular control of early forebrain development. The study of the mechanisms of cortical development through the use of mouse molecular genetics is still in its infancy but at this early stage it is still possible to appreciate the potential of the tools that are now available to identify, clone, characterize, and experimentally manipulate genes that regulate cortical formation. It is likely that the use of the mouse as an experimental model for the study of all aspects of cortical formation will continue to increase enormously.

Large numbers of mouse mutants have been found, some by chance and others as a result of systematic strategies for inducing and identifying new mutations. Some mutants were discovered as recessive mutations during the early days of mouse inbreeding; some were identified as spontaneous mutations in laboratory stocks of inbred mice; others were deliberately induced by exposure of mice to X-rays or chemical mutagens. Many mutations affect neural development; some of these disrupt cortical development, a good example being the reeler mouse, described later in this chapter. Mouse mutants have been used as start-points for the identification of novel genes regulating development, on the grounds that the site of genetic disruption in a mutant with an interesting developmental defect is likely to be in a gene that normally regulates that process. In many cases this assumption has been borne out. An example is the cloning of the Brachyury gene. Earlier this century, a mutant mouse with a short tail was identified following X-irradiation and was named T or Brachyury. Following the discovery of other T mutations in wild mouse populations and extensive genetic analysis of what is now known to be a complex of genes (the t complex), the Brachyury gene was finally cloned in 1990 (Herrmann *et al.*, 1990). The product of this gene turned out to be a DNA-binding protein, which is a transcription factor, a molecule with the potential to regulate the expression of other genes. It is required for mesodermal development and is expressed in the notochord (see Chapter 2) and tailbud.

The identification of the Brachyury gene illustrates some important points about the use of mouse mutants for the study of development. First, the isolation of novel genes by this method can take a very long time and can demand considerable resources. This disadvantage may lessen to some extent as the chromosomal positions of more and more genes are mapped in the mouse, since the locations of genes disrupted by mutagens (in so-called large scale mutagenesis screens) are likely to be found more quickly and their cloning is likely to become increasingly cost-effective. Reviews of the methods that can be used to find the disrupted genes, for example by positional cloning (the method used to identify the Brachyury gene, Herrmann *et al.* 1990), can be found elsewhere (Reith and Bernstein, 1991; Meisler, 1992; Magnuson and Faust, 1993). A second point is that one reason why the identification of Brachyury is a success story is that the gene encodes a transcription factor. Such regulatory genes are seen as having more potential to explain the control of development than genes encoding many other types of cellular protein. When setting out to identify a disrupted gene in a new mutant, there is no guarantee that such an interesting gene will be found. A third point is that genes that regulate key developmental processes are often conserved between species or, in an individual species, are members of a family of related genes (that may have arisen through gene duplication in evolution). The cloning of one gene can lead to the identification of other similar genes in the same or other species. Not only have homologues of Brachyury been found in other species but related genes have been identified in the mouse itself; one of these (T-brain-1, see below) plays an important role in cortical development.

This final point brings us to consider an alternative strategy that has been very successfully employed during the past decade for the cloning of mouse genes that control development. This involves the identification of mouse genes related to genes that regulate growth and development in other organisms such as *Drosophila melanogaster* or *Caenorhabditis elegans*. In these invertebrate species, the cloning of genes disrupted in mutagenesis screens is much more straightforward than in the mouse and so most knowledge of the molecular regulation of *Drosophila* and *Caenorhabditis* development comes from studies that begin with an analysis of mutants.

Despite the possibility that a similar approach can be adopted in mice, as described above, many studies on the control of mouse development begin from the cloning of potentially interesting mouse genes rather than from an analysis of mutants (this is sometimes called reverse genetics). This approach is possible because, as described later in this chapter, there is a remarkable degree of structural and functional conservation between many genes in invertebrates and in mammals. It is now relatively easy to use standard recombinant DNA methods to make a probe from one gene that will identify and allow the cloning of structurally related genes in the same or other species (accounts of these methods can be found in standard textbooks on molecular biology). The assumption underlying this approach is that structurally related genes will have similar functions; this is often but not always the case. The ability to test the functions of mouse genes isolated in this way has rested on the revolutionary discovery of methods for manipulating the mouse genome so as to alter the expression of specific genes of interest. These methods are outlined in the next section.

In conclusion, it is likely that the analysis of the genetic control of development in mammals will continue to exploit the advantages of the mouse for the foreseeable future. The identification of novel genes on the basis of homology to developmental genes in other species, and the testing of their functions with transgenic methods, is a powerful approach, although it suffers from the problem that some important genes may be unique to mammals. Therefore, more laborious analyses of natural and induced mutations are also essential.

2 METHODS FOR MANIPULATING THE MOUSE GENOME

The creation of transgenic mice (i.e. mice with specific alterations to their genetic constitution) is now a huge industry. There are various ways in which the genome can be manipulated, but all involve the application of DNA to mouse or mouse-derived cells. The idea is to achieve incorporation of the applied DNA into the DNA of the host cells, so that it will be transmitted through the germ cells to subsequent generations. In some methods, the applied DNA incorporates at random sites in the genome. This technique results in the addition of genetic material to the genome (sometimes called addition transgenics). Others are designed to target the applied DNA to a specific site and replace an endogenous gene. This method, gene targeting) can be used to substitute a non-functioning form of a gene and so delete the function of the gene in the resulting transgenic animal (a knock-out). Two main ways in which these outcomes can be achieved are summarized in Fig. 3.1.

Addition transgenics can be made by directly injecting DNA into the pronu-cleus of the fertilized egg (Fig. 2.1). The injected DNA will integrate into the genome, although the sites at which it integrates may alter its function in unpre-dictable ways (generating what are referred to as position effects). Gene replace-ment by the targeting of specific genes is a more involved procedure that makes use of cells derived from the mouse blastocyst, called embryonic stem cells. These cells are totipotent, i.e. they are capable of generating all the tissues of the body (Gearhart, 1998). They can be cultured and their genome can be manipulated *in vitro*. This manipulation makes use of the process of homologous recombina-tion, in which two molecules of DNA with very similar DNA sequences align, break, and cross-over. When DNA with nucleotide sequences similar to those in the embryonic stem cells is introduced into these cells, it recombines with the DNA at the site of the target gene and can substitute for the endogenous DNA. Embryonic stem cells in which this has been achieved can be selected in culture and used to make mice carrying the altered gene. This process is summarized in Fig. 3.1b. Although these methods have given us considerable insights into the functions of specific genes in development, they have limitations. The main one is that often it is very difficult to study the roles of genes at any but the earliest times at which they are expressed. As development proceeds beyond the point at which the altered gene is normally first expressed, phenotypic abnormalities aris-ing from the mutation may accumulate as secondary defects arise. Recent years have seen the introduction of new methods for generating mutations in specific tissues and at specific times of development, but as yet these methods have not been widely used. Another problem with the generation of targeted gene knock-outs is that other similar genes may substitute for the missing gene; in other words, many genes show a degree of redundancy in their actions at particular sites and times. One way around this difficulty is to breed mice with more than one gene deletion. Thus, although the production and use of transgenic mice is a very pow-erful methodology for studying the molecular mechanisms of development, an appreciation of the difficulties of interpretation associated with the approach is essential.

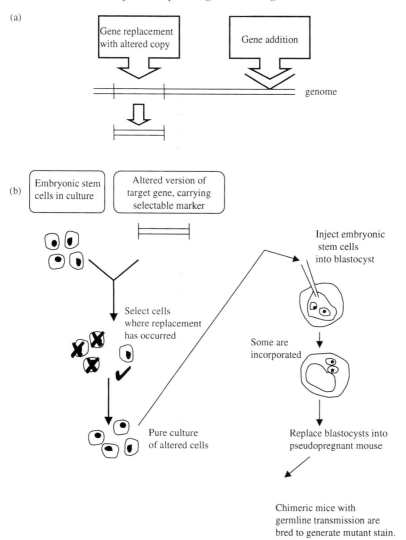

(a)

Gene replacement with altered copy

Gene addition

genome

(b)

Embryonic stem cells in culture

Altered version of target gene, carrying selectable marker

Inject embryonic stem cells into blastocyst

Select cells where replacement has occurred

Some are incorporated

Pure culture of altered cells

Replace blastocysts into pseudopregnant mouse

Chimeric mice with germline transmission are bred to generate mutant stain.

F I G . 3 . 1 . (a) Summary of the two main methods for generating transgenic mice: either specific genes are replaced by altered ones, or new genes are added to the genome. (b) Outline of the methods used to make alterations of specific genes, e.g. for the creation of knock-out mice. In culture, an endogenous gene in the embryonic stem cells is replaced by an altered copy of the gene. The altered copy carries a selectable marker, usually a gene conferring resistance to an antibiotic. When the antibiotic is added, all cells that have failed to integrate the altered version will be killed, since they will not have developed resistance. The engineered embryonic stem cells can then be used to generate mice.

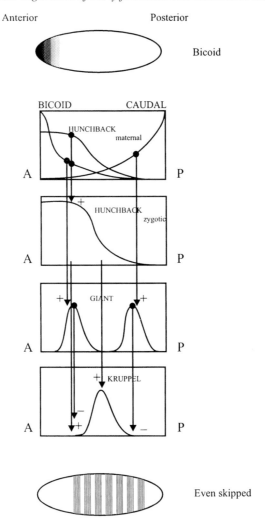

F I G .   3 . 2 . A schematic representation of *Drosophila* pattern formation along the anterior–posterior axis. Up to the blastoderm stage, the *Drosophila* embryo is a syncytium in which nuclei divide without being separated by cell membranes. This feature, which is not mirrored in mammals, facilitates the diffusion of regulatory factors. Communication between the oocyte and surrounding cells results in the localization of mRNA for bicoid (a transcription factor gene) to the anterior pole of the oocyte. BICOID diffuses from the anterior pole and forms a concentration gradient. BICOID controls the formation of an opposing concentration gradient of CAUDAL by translation suppression. BICOID also interacts synergistically with a gradient of maternal HUNCHBACK to define the spatial limit of zygotic HUNCHBACK expression. Other regulators, such as GIANT, have expression domains determined through activation by bicoid and caudal; the mechanisms establishing the expression domain of giant are not yet known, but may involve the sensing of a particular concentration of BICOID and CAUDAL. KRUPPEL expression is activated by HUNCHBACK and BICOID

3 GENES THAT REGULATE DEVELOPMENT IN *Drosophila* HAVE HOMOLOGUES IN MAMMALS

The fruit fly, *Drosophila melanogaster*, has been used intensively in genetic research for many decades. It is small, has a short life cycle of two weeks, and large numbers of mutants have been identified and studied. The combination of the extensive knowledge of *Drosophila* mutants with experimental embryological and molecular biological techniques has provided a profound understanding of the genetic regulation of development in this species. Remarkably, not only have many of the control mechanisms that operate in *Drosophila* been conserved in mammals, but so have many of the genes themselves. It is now commonplace to use information obtained from studies of *Drosophila* to search for specific regulatory genes in higher species and to formulate hypotheses regarding the general principles that underlie development in all organisms. In particular, work on *Drosophila* has provided a comprehensive understanding of how different regions of a developing organism can develop regional specificity. As shown in Fig. 3.2, morphogens (such as BICOID and CAUDAL) are distributed in gradients in the early *Drosophila* embryo. They evoke different cellular responses at different concentrations, specifying the expression patterns of other genes that themselves regulate later-expressed genes (Fig. 3.2). In this way, complex patterns of later-expressed genes emerge to confer positional identity on cells at each position in the embryo. The combined action of the specific cocktail of regulatory genes that each cell expresses is essential for conferring on each cell a particular phenotype appropriate for its position.

The work of many groups has shown that vertebrates have genes that are similar to those of *Drosophila* (Graham *et al.*, 1989; Wilkinson *et al.*, 1989; Krumlauf *et al.*, 1993). Vertebrate homologues have been found for *Drosophila* genes that act within cells to regulate the expression of other genes (transcription factors, see the following section) or that signal between cells to control processes such as axonal guidance (see Chapter 4). For transcription factors, a good example is the large family of Hox genes in mouse which have homology to the genes of the Antennapedia complex of *Drosophila*. Antennapedia genes regulate the identity of segments of the *Drosophila* body (they are known as homeotic genes) (Akam, 1987); Hox genes are expressed in and regulate the identity of regions of the murine hindbrain known as rhombomeres (Wilkinson *et al.*, 1989; Krumlauf *et al.*, 1993). The rhombomeres have similarity to *Drosophila* compartments (see Chapter 2) in that, after a certain stage of development, the movement of cells between them

---

but repressed by GIANT and other anterior repressors such as TAILLESS (not shown). The composition and concentration of transcription factors at each point in the embryo will determine the expression domains of later-expressed genes, such as even-skipped, through a combination of activation and repression. Thus, increasingly complex patterns of spatially restricted gene expression emerge and confer positional information on the nuclei in the blastoderm. In this diagram, capitalized names indicate proteins and lower-case names indicate genes. (After Rivera-Pomer and Jackle, 1996)

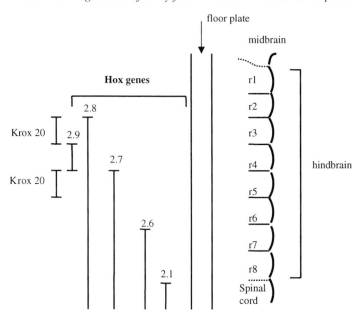

FIG. 3.3. Diagram of the right side of the rhombencephalon with its rhombomeres (r1–8). Mouse homeobox genes (Hox genes) and genes for other types of transcription factor (Krox20 encodes a zinc finger protein) are expressed in rhombomere-specific patterns. Examples are shown; domains of expression for Hox2.1, 2.6, 2.7, 2.8, and 2.9 are indicated by vertical lines.

The homeotic genes of *Drosophila* are expressed later in development than those that regulate early regionalization (Lewis, 1978; Gehring, 1986; Akam, 1987). *Drosophila* homeotic genes grouped together in a complex called HOM-C have vertebrate homologues, called Hox genes, whose primary site of expression is the developing nervous system (Krumlauf *et al.*, 1993). Anatomical, cellular, and molecular data demonstrate that the vertebrate hindbrain is segmented (Lumsden and Keynes, 1989; Lumsden, 1990) and recent work has examined the relationship between this segmentation and Hox gene expression. The schematic shows the patterns of expression of Hox genes in the vertebrate hindbrain (Krumlauf *et al.*, 1993). The overlapping expression patterns provide a means of specifying the identity of each rhombomere. Gene targeting in the mouse has generated numerous loss-of-function and gain-of-function mutations that provide clear evidence for the Hox clusters being vertebrate homeotic complexes. These mutations generate changes in the phenotypes of specific rhombomeres, such that they adopt the identities of more anterior or posterior rhombomeres (Wilkinson, 1989).

is prevented (Fraser *et al.*, 1990). The region-specific expression of some transcription factor genes in the rhombencephalon is illustrated in Fig. 3.3. Another good example of conservation of developmental mechanisms is in the guidance of axons. Many of the ligand–receptor systems that have been implicated in this process are highly conserved between *Drosophila* (and other species of invertebrate) and mammals (Tessier-Lavigne and Goodman, 1996; Goodman and Shatz, 1992). This is discussed further in Chapter 4.

4   TYPES OF MOLECULE THAT REGULATE FOREBRAIN DEVELOPMENT

It is useful to divide the molecules that regulate the development of the forebrain into two groups: (i) those that act intracellularly by binding directly to DNA to control the expression of other genes (transcription factors) and (ii) those that are released by one cell and affect the development of others (extracellular signalling molecules). Molecules in the second group are of many different types. Some are secreted molecules that are relatively small and can diffuse away from the cell to affect cells at a distance (perhaps several cell diameters or more away). Others, which may be larger or may be anchored to the cell surface, are not so free to diffuse and may operate at close range or may require cell–cell contact. Such molecules may be ligands, receptors, or both. For some extracellular molecules, their freedom to diffuse depends on the extracellular conditions and can be affected by interactions with the extracellular matrix or cell surfaces.

Table 3.1 lists many of the transcription factors currently known to regulate forebrain development. Table 3.2 lists some of the extracellular signalling molecules that currently are thought to be important in controlling key events in early forebrain development. Table 3.3 lists some of the major components of the extracellular matrix; these very large and relatively immobile molecules are listed separately, even though they are crucial components of the extracellular signalling processes.

Clearly, a full molecular explanation of the biochemical pathways that regulate forebrain development will involve other types of molecule, such as intracellular secondary messengers and cytoskeletal proteins. Once determined, these biochemical pathways are likely to link many of the molecules listed in Tables 3.1–3.3. Although a fair amount is known about intracellular messengers and cytoskeletal elements, many of them, and the ways they act, are not unique to forebrain and so their analysis may not provide the most useful clues to the way in which the unique characteristics of the forebrain develop. Therefore, we do not intend to review all of the potentially relevant literature regarding these molecules (although some issues are touched on throughout the book); rather, we shall focus on the effector molecules themselves, which have received enormous attention in recent years.

4.1   Transcription factors

The enzymes that generate RNA (RNA polymerases) do not recognize their promoters on purified DNA molecules. In order for the enzymes to recognize the promoter, one or more sequence-specific DNA-binding proteins must be present. These DNA-binding proteins are transcription factors, and there are several types that are involved in the regulation of developmental events. Three major classes of binding domain are illustrated in Fig. 3.4; these are the homeodomain, the zinc finger, and the leucine zipper. The analysis of mutant mice has given indications of the functions of many such transcription factors in development (Table 3.1). However, the gene or genes that are targeted by each transcription factor *in vivo* are

Table 3.1 Regulatory genes encoding transcription factors expressed in the developing murine forebrain.

Arx A homeobox-containing gene, expressed in the dorsal telencephalon (presumptive cerebral cortex) from E9.5, as well as in the ganglionic eminence, ventral thalamus, hypothalamus, and floor plate. (Miura *et al.*, 1997)

BF-1 and **BF-2** Encode winged helix (WH) proteins (previously called HNF-3/fork head proteins) characterized by a DNA-binding domain called the winged helix. BF-1 expression is restricted to the telencephalon. BF-2 expression is restricted to a region of the diencephalon. Mutation of BF-1 causes severe defects of telencephalic development, thought to be due to reduced mitotic rates. (Hatini *et al.*, 1994; Xuan *et al.*, 1995)

Brn1 and **Brn2** Homeobox genes expressed in the embryonic cortex. (Wegner *et al.*, 1993)

Dbx (formerly MmoxC) A homeobox-containing gene whose transcripts are detected within a region of the prospective cerebral cortex of the mid-gestation telencephalon, as well as in the diencephalon, hindbrain, and spinal cord. Expressed in regions of mitosis, where it may act to specify subsets of neuroblasts. (Lu *et al.*, 1992; Murtha *et al.*, 1991)

Dlx genes
Family of homeobox-containing genes with homology to *Drosophila* Distal-less (Porteus *et al.*, 1994; Price *et al.*, 1991; Price, 1993).
Dlx-1 Expressed in developing diencephalon. (Price *et al.*, 1991)
Dlx-2 (formerly Tes-1) Early in development (E9.5-E12.5), there is a border of expression between the lateral ganglionic eminence and the cerebral cortex. Later, by E16.5, expression extends into the cerebral cortex. (Bulfone *et al.*, 1993; Porteus *et al.*, 1991). Deletion of both Dlx-1 and Dlx-2 prevents migration of cells from lateral ganglionic eminence to neocortex. (Anderson *et al.*, 1997)
Dlx-5 Expressed in the diencephalon and telencephalon; telencephalic label is in the primordia of the ganglionic eminences. At E11.5, Dlx-5 expression is complementary to that of Lhx5. (Sheng *et al.*, 1997)

Emx-1 and **Emx-2** Mouse cognates of genes that regulate development of the *Drosophila* head (empty spiracles). They are homeobox-containing genes. Their expression patterns have suggested their involvement in regional patterning of the forebrain. They are expressed in very similar but not completely overlapping domains from E8.5-9 onwards. Mutation analysis has indicated that Emx-2 has roles in evagination of the cerebral hemispheres and specification of the limbic region of the telencephalon. (Briata *et al.*, 1996; Simeone *et al.*, 1992a,b; Boncinelli *et al.*, 1993; Gulisano *et al.*, 1996; Yoshida *et al.*, 1997)

Gli-3 A zinc finger gene expressed in the developing telencephalon and diencephalon; mutation of Gli-3 causes the extra-toe mutation (Xt), in which olfactory bulbs and the choroid plexus in the lateral ventricles fail to develop and cortical lamination is absent. (Franz, 1994; Grove *et al.*, 1998)

Gsh-2 A homeobox-containing gene resembling the *Drosophila* gene, Antennapedia, expressed in the ganglionic eminences of the telencephalon, the diencephalon, and the hindbrain. (Hsieh-Li *et al.*, 1995)

Heir-1 Helix-loop-helix transcription factor. (Ellmeier *et al.*, 1992)

Hfh 4 Winged helix gene. (Furuta *et al.*, 1997)

Id-2 Regulatory helix-loop-helix gene expressed in a laminar-specific pattern in the developing cortex. (Bulfone *et al.*, 1995; Neuman *et al.*, 1993)

Table 3.1

Lhx genes
Members of a family of genes each encoding two LIM domains (which bind zinc ions and may be involved in protein–protein interactions) and a homeodomain. LIM domains may modulate the functions of the homeodomain.

Lhx-1 (formerly Lim-1) Expressed in developing forebrain regions (both telencephalon and diencephalon). Targeted deletion results in embryos lacking anterior head structures. (Shawert and Behringer, 1995)

Lhx-2 (formerly LH-2) Expressed from mid-gestation in cells surrounding the telencephalic ventricles. At birth, it is expressed in cortical layers 2–6. Lhx-2 –/– embryos show neocortical hypoplasia. (Porter *et al.* 1997; Xu *et al.*, 1993)

Lhx-3 (formerly Lim-3/P-lim)

Lhx-4 (formerly Gsh-4)

Lhx-5 (formerly Lim-2) At E9.5, Lhx-5 is expressed in the telencephalon and diencephalon. At E12.5, Lhx-5 expression in the telencephalon is less apparent (whereas Lhx-1 expression appears strong). (Sheng *et al.*, 1997)

Msx-1 Homeobox gene expressed in the dorsal telencephalon; possible downstream target of bone morphogenetic proteins. (Furuta *et al.*, 1997; Davidson, 1995)

Nkx-2.1 and **Nkx-2.2** Members of the Nkx2 family of homeobox-containing genes, expressed from about E9 in restricted regions of developing forebrain, including the diencephalon and, in the case of Nkx-2.1, in the developing striatum of the telencephalon. (Lazzaro *et al.*, 1991; Price *et al.*, 1992; Price, 1993)

Nkx2.1 (also known as T/ebp and TTF-1) is essential for ventral forebrain development, including development of the hypothalamus and pituitary gland. (Kimura *et al.*, 1994)

Otx-1 and **Otx-2** Mouse cognates of *Drosophila* orthodenticle gene (which is involved in head development). They are homeobox-containing genes. Otx-2 is expressed within the forebrain and the midbrain with a posterior limit at the midbrain/hindbrain junction. Mutation of Otx-2 causes absence of forebrain and midbrain regions. Otx-1 expression largely overlaps with Otx-2 expression in the forebrain and midbrain. Mutation of Otx-1 causes subtle defects, including poor cortical differentiation. (Acampora *et al.*, 1995; Millet *et al.*, 1996; Simeone *et al.*, 1992a,b; Suda *et al.*, 1996; Boncinelli *et al.*, 1993; Frantz *et al.*, 1994b; Ang *et al.*, 1996; Ba-Charvet *et al.*, 1998)

Pax-6 Member of a family of genes (Pax genes) that contain a paired-box. The paired-box has been highly conserved during evolution and encodes a protein domain of 128 amino acids which binds DNA. Most Pax genes are expressed in the CNS in temporally and spatially restricted patterns. Pax-3, Pax-6, and Pax-7 are expressed from E8–E8.5 in the prosencephalon and its derivatives, including the telencephalon and diencephalon. Pax-6 is expressed in the developing cortex. Its mutation causes defects of cortical proliferation, migration and differentiation. (Stoykova *et al.*, 1996; Walther and Gruss, 1991; Stoykova and Gruss, 1994; Mastick *et al.*, 1997; Caric *et al.*, 1997; Gotz *et al.*, 1998; Warren and Price, 1997; Ericson *et al.*, 1997)

Prox-1 A homeobox gene related to *Drosophila* prospero expressed in developing cortex. (Oliver *et al.*, 1993; Torii *et al.*, 1999)

Prx-1 Prx genes encode homeodomain-containing proteins with homology to *Drosophila* genes (paired and gooseberry). Prx-1 is expressed from E10.5 in the telencephalic vesicles, as well as in other developing brain regions. (Leussink *et al.*, 1995)

Table 3.1 (*Continued*)

Sox Related to the sex determining gene SRY; possess DNA-binding domains that are sequence specific although they are related to those of DNA-binding proteins that are not specific. Members of the family are expressed in the cortical ventricular zone. (Uwanogho *et al.*, 1995)

Tbr-1 (T-brain-1) Encodes a putative transcription factor related to the Brachyury gene; expressed only in postmitotic cells. Expression largely restricted to the cerebral cortex, where it distinguishes domains that may give rise to paleocortex, limbic cortex, and neocortex. In adult, it is expressed preferentially in specific layers of the cerebral cortex and is involved in their development, perhaps by regulating reelin gene expression. (Bulfone *et al.*, 1995)

Tst-1 (SCIP) Homeobox gene expressed in the developing cortex in a laminar specific pattern. (Frantz *et al.*, 1994a; He *et al.*, 1989)

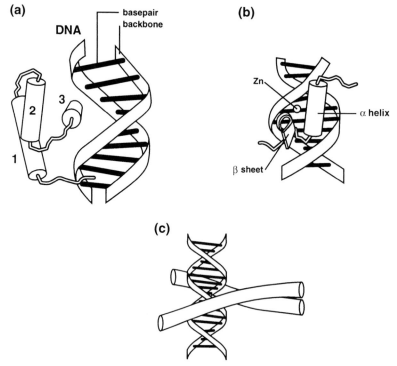

FIG. 3.4. Diagram showing three types of transcription factor that regulate the expression of other genes by interactions with specific sequences in their regulatory regions. (a) Homeodomain proteins comprise three alpha helices (shown as cylinders). Most of the binding with the DNA occurs through helix 3. (b) Zinc finger proteins comprise an alpha helix and a beta sheet held together by a zinc atom (Zn). The alpha helix fits into the major groove of the DNA. (c) Leucine zipper proteins comprise two alpha helices that dimerize.

Table 3.2 Some of the extracellular signalling molecules that may regulate forebrain development (excluding extracellular matrix molecules which are given in Table 3.3). Neurotrophic factors, which have major actions in cell survival, and molecules involved in axon guidance are discussed in more detail in later chapters.

1. *Proteins*

A. **Members of the transforming growth factor beta superfamily**

The peptides encoded by the genes of this family homodimerize or heterodimerize and are secreted from the cell. The receptors that bind these molecules transmit the signal to the nucleus by activation of specific cytoplasmic proteins called smads. Once activated, the smads are converted into transcription factors that enter the nucleus and activate specific genes. (Graff *et al.*, 1996; Hoodless *et al.*, 1996; Liu *et al.*, 1996)

One large subgroup of this family, containing the bone morphogenetic proteins (BMPs) (Hogan, 1996), is thought to be important for the regulation of gene expression, cell proliferation, and cell death in the developing dorsal telencephalon (Furuta *et al.*, 1997). BMPs were originally discovered for their ability to induce bone growth, but are now known to regulate diverse developmental processes including proliferation, cell death, cell migration, cell differentiation, and morphogenesis, at many sites.

B. **Members of the Wnt family**

The Wnts are a family of glycoproteins. Their name comes from a fusion of the name of the *Drosophila* segment polarity gene wingless with that of one of its vertebrate homologues, integrated. They have multiple roles in development and have been implicated in cell–cell signalling in the developing forebrain. (Salinas and Nusse, 1992; Grove *et al.*, 1998)

C. **Members of the hedgehog family**

Hedgehog proteins play crucial roles in patterning the developing *Drosophila*. It acts in a concentration-dependent manner. Vertebrates have at least three homologues, sonic hedgehog (shh), desert hedgehog (dhh), and indian hedgehog (ihh). Of these, Shh is most important for CNS development. It is produced by the notochord and induces floor plate cells. It often works with other signalling molecules such as Wnts and FGFs. (Ericson *et al.*, 1995, 1997)

D. **Fibroblast growth factors (FGFs)**

FGFs are associated with several developmental processes, such as angiogenesis, mesoderm formation, induction of specific neural structures, axonal extension, and cell survival. The family and its receptors are discussed further in Chapter 6.

E. **Epidermal growth factor (EGF)**

Recently implicated in fate determination in the developing cortex (Burrows *et al.*, 1997). Expression pattern is compatible with the idea that its receptor is important for the generation of predominantly glial cells later in development (Burrows *et al.*, 1997; Eagleson *et al.*, 1996; Kornblum *et al.*, 1997).

F. **Neuregulins**

Implicated in glial-guided migration of neuronal precursors; these secreted growth factors act on receptors erbB2, erbB3, and erbB4 (Rio *et al.*, 1997; Anton *et al.*, 1997).

G. **Notch and Delta**

Most known regulators of neural induction are diffusible proteins. Some, however, remain bound to the cell surface. This occurs in the Notch–Delta signalling pathway. The Notch receptor protein on one cell binds to the Delta protein on another cell only when the cells are juxtaposed. The functions of Notch and Delta in cell fate determination in *Drosophila* are better understood than their roles in mammalian development. Notch is expressed in the cortex where it has been proposed to have a role in neuronal fate determination (Chenn and McConnell, 1995).

Table 3.2 (*Continued*)

H. Cerberus, Chordin, Follistatin, Noggin
Secreted proteins implicated in early neural induction by mesodermal and endodermal tissues (Lamb *et al.*, 1993; Sasai *et al.*, 1994; Doniach, 1995; Bouwmeester *et al.*, 1996; Hemmati-Brivanlou and Melton, 1997). See Section 5.

2. Neurotransmitters
Glutamate, GABA, and serotonin (5-hydroxytryptamine) are neurotransmitters that have been implicated in the regulation of cortical developmental processes, such as proliferation, migration, and thalamocortical innervation (LoTurco *et al.*, 1995; Cases *et al.*, 1996; Komuro and Rakic, 1993; Rakic, 1997; Vitalis *et al.*, 1998). See this chapter (Sections 8 and 9) and Chapter 5.

3. Molecules involved in axon guidance
Includes (i) cell adhesion molecules and receptors of the immunoglobulin superfamily and (ii) diffusible and membrane-bound molecules of the netrin and semaphorin families. These are discussed in Chapter 4 (and listed in Table 4.2).

4. Neurotrophic factors
Includes (i) growth factors (such as the neurotrophins and fibroblast growth factors) and (ii) cytokines (such as ciliary neurotrophic factor). These are discussed in detail in Chapter 6 (and listed in Table 6.2).

---

mostly unknown. Some experiments have pointed to genes that may be directly or indirectly regulated by particular transcription factors (Edelman and Jones, 1995; Holst *et al.*, 1997; Chalepakis *et al.*, 1994), but many of these indications remain unproven.

4.2   Extracellular signalling and cell adhesion

During development, cells communicate with each other by diffusible signalling molecules (e.g. those listed in Table 3.2) that mediate processes such as inductive signalling in early neural development (this chapter), axonal guidance (Chapter 4), and cell death (Chapter 6). Developing cells are also influenced by molecules that mediate their adhesion to each other. Some such molecules generate the specialized cell junctions (occluding junctions, anchoring junctions, and communicating junctions) that form between cells in many tissues, including the neuroepithelium (Nadarajah *et al.*, 1997, 1998). In addition, cell adhesion molecules form a major component of the extracellular matrix. Until recently, this matrix was viewed as a relatively inert scaffolding but it is now known to play an active and complex role in regulating tissue development. There are two main classes of macromolecule that constitute the extracellular matrix. The first comprises polysaccharide glycosaminoglycans (GAGs), which are normally linked to protein, forming proteoglycans. The second comprises fibrous proteins that are structural (e.g. collagen) or adhesive (e.g. laminin or fibronectin).

Table 3.3 Some of the major classes of molecule secreted in their entirety into the extracellular matrix.

A. **Proteoglycans** Diverse family of molecules characterized by a core protein to which is attached one or more polysaccharide glycosaminoglycan (GAG) side chains. The heterogeneity of proteoglycan structure reflects variation in the core protein and in the type and size of the GAG side chains. Cells at different stages of development express different variants of the same proteoglycan. The GAG group of complex carbohydrates includes the following.

● Chondroitin sulphate: Composed of a repeated basic unit comprising two different sugars (glucuronic acid joined to acetylgalactosamine).

● Dermatan sulphate: Similar to chondroitin sulphate expect for conversion of some glucuronic acid residues to iduronic acid.

● Keratan sulphate: Repeating unit is galactose joined to acetylglucosamine.

● Heparan sulphate: Repeating unit is glucuronic acid or iduronic acid joined to acetylglucosamine.

● Hyaluronan (hyaluronic acid): Repeating unit is glucuronic acid joined to acetylglucosamine; this is a unique member of the GAGs since it functions *in vivo* as a free carbohydrate and individual molecules can self-associate and form networks. It can support both cell proliferation and migration.

B. **Glycoproteins** A variety of extracellular glycoproteins have been isolated. They interact not only with cells but also with other macromolecules in the extracellular matrix into which they are secreted. The following are some well-known examples.

● Collagen: A highly specialized family of glycoproteins of which there are at least 16 types; has a triple helical structure; major component of connective tissue.

● Fibronectin: Widely distributed, prominent adhesive protein that mediates various aspects of cellular interactions including migration; is a dimer of two non-identical subunits.

● Laminins: Family of large glycoproteins distributed ubiquitously in basement membranes; they are multifunctional, with roles in processes such as growth of neurites, differentiation, and migration; can interact with cells via cell surface receptors including integrins, with collagen, and heparan sulphate proteoglycan. Composed of three distinct chains that assemble into a cruciform molecule.

Glycosaminoglycans are long chains of sugar residues. They are highly negatively charged. On the basis of differences in their sugar residues and the nature of the linkage between the residues and the location of sulphate groups, they have been divided into four groups: (i) hyaluronic acid; (ii) chondroitin sulphate and dermatan sulphate; (iii) heparan sulphate and heparin; (iv) keratan sulphate. All glycosaminoglycans except for hyaluronic acid are attached to a protein core to form proteoglycan molecules that can contain as much as 95% carbohydrate by weight and have the potential for enormous heterogeneity. Proteoglycans may be secreted components of the extracellular matrix or may have their core protein anchored in the cell membrane. Fibrous protein such as collagen, the most abundant protein in mammals, is found in all multicellular animals, with most being in connective tissue. Adhesive glycoproteins such as fibronectin, tenascin, and laminin are secreted into the extracellular matrix; some are involved not only in cell adhesion but also in cell migration. Cells bind extracellular matrix molecules via specific receptor glycoproteins on their surface, for example the fibronectin receptor or the integrins.

There are other adhesive interactions between cells that are mediated by cell surface glycoproteins. These interactions are important for the ability of cells not only to adhere to other cells but to do so in a selective fashion. When cells from two tissues are dissociated and mixed, cells are often found to adhere more readily to cells of their own tissue than to cells of the other tissue; for example, this approach has been used to demonstrate selective adhesion of cells from different telencephalic regions (Gotz *et al.*, 1996). Glycoproteins differ from proteoglycans in several ways: (i) they usually contain less carbohydrate (1–60%); (ii) they have relatively short carbohydrate chains of less than 15 sugar residues; (iii) their sugar side chains have a different composition and arrangement. Cell surface glycoproteins mediate two classes of cell–cell adhesion mechanism, one that is calcium dependent and one that is calcium independent.

One of the best examples of a cell surface glycoprotein that mediates calcium-independent cell–cell adhesion is neural cell adhesion molecule (N-CAM), which is expressed on the surface of nerve and glial cells. This is a member of the immunoglobulin superfamily of recognition proteins to which antibodies belong. Homophilic interactions between N-CAM molecules on two cells bind the cells together. N-CAM has a large extracellular polypeptide chain that is folded into domains that are homologous to the immunoglobulin domains of antibodies. There are several forms of N-CAM, that differ mainly in their membrane associated and cytoplasmic portions. Many other similar cell surface glycoproteins with immunoglobulin domains that mediate calcium-independent cell–cell adhesion have been discovered.

Calcium-dependent cell–cell adhesion involves cell surface glycoproteins called cadherins. Cadherins are homologous transmembrane glycoproteins that undergo a large conformational change and are degraded enzymatically in the absence of extracellular calcium. It is likely that cadherins play important roles in neural development; for example, the neural tube expresses different forms of cadherin at different times in its development. Cadherins may be involved in the case, cited above, of the selective adhesion of cells from different telencephalic regions, a phenomenon that has been shown to be calcium dependent (Gotz *et al.*, 1996).

5 INDUCTIVE INTERACTIONS IN FOREBRAIN DEVELOPMENT

A central aim of developmental biology is to understand how, at each stage in the maturation of an organism, cells in different positions develop differently; i.e. how regional specification is achieved. This is as true for the development of a structure as complex as the cerebral cortex, where each point in the dorsal telencephalic wall aquires a unique functional property, with relative invariance in the layout of these properties between the individuals of the same species, as it is for the earliest embryos and their components. In fact, many of the principles that govern the ways in which regional specification arises during development have been identified in studies of early embryogenesis. It is useful to have a grasp of these concepts when thinking about the ways in which regional specification of the cerebral cortex might be controlled. Our relative ignorance of the mechanisms that control cortical regionalization makes it all the more important to generate hypotheses with knowledge of principles deduced from studies of earlier developing systems.

Two terms used to describe complementary mechanisms that can generate regional specification are mosaicism and regulation. The recognition of whether a developing system is mosaic or regulated requires experimental interference. If cells are manipulated (by, for example, separation from one another), and yet they continue to follow the developmental pathways that normally they would have followed, they are said to be mosaic. Conversely, if after experimental manipulation cells follow a different developmental pathway from normal, they are said to display regulative behaviour. Both types of behaviour can occur in a single embryo or system, or one type can precede the other (Slack, 1991). We shall return to these ideas in later chapters that consider the generation of cortical maps.

Commonly, regulative behaviour is found among cells undergoing regional specification in the developing mammalian nervous system. Where it occurs, it indicates that the mechanism of specification involves intercellular signalling. In early embryogenesis, major sources of such signals are well defined, and include the dorsal lip of the blastopore formed at gastrulation (Fig. 3.5; the so-called Spemann organizer; Spemann, 1938) and mesodermal derivatives such as the prechordal mesoderm and notochord (Fig. 3.6). The signals that affect the developmental pathway taken by the responsive cells (so-called competent cells) receiving

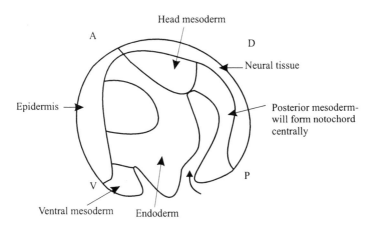

FIG. 3.5. Section of a midgastrula *Xenopus* embryo showing the layout of ectodermal, mesodermal and endodermal tissues. The curved arrow shows the direction of mesodermal ingression. Abbreviations: A, anterior; D, dorsal; P, posterior; V, ventral.

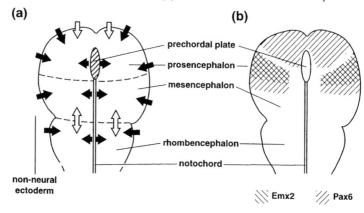

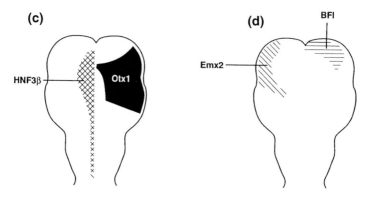

F I G .   3 . 6 . (a) Diagram showing the anterior neural plate illustrating a hypothesis for the generation of regional specification in the anterior neural plate by inductive signalling. Inductive signals mediated by diffusible molecules are indicated: filled arrows mark signalling from the neural ridge by bone morphogenetic proteins; open arrowheads mark signalling from the anterior neural ridge and the mesencephalon/rhombencephalon border (the isthmus) by fibroblast growth factor 8; arrowheads mark signalling from the notochord, floor plate, and prechordal plate by sonic hedgehog. (b) The expression of regulatory genes is regionally restricted in the anterior neural plate. Early expression of two such genes, Pax6 and Emx2, is shown. (c) Two further examples of the region-specific expression of regulatory genes in the anterior neural plate. (d) At a slightly later stage of neural plate development, there is a change in the expression of Emx2 (shown at an earlier stage in b). The gene BF1 is expressed in the telencephalic primordium. (After Rubenstein and Beachy, 1998; Rubenstein *et al.*, 1998)

them are termed inductive signals. Although inductive signalling is almost certainly a widespread mechanism in the later stages of cortical regionalization, its clearest roles are in the early stages of forebrain development where it is mediated by molecules that include some of those listed in Table 3.2.

Early in embryogenesis, signals from the dorsal mesoderm induce neural development in the overlying dorsal ectoderm (Chapter 2). Much of the work on this process has been carried out in *Xenopus laevis*. Neural induction occurs during gastrulation, at which stage mesoderm ingresses beneath the ectoderm (Fig. 3.5). The first mesoderm to ingress gives rise to the anterior head mesoderm; the mesoderm that follows will form the notochord centrally (the chordamesoderm) and more lateral mesodermal structures (blocks of segmented tissue called somites, that will give rise to the vertebrae and ribs, skeletal muscle, and part of the skin). The anterior mesoderm differs from the chordamesoderm not only in the time of its development but also in the genes that it expresses: for example, it expresses the goosecoid homeobox gene, whereas the chordamesoderm does not (Filosa *et al.*, 1997). It has been proposed that:

1. Signals from both the anterior mesoderm and the chordamesoderm initiate neural development by inducing neural tissue of an anterior type (i.e. characteristic of forebrain and midbrain) in the overlying ectoderm along its entire anteroposterior length.

2. A second signal from chordamesoderm alone converts the overlying neurectoderm induced by the first signal into neural tissue of a more posterior type (i.e. hindbrain and spinal cord).

These ideas were proposed in the 1950s by Nieuwkoop and by Saxen and Toivonen (reviewed by Nieuwkoop and Albers, 1990; Saxen, 1989; Doniach, 1995) and led to the search for possible neural-inducing molecules. Several secreted proteins expressed in dorsal mesoderm have been proposed as candidates for the first signal (the inducer of anterior neurectoderm), including noggin, follistatin, and chordin; mesoderm-derived molecules that may posteriorize neural tissue over the chordamesoderm include fibroblast growth factors (reviewed in Doniach, 1995).

Although the role of the mesoderm in neural induction is well accepted, recent work in the mouse has indicated that anterior endodermal tissue may in fact be responsible for the very first induction of anterior neural structures and for the correct definition of the prosencephalic neurectoderm (Thomas and Beddington, 1996). The evidence is that initial anterior neural induction by endoderm occurs before axial mesoderm is formed, although it may rely on axial mesoderm for its maintenance since the endodermal structures that induce anterior neurectoderm do not persist in the embryo. Further work on *Xenopus* has identified an endodermally-expressed gene, Cerberus, that encodes a secreted protein capable of inducing head structures, including anterior CNS tissue (Bouwmeester *et al.*, 1996). The targets of secreted proteins such as Cerberus are not yet known. The biochemical pathways that these molecules activate are likely to involve other molecules required for head and anterior neural development, such as the homeobox-containing genes Otx-2 and Lim-1 (also called Lhx-1; refer to Table 3.1 above). Lim-1 is normally expressed in the anterior organizing tissues of the early embryo, including the anterior mesoderm. Its targeted deletion results in embryos lacking anterior head structures, although the rest of the body develops relatively normally (Shawert and Behringer, 1995). Otx-2 expression is found in anterior ectoderm, where it depends on interactions with the underlying anterior mesoderm; it is also found in anterior mesodermal and endodermal tissue. Targeted deletion of Otx-2 results in severe defects of gastrulation and mesodermal formation and in the loss of anterior neural tissue (Ang *et al.*, 1996).

As we have seen in Chapter 2, the ventral forebrain arises from the medial part of the anterior neural plate. The optic stalks and hypothalamus develop in this region. The medial part of the prosencephalic neural plate directly overlies anterior meso-dermal and endodermal tissues (called the prechordal mesendoderm or prechordal plate; Fig. 3.6) and it has long been recognized that these tissues are essential for correct development of the optic stalks and hypothalamus (Adelmann, 1936a,b). More recent studies of zebrafish have shown that development of the anterior cen-tral nervous system depends on a small group of ectodermal cells located in the prospective head region; removal of these cells during gastrulation perturbs sub-sequent neural patterning (Houart *et al.*, 1998). Work in the mouse has shown that cultured explants of prechordal plate can induce ventral forebrain properties (such as expression of Nkx2.1, a homeobox-containing gene whose expression domain in the neural plate is restricted to medial, i.e. putative ventral, tissue) (Table 3.1) in prosencephalic neural plate (Shimamura and Rubenstein, 1997). Transplantation of the prechordal plate to ectopic locations in extraembryonic ectoderm in chicks induces the formation of ventral forebrain tissue (Pera and Kessel, 1997). Other experiments have indicated that the secreted factors BMP7 and SHH (Table 3.2) are involved in the induction of ventral forebrain by the prechordal plate (Dale *et al.*, 1997).

A current hypothesis for inductive signals that generate regional specification in the anterior neural plate is shown in Fig. 3.6a. The secreted signalling protein encoded by Sonic hedgehog (Shh) is expressed along the anteroposterior length of the axial mesoderm, including the prechordal plate, and induces ventral properties in the overlying neural tube (Fig. 3.6; Echelard *et al.*, 1993). In mice lacking Shh function (Chiang *et al.*, 1996), there is a loss of ventral neural fates throughout the anteroposterior length of the neural tube. In the forebrain, these include an absence of ventral forebrain structures and a failure to subdivide the region that will develop into the eyes, leading to the production of a single (cyclopic) eye. The rest of the forebrain expresses molecules characteristic of dorsal telencephalon and develops as a single vesicle. Transduction of SHH protein, which may involve transmembrane proteins called Patched and Smoothened (Marigo *et al.*, 1996; Van den Heuvel and Ingham, 1996), appears directly or indirectly to regulate the expression of a number of transcription factor genes that confer regional identities on the anterior neural plate. These include the winged-helix transcription factor HNF3b, which may be indirectly regulated via Shh-induced changes in the activity of Gli proteins (Sasaki *et al.*, 1997), and homeobox-containing genes of the Nkx and Pax families (Table 3.1; Rubenstein and Beachy, 1998). It is very likely that, as in the developing spinal cord, the concentration of SHH plays a part in determining which transcription factors are expressed at different sites in the anterior neural plate (Ericson *et al.*, 1995, 1997).

There is now evidence that inductive interactions are also involved in the specification of the dorsal and anterior forebrain. These inductive signals may originate from cells at the boundary between the neurectoderm and the surface (non-neural) ectoderm (Fig. 3.6). BMPs (Table 3.2) are among the possible mediators of these interactions (Furuta *et al.*, 1997). There is strong evidence that, in more posterior neurectoderm, BMPs from the surrounding surface ectoderm induce lateral neural plate, which later becomes dorsal spinal cord (Tanabe and Jessell, 1996). It has been proposed, on the grounds that some Bmp genes are also expressed in and around the early prosencephalic neurectoderm (Furuta *et al.*, 1997), that they play a similar role in specification of dorsal forebrain (Shimamura and Rubenstein, 1997; Rubenstein and Beachy, 1998). How these molecules might act to specify regional identity is not yet clear, although there is evidence that they can induce expression of transcription factor genes such as Msx1 (Table 3.1) that are expressed in the dorsal midline and repress other genes that are regionally expressed, such as BF1 (Table 3.1) (Furuta *et al.*, 1997).

In addition to these inductive signals from midline and lateral issues, the anterior neural ridge of the neural plate (Fig. 3.6) is proposed to be an inducing centre for the anterior neural plate (Shimamura and Rubenstein, 1997). When the anterior neural ridge is removed, expression of BF1 is eliminated (Shimamura and Rubenstein, 1997). This gene is normally expressed in the anterolateral neural plate and, as described below, is essential for the development of the telencephalon from that region (Fig. 3.6, Table 3.1). The anterior neural ridge expresses FGF8, a molecule known to have inducing properties at another site of its expression at the boundary between the midbrain and hindbrain (Crossley *et al.*, 1996). When the anterior neural ridge is removed, beads soaked in FGF8 can restore the expression of BF1 in the anterior neural plate (Shimamura and Rubenstein, 1997). At the boundary between midbrain and hindbrain, FGF8 induces expression of a different homeobox-containing gene called En2 (Crossley *et al.*, 1996; Lee *et al.*, 1997), indicating that, as is the case with Shh induction (Shimamura and Rubenstein, 1997), different regions of the neural plate respond differently to the same molecules. In other words, the competence of different regions of the neural plate to respond to the same inducing signal appears to differ. Regional differences in terms of regulatory gene expression are present in the neural plate, and they are almost certainly responsible for at least some aspects of differing competence (Fig. 3.6). How these differences in competence are established is unclear (possibilities are discussed below). As described in the next section, these patterns of gene expression become increasingly elaborate as the forebrain develops.

Induction of anterior neural tissue by other surrounding structures is likely to be involved in early forebrain regionalization. For example, embryological experiments have indicated an inductive influence of the olfactory placode (Fig. 2.1) on the subsequent development of the olfactory bulb and other forebrain regions (Stout and Eraziadei, 1980). It has been suggested that the relevant morphogenetically active substance produced in the olfactory placodal neuroepithelium may be the simple molecule retinoic acid. This molecule has received much attention and is known to be a potent morphogen in limb development (LaMantia *et al.*, 1993). The work on limb bud development arose out of observations of the effect of surgical disruption during development. On the basis of experiments on the salamander *Ambystoma* at tailbud stage (Harrison, 1918), it has long been known that half of the limb disc (the cells that normally give rise to the limb) will generate an entire limb if transplanted to a new site or left *in situ*. Following experiments involving grafting a small part of the chick limb bud, called the Zone of Polarising Activity (Saunders and Gasseling, 1968) into another limb which gave rise to supernumerary digits, it was speculated that a morphogen would diffuse from the ZPA to form a gradient and thereby specify the anterior–posterior axis giving rise to the digits of the limb (Tickle *et al.*, 1975). Naizi and Saxena (1978) found that application of retinal palmitate to amputated toad limbs led to several reduplicated regenerates. This type of experiment was repeated by Maden (1982) on *Ambystoma* with more extensive and broadly similar results. Tickle *et al.* (1982), and Summerbell (1983) established that the action of retinoic acid could mimic the action of an additional ZPA. Conversely, blocking the synthesis of retinoic acid pharmacologically prevents limb bud initiation (Stratford *et al.*, 1996). It has been suggested that the establishment of a gradient of retinoic acid activates certain homeotic genes in cells in the limb field.

As yet, it is not clear how inductive signals combine to generate regional differences in patterns of regulatory gene expression (Fig. 3.6) and morphological specification in the anterior neural plate. The patterning of the developing forebrain by regulatory genes is described in the next section. The subsequent section describes models that may link inductive signalling with regionalization.

6   Generation of Regional Diversity in Forebrain

The very early regionalization of the prosencephalon can be detected by morphological criteria, such as characteristic constrictions or evaginations of the tissue, and also by analysis of the discrete domains of expression of regulatory genes (Puelles and Rubenstein, 1993; Shimamura *et al.*, 1995). Figure 3.7 summarizes expression patterns of a number of regulatory genes that are thought to play a role in the specification of the different regions of the forebrain. It is possible that these genes, probably through combinatorial actions, give each region of the developing forebrain a unique identity. They may do this by controlling the expression of numerous other genes required for the characteristic morphological differentiation of that region. At present, the known regulatory genes that are regionally expressed in the embryonic forebrain include members of several groups, such as the Pax,

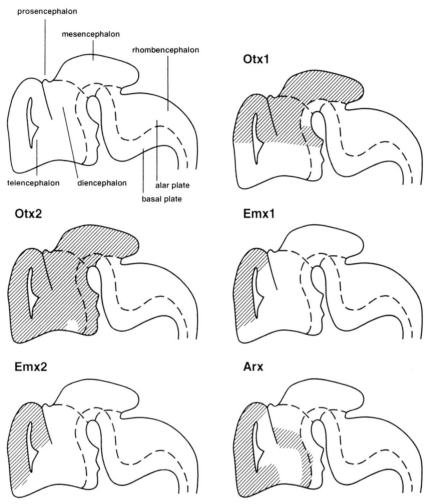

F I G . 3 . 7 . Diagrams showing the expression patterns of several of the genes known to regulate forebrain development. Cross-hatching shows the main domains of expression on a schematic view of the forebrain of an embryonic mouse. For some genes, the domains of expression can alter in detail during embryogenesis: a good example of this is Pax6, whose expression is shown at around mid-gestation (marked 'early') and a few days later (marked 'late'). The discovery of further genes is anticipated and blank diagrams are included for the reader to add further information.

Gbx, En, Wnt, Dlx, Nkx, Emx, and Otx families (Table 3.1; Fig. 3.7) (Puelles and Rubenstein, 1993; Shimamura *et al.*, 1995); the list continues to increase.

In recent years, the correspondence between morphological features of the developing forebrain and the domains of expression of regulatory genes has been studied. It has been found that the boundaries between domains of regulatory gene

Pax6 (early)   **Pax6 (late)**

BF1   **BF2**

Dlx2   **Dlx5**

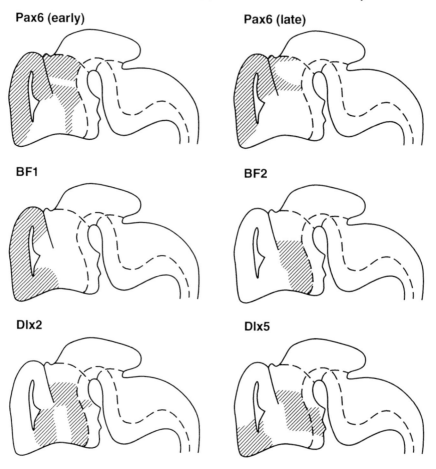

F I G .   3 . 7 . (*Continued*)

expression often correspond to anatomical boundaries between morphologically distinct structures. These anatomical boundaries appear as regions of the forebrain (i) evaginate (e.g. to form the paired telencephalic vesicles, optic vesicles, and olfactory bulbs), (ii) enlarge inwardly (e.g. to form the ganglionic eminences), and (iii) bend (e.g. at the junction between the midbrain and the forebrain). This work has led to the proposal that the early forebrain can be subdivided into a number of transverse domains, or prosomeres, as summarized in Fig. 3.8 (Puelles and Rubenstein, 1993). There is similar evidence that the prosencephalon can also be subdivided longitudinally (Fig. 3.8), into regions that correspond to longitudinally oriented regions in the spinal cord, called (from ventral to dorsal) the floorplate, basal plate, alar plate, and roof plate. In the spinal cord, these regions can be distinguished on the basis of morphological landmarks and patterns of gene expression;

Lhx1 (Lim1)   Tbr1

Id2

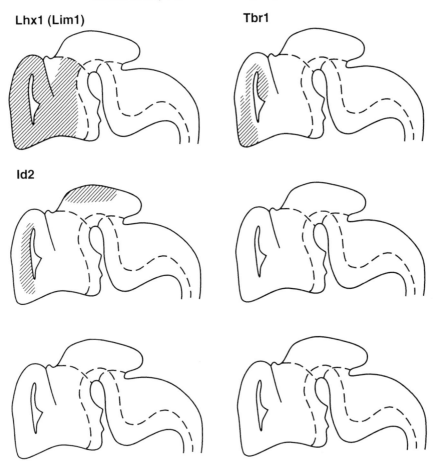

FIG. 3.7. (*Continued*)

in the forebrain, gene expression studies have indicated the existence of correlated regions (Puelles and Rubenstein, 1993; Shimamura *et al.*, 1995; Shimamura
and Rubenstein, 1997). In this way, the neuroepithelium of the forebrain can be
subdivided by a grid of expression domains into histogenic primordia.

The regional specificity of gene expression in the prosencephalon has a parallel
in the mammalian hindbrain (rhombencephalon: Fig. 3.3), where the expression
of each of a family of Hox genes ends at a specific boundary between hindbrain
neuromeres (rhombomeres) (Krumlauf, 1994). As in the rhombencephalon, it is
to be expected that recent advances in transgenic methods will help elucidate
the roles of the regionally expressed prosencephalic regulatory genes in defining
the morphological characteristics of each forebrain region. Some of the proposed
activities of forebrain-expressed regulatory genes are given in Table 3.1.

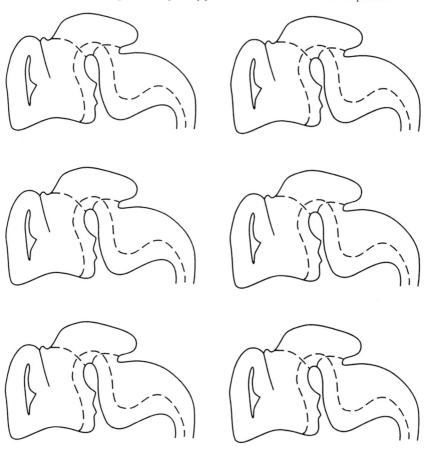

FIG.   3.7. (*Continued*)

Assuming strict parallels between regionalization of the hindbrain and forebrain is premature. One possible difference between the segmentation process in the two regions might be the behaviour of cells at the boundaries between the neuromeres, i.e. the rhombomeres in the hindbrain and the prosomeres in the forebrain. Cell lineage analysis has shown that cells can only cross the inter-rhombomeric boundaries before a certain stage of development, and never after (Fraser *et al.*, 1990). In other words, the developing rhombomeres become cellular compartments whose boundaries are respected by the cells within them, and their descendants. It is not yet known whether the same is true for interprosomeric borders; what evidence there is hints that this may not be the case (Golden and Cepko, 1996).

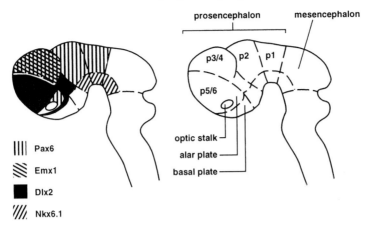

F I G .   3 . 8 . The Prosomeric Model (Rubenstein and Beachy, 1998; Rubenstein *et al.*, 1998) in which the forebrain is divided into regions, labelled p1, p2, p3/4, and p4/5 on the basis of morphology and patterns of gene expression. Some examples of genes whose expression borders fit the prosomeric boundaries are shown (Pax6, Emx1, Dlx2, Nkx6.1).

7 FORMAL MODELS OF REGIONAL SPECIFICATION

Regional specificity of regulatory gene expression in the prosencephalon is likely to control regional differences in morphological characteristics, through actions on the cellular processes of proliferation, migration, and differentiation. These controlling influences of regulatory genes on morphology will be discussed later. In this section we consider how different regions of the forebrain come to express different genes in the first place. This remains a subject of speculation. One simple possibility is that a small number of regulatory genes distributed over the neural plate and very early neural tube may generate morphogen gradients. The existence of such molecules with graded distributions may create domains of gene expression with sharp boundaries. This type of process is known to generate regionalized domains of gene expression in the early embryo of the fruit fly, *Drosophila melanogaster*, as shown in Fig. 3.2. Although homologues of these genes exist in the mammalian forebrain, drawing close parallels between mammalian forebrain and *Drosophila* development may be dangerous given the differences between them at a cellular level. None the less, the principle that continuous morphogen gradients may be read-out to create domains of expression of other genes distributed with discrete levels is now well established.

The problem is usually formulated in terms of how a mass of cells acquire differences that are used to determine their different fates. The fundamental conceptual problem is how each cell acquires the collection of all its chemical constituents, reaction constants, etc. that distinguishes it from another cell (Slack, 1991). One obvious way in which cells can be distinguished from one another is if they carry a different value of some substance, or morphogen. Many different formal models have been proposed for how such patterns of morphogens can be generated. These models are usually formulated in the light of the concept of positional information and are constrained by the regulatory phenomena often seen in embryogenesis.

1. Positional information

Evidence from classical embryological experiments on the properties of a mass of cells which involved the removal of some cells or the transposition of cells to a new position resulted in the notion that the fate of cell is determined by its position within the morphogenetic field of cells. A set of cells that makes a morphogenetic field can form its own organ when transplanted to a foreign site and cells within the field can regulate to take over the function of other cells that are removed from it. How is each cell within the field instructed or, as expressed by Wolpert (1969, 1971), how does the cell acquire its positional information? One fundamental way in which information is supplied in development is through inducing signals supplied through extracellular means and various ways of assigning differences amongst cells by means of morphogens have been considered. In the simplest case of a one-dimensional field of cells that specifies the digits of the hand, for example, a gradient of morphogen would enable different parts of the field to be distinguished; specifying particular threshold values of morphogen would determine which cells would develop into which digit.

2. Simple gradient models

The simplest way of producing a spatially varying profile of some putative morphogen is that for the one-dimensional case. At one end of the line of cells there is a source of morphogen; at the other end there is a sink and morphogen flows from source to sink to set up a graded variant of morphogen down the line of cells (Crick, 1970). For two-dimensional sheets of cells, a single source is replaced by a line of sources, and there are two different types of source to correspond to the two different dimensions of variation. Whereas in principle such a system can produce satisfactory gradients, it is unlikely to operate in developing systems. It relies too heavily on specific cells to be sources and sinks and furthermore it takes an unrealistically long time to set up the gradients.

3. Distributed sink model

One variation of this scheme is that there is a single source (for one dimension) but all cells acts as sinks through leakage and other forms of loss (Fig. 3.9a) (Slack, 1991; Meinhardt, 1982). According to this scheme, gradients of 1 mm can be set up within 1 hour, which is a satisfactory speed. Rearrangement of cells within the field leads to regulation, i.e. the original gradient being restored. However, this system has three main disadvantages: (i) following changes in size of the field, the full gradient is not restored, so that an incomplete structure will be generated; (ii) regulation of the source is impossible; i.e. following removal of the source cells a new source cannot be generated; (iii) the system is too self-regulating in that it is insensitive to small perturbations, which, it is thought, are needed to introduce essential asymmetries into the system.

4. Reaction-diffusion model

Gierer and Meinhardt (1972) proposed a model in which both source and sink are distributed. In this model there are two molecules with different properties: an activator, which stimulates its own production together with that of a second molecules called an inhibitor. The inhibitor diffuses at a faster rate than the activator and represses the production of activator. A small local increase in the amount of activator will result in more activator being produced there, this giving rise to a local source of activator, which can be regarded as the morphogen. The inhibitor produced as a result will diffuse out more quickly than the activator and so a sink for activator will be established nearby. In this way, spatial patterns of activator and inhibitor become distributed across the array of cells (Fig. 3.9b). There is a class

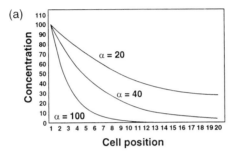

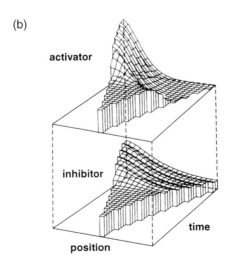

FIG. 3.9. Plots of morphogen concentration as a function of position along one dimension according to various models for assigning positional information to a group of cells. (a) Steady state plots for the distributed sink model. The slope of the gradient is determined by the value of α, which is a measure of the spatial and temporal character of the diffusion process. From Stack (1991) with permission. (b) Steady state plots for the reaction-diffusion model. Initially flat distributions of activator and inhibitor give rise to pronounced gradients, in this case with a peak at one end. (Reproduced with permission from Meinhardt, 1982)

of models of this type, the first being that due to Turing (1952). In these reaction-diffusion models, a crucial parameter is the size of the field compared with the spatial scale of diffusion of the two molecules. If the size of the morphogenetic field is very much smaller than the diffusion length scale, periodically repeating patterns will be produced; if the values of these two parameters are comparable, a single gradient of morphogen results. Imposing a weak gradient of activator production to determine polarity yields a single gradient. The extent of the gradient is preserved following artificial diminution of field size, up to a limit. Reduction of the field to one-half of full size preserves the almost complete range of the gradient but when the field is further reduced only a fraction of the gradient is preserved.

5. Role of gradients

The primary role to be fulfilled by systems of gradients is to provide a way for cells to be distinguished one from another. The reaction-diffusion scheme at least provides a way of doing this which is resistant (within limits) to changes in morphogenetic field size. It is assumed that a separate mechanism exists that translates an amount of morphogen into an instruction to build a cellular structure. In some cases, patterns of morphogens are required to specify the coordinate systems of developing organs. In these cases, it is natural (although not necessary) to assume that the axes of the morphogens will match those of the required coordinate system; for example a rectangular coordinate system might be provided by two morphogens each identified with one axis. In cases where there is no such requirement, as long as cells can be distinguished one from another, the pattern of morphogens can be arbitrary.

6. Clock and wave front model

An example of how time is used in the generation of a spatial pattern is provided by the clock and wave front model due to Cooke and Zeeman (1976). Their model was advanced to account for how the vertebrate somites are formed sequentially and they proposed that there is an interaction between a signal advancing from head to tail (the wave front) and an oscillatory signal generated within the cells themselves with a much shorter time scale (Winfree, 1970, 1972). The idea is that the passage of the wave front through the tissue sequentially recruits cells into the activities of somite formation. Whether a cell does become part of a somite will depend on the phase of the oscillation at that particular time. In this way successive populations of cells arranged in small groups undergo change almost syncronously amongst themselves, giving rise to the generation of a series of somites in a discontinuous fashion. This model is of interest as it is one example of what other types of schemes are available for the generation of pattern. However it has not yet been clearly worked out and perhaps for this reason it has not been tested experimentally.

8 REGULATION OF SIZE DIFFERENCES BETWEEN MAJOR FOREBRAIN STRUCTURES

Clearly, an important feature of each region of the forebrain is its size. The major components of the forebrain grow at different rates. How is this controlled? At present, there are relatively few explicit links between what is now an extensive body of literature on the mechanisms that regulate the cell cycle in eukaryotic cells and the control of proliferation in cortical progenitors. It is likely that these links will strengthen significantly in the next few years. Without doubt, our understanding of the control of the cell cycle in other cell types will provide essential background to future research on early cortical neurogenesis. Here, we provide a brief overview of our current understanding of how the cell cycle is controlled; there are many extensive reviews (Hartwell and Weinert, 1989; Murray and Kirschner, 1989; Nurse, 1990; Murray and Hunt, 1993).

It is now recognized that cells possess a set of interacting proteins that induce and coordinate each stage of the cell cycle. These proteins can be grouped into two key classes, the cyclin-dependent protein kinases (Cdks) and the cyclins. The cyclins bind to Cdks and regulate their ability to phosphorylate target proteins. The cell cycle is driven by the cyclical assembly, activation, and breakdown of the Cdk–cyclin complexes. Some cyclins bind to Cdks during G2 phase, and are required for entry into M phase; other cyclins bind to Cdks during G1 phase, and are required for entry into S phase. It is also known that there are mechanisms for stopping the cell cycle at particular points, called checkpoints. There are three well-recognized checkpoints: one in G1 phase, shortly before the entry into S phase (called the G1 checkpoint); one in G2 phase, before entry into M phase (the G2 checkpoint); and one in M phase (the metaphase checkpoint). It is at these checkpoints that signals from the cell's environment can act on the cell cycle machinery. Thus, the length of the G1 phase can be modulated by influences from outside the cell (Massague and Polyak, 1995) and, in higher eukaryotic cells, signals that stop the cell cycle usually do so by acting on the G1 checkpoint.

As discussed in Chapter 2, the overall length of the cell cycle increases progressively throughout cortical neurogenesis and, as in other cell types, this is due to a lengthening of the G1 phase (Waechter and Jaensch, 1972; Schultze and Korr, 1981; Schmahl, 1983; Takahashi *et al.*, 1992a,b, 1993, 1994, 1995a, 1996; Miller *et al.*, 1995; Caviness *et al.*, 1997). This indicates that regulating the length of the G1 phase is crucial for coordinating neocortical histogenesis. It is known that both growth factors and transcription factors can influence rates of proliferation in cortical cells, and it is possible that they do so by acting on the G1 checkpoint.

8.1   Growth factors

To date, a few molecules that have the potential to regulate the proliferation of neocortical stem cells have been identified, although how they might act *in vivo* is unresolved. These include members of the fibroblast growth factor (FGF) family, the neurotrophin family (specifically, neurotrophin-3), and neurotransmitters (γ-aminobutyric acid, GABA, and glutamate) (LoTurco *et al.*, 1995; Ghosh and Greenberg, 1995). FGF-2 has been shown to have a mitogenic effect on dissociated cells from the cortical proliferative zone (Kilpatrick and Bartlett, 1993; Ghosh and Greenberg, 1995; Antonopoulos *et al.*, 1997; Cavanagh *et al.*, 1997). A more recent study *in vivo* has shown that injecting FGF-2 into the cerebral ventricles of rat embryos increases the number of rounds of division of cortical progenitors (Vaccarino *et al.*, 1999). A particularly intriguing observation by Ghosh and Greenberg (1995) is that exogenous mitogens such as FGF-2 may exert different effects on cortical progenitors of different ages. In their study, FGF-2 induced the proliferation of progenitor cells for 10–12 days in culture, but after this period the cells differentiated to form glia. It is possible that progenitors have some intrinsic timing mechanism that alters the way in which they respond to the same factors and this may contribute to the transition from neurogenesis to gliogenesis (Chapter 2). Some recent evidence indicates that, while addition of FGF-2 has mitogenic effects, FGF-2 may not be essential for proliferation in the cortex *in vivo*. Mice lacking FGF-2 show defects in cortical cell fates, migration and differentiation, but not proliferation (Dono *et al.*, 1998).

Neurotrophin-3 (NT-3), transforming growth factor-β (TGF-β), glutamate (acting via kainate receptors), and GABA (acting via GABA-A receptors) have an opposite effect. They are anti-mitogenic, causing cells to leave the cell cycle and slowing proliferation (LoTurco *et al.*, 1995; Ghosh and Greenberg, 1995; Massague and Polyak, 1995; Antonopoulos *et al.*, 1997). It is proposed that these effects involve a lengthening of the G1 phase of the cell cycle.

8.2   Transcription factors

Some of the regulatory genes that define the telencephalon and its subdivisions are given in Figs. 3.7 and 3.8 and Table 3.1. They include BF-1 (Tao and Lai, 1992; Shimamura *et al.*, 1995), Emx-1 and Emx-2, Otx-1 and Otx-2 (Simeone *et al.*, 1992a,b; Frantz *et al.*, 1994c), and several other genes whose primary sites of expression are elsewhere and whose telencephalic expression patterns are less well defined (e.g. Pax-6; Walther and Gruss, 1991). BF-1 is a member of a family of genes called HNF-3, whose proteins bind DNA and are homologous to a *Drosophila* transcription factor, fork head (Tao and Lai, 1992). BF-1 expression is restricted to the telencephalon from the time when this structure first emerges (Tao and Lai, 1992; Shimamura *et al.*, 1995). This suggests a role for BF-1 specifying the telencephalon, and more recent knock-out experiments have indicated that its primary role may be to regulate proliferation rates in this structure (Xuan *et al.*, 1995). Clearly, an exceptionally high rate of proliferation is one of the defining features of the telencephalon, but it seems likely that other, perhaps as yet unidentified genes, must also contribute to its specification. Other genes expressed in the telencephalon are less compelling as candidates for specifying this structure and its proliferative rates, since they are either expressed more widely both inside and outside the telencephalon or their expression is restricted to only a part of the telencephalon (Figs. 3.7 and 3.8). These genes may be important for the specification of regions within the telencephalon. Data on this issue are incomplete at present, but it is hypothesized that genes such as Emx-1 and Emx-2 or Otx-1 and Otx-2 define different regions and/or different layers of cells within those regions (Boncinelli *et al.*, 1995). For example, Otx-1 is expressed in the ventricular zone and the deep layers of the neocortex (Franz *et al.*, 1994). It is conceivable that such genes might also play roles in regulating proliferation, although this remains to be tested.

In a recent study we used a mouse with a mutation of Pax-6 (small eye) to study the role of this gene in the development of the diencephalon (Warren and Price, 1997). Pax-6, isolated independently by homology to gooseberry-distal (Walther and Gruss, 1991) and from positional cloning at the aniridia locus (Ton *et al.*, 1991), encodes two DNA-binding motifs, a paired domain (Bopp *et al.*, 1986; Treisman *et al.*, 1991), and a paired-like homeodomain (Frigerio *et al.*, 1986). Its mRNA is first detected on embryonic day 8.5 (E8.5) in the mouse and it is a prime candidate for a regulator of regionalization, differentiation, and/or maintenance of various parts of the CNS, including the forebrain (Stoykova and Gruss, 1994). There are several alleles of small eye, which are thought to be null mutations (i.e. lacking gene function) (Hill *et al.*, 1991). Studies of proliferation rates in the small eye mutants have shown alterations in regions of the developing central nervous system that express the gene (Warren and Price, 1997; Gotz *et al.*, 1998; Warren *et al.*, 1999). These effects are variable from region to region; in the diencephalon, loss of Pax-6 expression appears to reduce proliferative rates whereas in the developing cortex it may increase proliferative rates. In conclusion, there is evidence that several regionally expressed transcription factors regulate proliferative rates and may contribute to the generation of differences in size between different parts of the embryonic forebrain.

9 MOLECULAR CONTROL OF CELL MIGRATION

As discussed in Chapter 2, many neuronal precursors migrate from the proliferative zone to their eventual destination in the developing cortex along the processes of radial glial cells. It is likely that some migrating cortical neuronal precursors use other substrates, but as yet relatively little is known about the mechanisms that control such movements. More is known about the regulation of glial-guided migration. This process has several components: neurons must recognize and adhere to glial cells, move along them at an appropriate rate, and cease their migration at an appropriate point. The cessation of neuronal precursor migration during normal cortical development is near to the border of the cortical plate and marginal zone. In some mutants, such as the reeler mouse (see below), and following some heterochronic transplants of cortical precursors (see Chapter 2), cessation of migration may occur deeper in the cortical plate.

Figure 3.10 illustrates some of the events that may be involved in normal glial-directed migration. Migrating neurons have two processes, one called a leading process that follows the radial glial fibres, the other called a trailing process. These contain assemblies of microtubules and actin-like contractile proteins whose actions generate the forces that propel the neuron. One model of how these

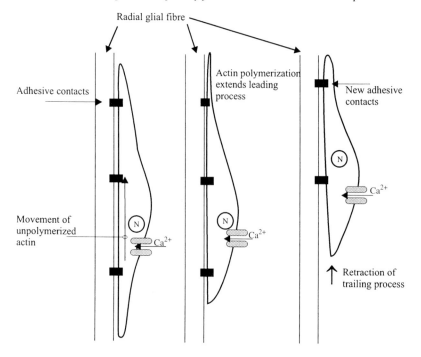

FIG. 3.10. Mechanisms of neuronal migration along glial fibres. Factors in the nucleus (N) and levels of intracellular calcium may contribute to regulating the process; the movement of actin and the formation and breaking of adhesive contacts are key components of the machinery itself (Rakic, 1997).

cytoskeletal proteins act is that unpolymerized actin is continually shifting forwards, towards the leading process of the cell, where it polymerizes. At the same time, microtubules and/or actin transport cell membrane to the leading process, in the form of intracellular vesicles. By forming new adhesive contacts with the glial fibre along the leading process and breaking adhesive contacts further back, where tension is generated by the forward flow, the cell body moves. This intracellular machinery is regulated by various intracellular, membrane-bound, and extracellular molecules. Knowledge of these molecules and the ways in which they act is still patchy; the following paragraphs summarize the major elements of our understanding to date.

Polymerization of cytoskeletal and contractile proteins may be triggered by the influx of calcium, which is regulated by voltage- and ligand-gated ion channels (in particular, the voltage-gated N-type calcium channel and the ligand-gated NMDA channel) on the leading process and cell body of migrating neurons (Komuro and Rakic, 1992, 1993, 1996). Correlations of fluctuations in intracellular calcium with rates of neuronal migration and studies of the effects of manipulating intracellular calcium fluctuations on migratory rates have indicated that changes in the levels of intracellular calcium may provide an intracellular signal regulating the rate of neuronal precursor migration (Komuro and Rakic, 1996).

A number of molecules present on the surface of migrating neurons have been implicated in the migration of neurons along glial processes (Rakic *et al.*, 1994). The most extensively studied is the neuronal protein astrotactin, blockade of which stops neuronal migration *in vitro* (Fishell and Hatten, 1991; Zheng *et al.*, 1996). The gene for astrotactin has recently been cloned (Zheng *et al.*, 1996), and its sequence indicates that astrotactin protein has regions with similarity to those in other adhesion molecules of the fibronectin family and in epidermal growth factors. Astrotactin mRNA is expressed in postmitotic neurons undergoing migration in the cortex of the developing brain (Zheng *et al.*, 1996). Perturbation of astrotactin with antibodies indicates that it is a ligand for neuronal binding to glial processes during migration. Since removal of astrotactin activity reduces the rate of neuronal precursor movement to less than half of normal, it is proposed that astrotactin contributes to controlling the rate of neuronal migration along radial glial fibres.

Other molecules implicated in glial-guided migration of neuronal precursors include neuregulins, which are secreted growth factors, and their receptors erbB2, erbB3, and erbB4 (Rio *et al.*, 1997; Anton *et al.*, 1997). These molecules appear to be important for the ability of glial cells to grow processes and to support the migration of neurons over them. In addition, the transcription factor Pax-6 has been implicated in neuronal migration in the developing cortex. Pax-6 regulates the expression of other genes; although no target genes have been identified for certain, there is evidence that its protein product binds to the promoter of cell adhesion molecules such as L1 (Edelman and Jones, 1995; Chalepakis *et al.*, 1994). Loss of Pax-6 leads to defective cortical migration; transplantation of neuronal precursors into a normal cortex has indicated that this is due to defects in the environment of the migrating neuronal precursors (Caric *et al.*, 1997). It is possible that defects of radial glial cells contribute to this environmental abnormality (Gotz *et al.*, 1998).

Studies of mutant mice with defects of migration have led to the discovery of molecules that, rather than regulating the process of cell movement itself, are involved in controlling the events that occur at the end of migration. Best-known of these mutants is reeler (Caviness and Rakic, 1978; Goffinet, 1984). In the cortex of reeler mice, cell proliferation and the initial elements of cell migration are normal. The preplate, however, is not split into two layers by the cortical plate cells, as occurs in normal development (refer to Fig. 2.6 in Chapter 2). Neurons of the cortical plate accumulate beneath the undivided preplate, which has been termed the 'superplate' in these mutants. The superplate contains Cajal–Retzius neurons and cells that would normally form the subplate. There is evidence that the layers of the cortical plate are formed in the opposite order to normal, with superficial parts being generated first and deep parts generated later, although this is against a background of general disordering of the cortical layers (Caviness and

Rakic, 1978). The reeler gene has recently been identified (D'Arcangelo *et al.*, 1995, 1997; Bar *et al.*, 1995; Hirotsune *et al.*, 1995; Royaux *et al.*, 1997). It encodes a large secreted extracellular matrix-like protein, called reelin, whose structural similarities with other growth factors and adhesion molecules suggest that it mediates cell adhesion. Reelin is produced by Cajal–Retzius neurons in the superficial part of the preplate; these neurons contribute to the marginal zone after the formation of the cortical plate (Schiffmann *et al.*, 1997).

Other extracellular matrix proteins that are known to be present in the pre-plate, such as fibronectin, chondroitin sulphate proteoglycans, and hyaluronectin (Table 3.3), remain associated with the preplate cells as they separate into the marginal zone and subplate (Miller *et al.*, 1995), and reelin is unusual in being specifically produced in the superficial preplate and the marginal zone. The way in which reelin functions is not yet clear but its distribution is intriguing; it raises the possibility that neuronal precursors entering the preplate might detect the difference in reelin concentration between its superficial and deep parts and position themselves accordingly. For example, reelin may act to stop migrating neurons below the marginal zone, preventing them from reversing their direction along the radial glia, or it may repel subplate cells, allowing a space to form for newly arrived neuronal precursors (Nakajima *et al.*, 1997; Schiffmann *et al.*, 1997; Sheppard and Pearlman, 1997). In addition to its role in cell migration, reelin has been proposed to influence the development of axonal connections between the entorhinal cortex and hippocampus (Del Rio *et al.*, 1997).

Recently, another gene whose mutation produces a reeler-like phenotype, without loss of reelin production, has been discovered. This gene, called mdab1, is a homologue of a *Drosophila* gene, disabled. The product of the gene is a cyto-plasmic protein that is expressed in migrating cortical neurons and that binds to non-receptor tyrosine kinases within the cell. A current hypothesis is that the product of mdab1 (called mDab1 p80) and the molecules that it binds to are a part of the signalling cascade that responds to reelin (Howell *et al.*, 1997; Sheldon *et al.*, 1997; Ware *et al.*, 1997).

10 MOLECULAR CONTROL OF DIFFERENTIATION

10.1 Regionalization

The areas of the cerebral cortex are distinguished on the basis of cytoarchitectural patterns and the specific connections that they make (see Chapter 2). As discussed earlier (Section 8.2), the development of distinct cortical regions is likely to involve a complex network of interactions between cells within the developing cortex and, via axonal connections, cells outside it. It is probable that cells become specified to particular fates early in corticogenesis, as a first step in a process of commitment that will eventually lead to their determination and, finally, their full differentiation. Thus, the region-specific, laminar-specific, or type-specific features of cortical cells will be determined by many different types of molecule, including such key players as transcription factors and intercellular signalling molecules. With regard to regional specification, very little is known about the molecules that confer region-specific identities on the areas of the cortex. This is in contrast to the much more extensive knowledge, reviewed earlier in this chapter, of the regulatory genes that act over broader domains to regionalize the forebrain or hindbrain. It is tempting to think that the lack of corresponding information for the cortex reflects the fact that areal specification in this region owes more to interactions between cortical cells and innervating axons than is the case elsewhere in the developing CNS. While this may be true, there is now preliminary evidence that regulatory genes (such as Pax-6) are expressed in a graded fashion in the early cortex (Warren *et al.*, 1999). Gradients of such regulatory proteins may confer unique identities on different regions of the cortex, but at present this is highly speculative. There are several clear examples of other types of molecule that are regionally-expressed in the cortex (Levitt, 1984; Zacco *et al.*, 1990; Hatanaka *et al.*, 1994; Cohen-Tannoudji *et al.*, 1994; Arimatsu *et al.*, 1999) and these may play a role in its parcellation. The best defined of these is limbic system-associated protein (Levitt, 1984; Zacco *et al.*, 1990). This cell adhesion molecule is a member of the immunoglobulin superfamily, is expressed in the prefrontal, perirhinal, entorhinal, and subicular cortex, and can selectively augment adhesion and outgrowth of limbic neurons (Pimenta *et al.*, 1995). It is suggested that the early expression of limbic system-associated protein is needed for the correct targeting of axons to the expressing regions of the cortex. A further consideration of the mechanisms of cortical regionalization, which includes discussion of the role of innervating axons, is in Chapter 5.

10.2 Lamination

Little is known about regulatory molecules that might control the development of specific cortical layers. There are examples of regulatory genes that are expressed in specific layers during development, including Tbr-1, SCIP, Id-2, and Otx-1 and Otx-2 (Table 3.1). Tbr-1 is expressed in all cortical layers but is more pronounced in subplate, layer 6 and possibly some of layer 5, and in superficial layers 1–3 (Bulfone *et al.*, 1995). SCIP is expressed in layers 2, 3, and 5, (Frantz *et al.*, 1994a). Id-2 is expressed in layers above and below layer 4 (Bulfone *et al.*, 1995; Neuman *et al.*, 1993). It has been hypothesized that differential expression of Otx-1 and Otx-2 could determine laminar fate. Otx-1 and Otx-2 expression has been studied at various stages of development and adulthood in an attempt to explore this hypothesis (Frantz *et al.*, 1994b). During early corticogenesis in rodents, Otx-1 expression is seen in the ventricular zone underlying the developing cerebral cortex and in the ganglionic eminence (the presumptive striatum). As development continues, Otx-1 expression is still visible in the ventricular zone. In addition, the cortical plate, which at this stage consists of layer 5 and 6 cells, also expresses Otx-1. Weak labelling is also detectable in the intermediate zone. Shortly before birth, Otx-1 expression is seen in the cortical plate, in which layer 5 and 6 have finished forming. However, there is a fall in Otx-1 expression in the ventricular zone, which at this stage is producing cells destined to become incorporated into the more superficial layers. Postnatally, Otx-1 is expressed in layer 5 cells of the posterior and lateral cortices, but not in the frontal, insular, or orbital cortex. In layer 6, Otx-1 is expressed in a uniform manner, but there seems to be a fall in the number of cells expressing Otx-1 as a function of time. Otx-2 is only expressed in the cerebral ventricular zone at the very early stages of development.

Thus, Otx-1 is expressed in a subpopulation of ventricular cells that will give rise to layer 5 and 6 cells. After layer 5 and layer 6 are produced, Otx-1 is no longer expressed in the ventricular zone, implying that in the cortex it is only important in the deep layer morphogenesis. Only layer 5 cells in the posterior and lateral cortices express Otx-1. These cells probably project to cortical targets (inferred from their size and location). Otx-1 expression occurs early on in development and may mark a subpopulation of ventricular cells which are biased to become layer 5 cells, even before the final cell division.

10.3   Cortical cell types

Understanding the structural and cellular development of the cerebral cortex involves the definition of the genetic and epigenetic events that control both neurogenesis and gliogenesis as well as the characterization of the competence of progenitors and precursors in the proliferative zone at different stages of development. This represents one of the major challenges for future research on cortical development. The aim of such research is to understand how the commitment of ectodermal cells in the neural plate to their ultimate fates is achieved (i.e. how they are specified and determined). To date, much work on the factors that control the differentiation of cortical precursors has been carried out *in vitro*, where access to the cells is enhanced and the response of cells to signalling factors can be readily assessed; in the future it is likely that more and more studies will be done *in vivo*, involving genetic manipulation of progenitor and precursor cells and/or manipulation of their environment through *in vivo* injections of signalling molecules, vectors producing such molecules, or cell transplants. In considering the interpretation of work in this area of research, we need to bear in mind the fact that *in vitro* studies alone can be misleading, since culture conditions are unlikely to mimic *in vivo* conditions precisely and even very subtle alterations in a progenitor or precursor cell's environment may cause it to change its fate. In addition, the limitations of current techniques for the analysis of the lineages of cortical cells mean that descriptions of the lines of descent of the major classes of cortical cell are controversial and, in any case, cover only accessible portions of the period of corticogenesis (see Section 2.7 in Chapter 2). The fact that our knowledge of the developmental pathways taken by neural plate cells *in vivo* as they progress towards fully differentiated cortical cells is inadequate hinders comparison of events *in vitro* with those *in vivo*, and can prevent a definitive assessment of the *in vivo* relevance of conclusions from culture work. Nevertheless, studies using *in vitro* methods have suggested that the precursor cells that generate the cerebral cortex need several growth factors to regulate their differentiation. Molecules that have been implicated in this process include fibroblast growth factor-1, heparan sulphate proteoglycan, leukaemia inhibitory factor receptors, bone morphogenetic protein 4, and epidermal growth factor receptor.

In culture, fibroblast growth factor-1 in the presence of heparan sulphate proteoglycan (which binds to fibroblast growth factor-1 and presents it to its receptor) stimulates the differentiation of embryonic cortical precursors into neurons (Nurcombe *et al.*, 1993). *In vivo*, fibroblast growth factor-1 expression in the embryonic telencephalon coincides with the onset of neurogenesis (Nurcombe *et al.*, 1993) and there is concomitant expression of heparan sulphate proteoglycan (Ford *et al.*, 1994). Other studies have suggested that signalling through a leukaemia inhibitory factor receptor may regulate the differentiation of astrocytes (Ware *et al.*, 1995). Experiments by Lavdas *et al.* (1997) have indicated that 5-HT promotes the differentiation of cortical glutamatergic neurons.

Some recent work has concentrated on the environmental signals that influence the relative abundance of specific subpopulations of progenitor cells in different regions and at different stages of development (for example in the cortical ventricular zone, where predominantly neuronal precursors arise, and the subventricular zone, where predominantly glial cells arise; see Chapter 2). Changes in the abundance of different types of progenitor are likely to underlie changes in the numbers of different types of cell produced in the developing cortex throughout development. Such changes may be caused by instructive signals that alter the potential of progenitor cells, or they may be caused by selective proliferation and/or death of subpopulations of progenitors with specific potentials (Lillien, 1998). For example, there is evidence that bone morphogenetic protein 4 promotes a glial cell fate in subventricular zone progenitor cells by affecting their potential (Gross *et al.*, 1996). Other work has shown that high levels of stimulation of the epidermal growth factor receptor in multipotential cortical progenitor cells alters their fate, leading to an increased probability of producing glial cells (Burrows *et al.*, 1997). Early in development, progenitor cells in the forebrain express lower levels of epidermal growth factor receptors than they do later on, which is consistent with the hypothesis that this receptor is important for the generation of predominantly glial cells later in development (Burrows *et al.*, 1997; Eagleson *et al.*, 1996; Kornblum *et al.*, 1997).

As well as searching for and analysing cell–cell signalling molecules that may control the differentiation of cortical progenitors, work has begun to find the molecules that act intracellularly to control the commitment of these cells. This work is in its early stages, but several interesting studies have been reported. Potentially important factors include the neurogenins (ngn-1 and ngn-2), which have homology to the *Drosophila* gene atonal. These are transcription factors expressed in subsets of progenitor cells in the cortex as well as in other regions such as the retina (Gradwohl *et al.*, 1996; Ma *et al.*, 1996; Sommer *et al.*, 1996). In *Xenopus*, misexpression of the *Xenopus* neurogenin-related 1 gene, even in non-neurogenic regions, results in premature and ectopic neurogenesis, an effect that is mediated by induction of another transcription factor, XneuroD (Ma *et al.*, 1996). Thus, these genes may act as regulators of competence and/or commitment to a neuronal fate; their expression may be regulated by intercellular signalling by factors such as Notch (Ma *et al.*, 1996; De la Pompa *et al.*, 1997).

4
Guidance of axons and innervation of cortical structures

To create the nervous system, precise synaptic connections must form between cells. This process involves the outgrowth of axons, their travel to distant sites, and their innervation of target structures. Axons travel together in discrete bundles, which in the adult can be several centimetres long. However, at the time of axonal outgrowth the distances to be travelled are very much shorter than this. There is a range of possible types of mechanism which can yield guidance with differing degrees of precision. At one extreme, growth cones may take routes at random and only those that happen to contact an appropriate target region are preserved. At the other extreme, the guidance mechanism results in growth cones being led to their targets with few or no errors.

There are two problems that the axon has to overcome: to navigate to the correct target structure; and then to make connections with the right cells within the target. The latter results in the formation in the target structure of a map of the cells of origin. In this chapter we concentrate on mechanisms for navigation and the next chapter deals with mechanisms of map formation. Clearly these two problems are not entirely independent of one another; the mechanisms for axon guidance may also contribute to map formation.

1   CORTICAL CONNECTIONS IN THE ADULT BRAIN

Figure 4.1 summarizes the major afferent and efferent axonal connections of the cerebral cortex. The main afferent input to the cortex comes from the thalamus (thalamocortical projections), which transmits almost all sensory information (olfaction is an exception). The adult thalamus can be divided into a number of anatomically distinct regions or nuclei (Fig. 4.2), each comprising a collection of neurons that have defined reciprocal interconnections with particular cortical

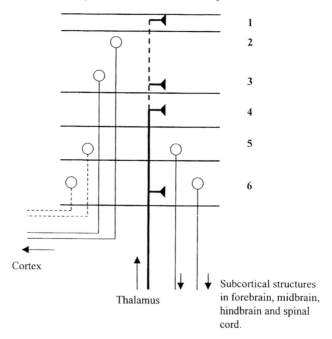

Cortex

Thalamus

Subcortical structures
in forebrain, midbrain,
hindbrain and spinal
cord.

F I G .   4 . 1 . Diagram showing the layers of origin and termination of major cortical afferents and efferents (note that layers 2 and 3 are hard to distinguish cytoarchitectonically in many species). Cortical afferents from the thalamus terminate mainly in layer 4, with some innervating layers 1, 3, and 6. Efferents to other cortical areas arise from layers 2, 3, 5, and 6. In cases where such corticocortical projections transfer information from cortical areas with less complex properties to areas with greater complexity (feedforward projections), these projections originate mainly in layers 2 and 3. In many reciprocal pathways (feedback projections), the origin is mainly in layers 5 and 6. (Kato *et al.*, 1991b; Ferrer *et al.*, 1988; Batardiere *et al.*, 1998). Efferents to subcortical structures in the forebrain (e.g. thalamus), midbrain (e.g. superior colliculus), hindbrain (e.g. medullary nuclei), and spinal cord arise from layers 5 and 6.

areas. Sense organs except the olfactory bulb and major subcortical motor centres send their afferents to one or more specific thalamic nuclei; the cortical projections of dorsal thalamic nuclei are listed in Table 4.1 (Jones, 1985). The order of axons in the thalamocortical projections from each nucleus generates maps of the sensory surfaces of the body in corresponding cortical areas. What is more, many adjacent areas of the neocortex receive their projections from adjacent thalamic nuclei, although there are examples of non-adjacent thalamic nuclei that project to adjacent but clearly distinct cortical areas (Caviness and Frost, 1980; Crandall and Caviness, 1984b; Jones, 1985; Caviness, 1988). Thus, as a general rule, neighbouring thalamic neurons preserve their relative positions as they project to the cortex and the spatial order of the nuclei in the thalamus, and of the cells in each nucleus, is transformed with considerable accuracy onto the neocortical sheet. The possible mechanisms that generate this mapping are discussed further in Chapter 5.

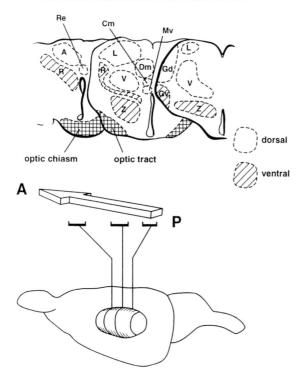

F I G .   4 . 2 . Diagram of three sections through the thalamus (from posterior, P, to anterior, A), showing the positions of major nuclei or groups of nuclei. Overall, nuclei fall into
two groups, those of the dorsal thalamus and those of the ventral thalamus. Thalamocortical
pathways arise in the dorsal thalamus. Abbreviations: A, anterior nuclei; Cm, centromedial
nucleus; Dm, dorsomedial nucleus; Gd, dorsal lateral geniculate nucleus; Gv, ventral lateral
geniculate nucleus; L, lateral nuclei; Mv, medial ventral nucleus; R, reticular nucleus; Re,
reuniens nucleus; V, ventral nuclei; Z, zona incerta.

Table 4.1 List of major groups of dorsal thalamic nuclei (Fig. 4.2) and their main cortical
targets.

1. Anterior complex: anterior and medial limbic
2. Dorsal lateral geniculate nucleus: visual
3. Intralaminar complex (e.g. centromedial nucleus): frontal (including motor) and parietal
   (including somatosensory)
4. Lateral group: parietotemporal, cingulate
5. Medial geniculate complex: auditory
6. Medial group (e.g. reuniens nucleus): frontal, hippocampal formation
7. Ventral group: frontal, somatosensory, cingulate, and other diffuse projections

In the adult, thalamocortical connections terminate mainly in cortical layer 4, although there are some inputs to other layers (mainly 1, 3, and 6) which vary between cortical area and species (Gilbert and Wiesel, 1981; Humphrey *et al.*, 1985). The major efferent pathways from the cortex to subcortical structures (referred to as corticofugal pathways) originate in deep layers (Fig. 4.1). Neurons in layer 6 project to the thalamus; neurons in cortical layer 5 project to targets in the midbrain, hindbrain, and spinal cord. Neurons in superficial layers 2 and 3 project intracortically. In primates and carnivores such as the cat, these neurons project mainly to other cortical regions on the same (called ipsilateral corticocortical connections) or the opposite (called callosal connections) side of the brain (Gilbert and Wiesel, 1981); these connections originate from neurons distributed more widely across all the cortical layers in rodents (O'Leary and Koester, 1993).

2   OBSERVATIONS ON THE DEVELOPMENT OF CORTICAL CONNECTIONS

Much of our knowledge of the events that occur as cortical connections develop has come from studies of the developing visual system. Many examples of such studies will be quoted in the following account. The intense interest in this system over the past decades probably stems in large part from the relative ease with which it can be analysed with electrophysiological and anatomical methods. Precise stimuli can be applied in functional tests and, in anatomical studies, the eyes are easily accessible for the application of neuronal tracers that can travel transneuronally as far as the cortex. Many of the earlier studies of developing visual cortical connections were carried out in large mammals, such as cats. Recent years have seen the development of new methods for high-resolution labelling of axons and cell bodies in fixed tissue, using fluorescent carbocyanine dyes which diffuse along the membranes of cells and their axons (Honig and Hume, 1986; Godement *et al.*, 1987). These techniques have greatly helped the analysis of developing cortical connections in fetal material from all types of mammal, including rodents, and they have made it easier to extend the analysis of cortical connections to non-visual areas. The enhanced ability to study rodent development brings obvious advantages in view of the potential for exploring the mechanisms of development through the use of mutant strains of mice (Chapter 3).

The major components of the mammalian visual system are the retina, lateral geniculate nucleus (LGN), which is in the thalamus, and the visual cortex, which is at the occipital (posterior) pole of the cerebral hemispheres (Fig. 4.3). Connections from the thalamus to the cortex are called thalamocortical connections; those from specifically the LGN are termed geniculocortical connections and they bundle together into a pathway called the optic radiation.

2.1   Geniculocortical development

The development of the LGN has been studied using [^{3}H]thymidine or the thymidine analogue, bromodeoxyuridine, to label geniculate cells as they are generated.

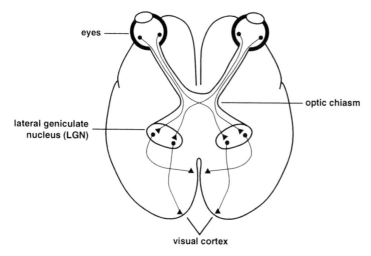

FIG. 4.3. Diagram of the visual system (human). Ganglion cells in the retinae of the eyes send their axons to the lateral geniculate nucleus (LGN) in the thalamus. Axons from ganglion cells on the medial (nasal) side of the retina project to the opposite side of the brain; they cross at the optic chiasm. Axons from ganglion cells on the lateral (temporal) side of the retina project to the same side of the brain. Ganglion cells synapse on LGN neurons and LGN neurons project to the visual cortex. All visual information from the left side of each eye (related to the right side of the visual field) is relayed to the left cerebral hemisphere and vice versa.

In the cat, neurons of the LGN are born between embryonic day 24 (E24) and E31, and the first-generated cells collect to form the anlage of the LGN at E29 (Hickey and Hitchcock, 1984). Gestation in the cat is 65 days and so these events occur from just before gestation to around mid-gestation. Similarly, in rodents, the LGN is born around mid-gestation (Altman and Bayer, 1989a,b).

Neuronal tracing methods have been used to time the growth of geniculocortical connections in several species. In the cat, axons from the LGN grow into the telencephalon early in fetal development, before E35, to begin forming the optic radiations within the intermediate zone (Fig. 4.4; Shatz and Luskin, 1986; McConnell *et al.*, 1989). Axons arrive in the vicinity of the developing visual cortex by E39, and accumulate in the subplate over the following three weeks. Between E46 and E55, geniculocortical axons invade the marginal zone (future layer 1), presumably by traversing the cortical plate without terminating in it. It is not until between E55 and birth (P0) that an appreciable number of terminals appear in the cortical plate itself. Initially, this ingrowth is through the deeper cortical layers, 5 and 6, but by P25 the adult-like laminar pattern of geniculocortical input can be discerned, mainly in layer 4 but also in layer 6 (Shatz *et al.*, 1988, 1991). The density of terminals in layer 5 and in the subplate decreases between P0 and P25. Many of the early projections from the LGN to layer 1 appear to be sustained only transiently. Kato *et al.* (1984) have demonstrated that the projection from the LGN to layer 1 of area 17 is dense in newborn kittens, but becomes very sparse after one month.

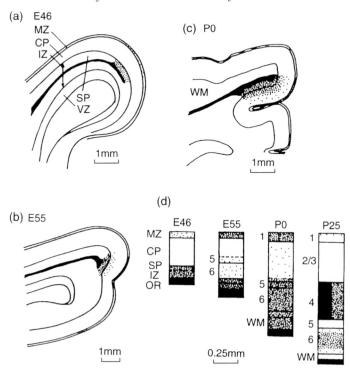

FIG. 4.4. The development of the geniculocortical pathway in the cat, as revealed by intraocularly injected tritiated proline, an anterograde transneuronal tract-tracer. (a) At embryonic day 46 (E46) geniculocortical axons have grown through the intermediate zone (IZ) forming the optic radiation. Most terminate below the presumptive visual cortex in the subplate (SP) although a few axons reach the marginal zone (MZ). CP, cortical plate; VZ, ventricular zone. (b) By E55, the penetration of the cortical plate begins and the density of terminals in the marginal zone increases. (c) By the time of birth (P0), there is substantial invasion of the deep cortical layers with a few terminals in the more superficial layers, which are still forming. WM, white matter. (d) Schematic diagrams illustrate these changes in more detail. By P25, the geniculocortical afferents terminate almost exclusively in layers 4 and 6 and segregation into ocular dominance columns is apparent anatomically. The earlier dense input to layer 1 is now reduced. OR, optic radiation. Based on Shatz and Luskin (1986).

A similar course of events occurs in other species. In rats, outgrowth from the LGN begins around E14–15 (gestation is around 21 days). By E16–17, geniculate axons are already in the internal capsule, and some have reached the developing cortex (Lund and Mustari, 1977; Altman and Bayer, 1989a; Catalano *et al.*, 1991; Blakemore and Molnar, 1990; Erzurumlu and Jhaveri, 1990; De Carlos and O'Leary, 1992; Molnar, 1998).

In the cat and primate, the developing geniculocortical axons wait in the subplate until the migration of cells into layer 4 is complete before penetrating the cortex (Rakic, 1976a; Lund and Mustari, 1977; Shatz and Luskin, 1986). There is controversy over whether there is also a waiting time in rodents. Earlier studies indicated that axons wait in the subplate for up to a week, but more recent work suggests either that it is only a few days or that there is no detectable wait (Dawson and Killackey, 1985; Wise and Jones, 1978; Catalano *et al.*, 1991; Lund and Mustari, 1977; De Carlos and O'Leary, 1992; Erzurumlu and Jhaveri, 1990; Reinoso and O'Leary, 1990; Molnar, 1998). It is possible that geniculocortical axons form temporary synapses with the cells that are present transiently in the subplate during this time (Chun *et al.*, 1987; Rakic, 1983; Crandall and Caviness, 1984a; Shatz and Luskin, 1986; Friauf *et al.*, 1990; Kostovic and Rakic, 1990). Once the geniculocortical afferents have penetrated the visual cortex, subplate neurons become much less numerous in the early stages of postnatal life (Kostovic and Rakic, 1980; Chun *et al.*, 1987; Wahle and Meyer, 1987; Luskin and Shatz, 1985b; Wood *et al.*, 1992).

Crucial questions about the way in which the geniculocortical projection develops remain unanswered. In particular, the degree of orderliness with which the axons grow is not clear. In many cases the only available evidence comes from observations of the maps of connections shortly after they have formed, from which only weak inferences about preceding developmental events within the growing pathway can be drawn. Numerous studies have shown that the retina is projected onto the cortex in at least a roughly topographically ordered fashion soon after geniculocortical axons have reached the cortex (for example Henderson and Blakemore, 1986; Bullier *et al.*, 1984; Price and Blakemore, 1985a,b) and this suggests that geniculocortical axons might grow through the intermediate zone in a topographically ordered fashion as well. The difficulty of supporting this suggestion with direct evidence is that the developing geniculocortical pathway is such a tight bundle that the identification of topographic organization will require the application of highly refined and technically difficult neuroanatomical methods. Recent studies on the hamster have demonstrated a refinement of topography in the geniculocortical projection, that could be due to the retraction of early collaterals that attempt to enter the cortex at inappropriate points (Naegele *et al.*, 1988). Similarly, Crandall and Caviness (1984a) made injections of retrograde traces into the cortex of neonatal mice and suggested that the divergence of their thalamocortical pathways may be greater than in adults.

2.2   Corticofugal and corticocortical systems

At around the time when geniculocortical axons begin to grow towards the developing cortex, the cortex starts to send its first projections back towards the LGN (McConnell *et al.*, 1989). These axons originate in the subplate, which projects not only to the thalamus but also to the superior colliculus and through the corpus callosum (McConnell *et al.*, 1989; Shatz *et al.*, 1991). Using the carbocyanine dye DiI in fetal cats, McConnell *et al.* (1989) showed that axons from the developing cortex first reach the thalamus between E26 and E30. They have suggested that the thalamic axons from the subplate are pioneers in that they are the first to form a pathway between these two structures. However, in the rat, corticothalamic and thalamocortical axons appear to grow simultaneously and to meet in the internal capsule (De Carlos and O'Leary, 1992; Blakemore and Molnar, 1990). There is some controversy over the extent to which axons of these two pathways fasciculate after they meet. Overall, the evidence indicates that the two pathways remain well-segregated throughout much of their extents, although fasciculation may occur where they first meet and immediately below the developing cortical plate (Molnar, 1998; De Carlos and O'Leary, 1992) (see next chapter for further discussion of this issue).

Layer 5 of the developing cortex sends projections to the midbrain, hindbrain, and spinal cord. In adults, the distribution of layer 5 neurons projecting to each subcortical target is restricted to particular neocortical areas. Corticotectal neurons, which send their axons to the superior colliculus in the midbrain, are located in the visual cortex. Corticospinal neurons are mainly in the sensorimotor cortex. However, at around the time of birth in rats, layer 5 neurons all over the neocortex project to the spinal cord and superior colliculus. Subsequently, axonal elimination without death of the inappropriately projecting cells removes some projections to leave the more restricted adult distribution (Stanfield *et al.*, 1982; Bates and Killackey, 1984; Thong and Dreher, 1986; O'Leary *et al.*, 1990). Recent work, illustrated in Fig. 4.5, has shown that the transient projections arise as branches from primary axons that run to the spinal cord (O'Leary and Terashima, 1988; De Carlos and O'Leary, 1992).

The development of connections between cortical regions (i.e. ipsilateral corticocortical and callosal) is described in more detail in Chapter 5 since much of what is known about their development concerns the development and subsequent refinement of projections after the initial period of growth. There is considerable evidence that when these pathways are growing, some axons are routed towards or into inappropriate regions of the cortex. For example, work by Price and Zumbroich (1989) on ipsilateral connections suggested that the initial outgrowth of these axons in the visual cortex of the cat might be random, with later validation of connections that link appropriate points in the developing cortical maps and removal of the other inappropriate connections. More recent work by Caric and Price (1996) has indicated that a detectable proportion of axons from discrete points in one cortical area may grow in bundles to appropriate points in another cortical area, suggesting that there may be guidance of at least some ipsilateral corticocortical axons as they are growing (Barone *et al.*, 1996). Overall, the events that occur as ipsilateral corticocortical axons grow are not clear; the production of misrouted axons is a commonly reported feature, although the proportions of such inappropriate axons appears to vary greatly depending on the region of cortex under study and the species (Dehay *et al.*, 1984, 1988b; Price and Blakemore, 1985a,b; Price, 1986; Kennedy *et al.*, 1989; Price and Zumbroich, 1989; Kato *et al.*, 1991b; Kennedy *et al.*, 1994; Price *et al.*, 1994a; Barone *et al.*, 1995, 1996; Caric and Price, 1996). One problem with studying the guidance of ipsilateral corticocortical connections

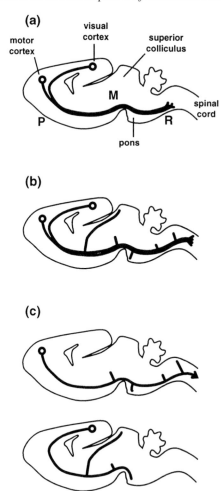

FIG. 4.5. Diagrams of parasagittal sections through the rat brain at various stages of development showing the targeting of subcortical structures by corticofugal projections. (a) Axonal extension: during late embryonic stages, cortical neurons send axons towards the spinal cord, bypassing their subcortical targets. P, prosencephalon; M, mesencephalon; R, rhombencephalon. (b) Collateral formation: branches form along the spinally directed axons. (c) Selective axonal elimination: specific collaterals or segments of the primary axon are selectively eliminated to generate projections that are appropriate for the cortical location of the cells of origin (i.e. motor cortex, *top diagram*, and visual cortex, *bottom diagram*). (After O'Leary and Koester, 1993)

is that many are very short-range and do not take long to grow, making it difficult to monitor their elongation phase *in vivo*.

The steps involved in the elongation of callosal axons may prove more tractable due to the greater length and discrete nature of the corpus callosum. In the rodent, layer 5 cells project either subcortically or across the callosum and there is evidence that this distinction between the two cell types is established early, before they form axons (Koester and O'Leary, 1993). The result of this early specification is that one set of axons from layer 5 travel ventrolaterally, towards the ventral telencephalon, whereas the other travels medially into the callosum. As is the case in the ipsilateral corticocortical pathways, the newly formed callosal pathways show considerable exuberance of connections. In adults, certain areas of the cortex do not have callosal connections; others (e.g. around the borders of cortical areas) have a patchy distribution of callosally projecting neurons (Innocenti, 1981; Dehay *et al.*, 1988b). In many of the developing callosal pathways examined to date, although not all (Dehay *et al.*, 1988b), these restricted patterns of projection have been found to arise from initially more widespread distributions (Innocenti, 1981; O'Leary *et al.*, 1981; Ivy and Killackey, 1981; Innocenti and Tettoni, 1997).

3   MECHANISMS CONTROLLING THE DEVELOPMENT OF AXONAL CONNECTIONS

To achieve the precise connectivity of the cerebral cortex, afferent and efferent axons must grow along specific pathways, select appropriate target areas, and establish synaptic contacts with appropriate subsets of neurons in those regions, as outlined in the preceding section. The mechanisms that regulate these processes are far from clear. Work in the past decade has indicated some possibilities and has generated strong controversies. It is very likely that there are many different types of mechanism that combine to guide axons to their target. The basic question concerns how the structure at the tip of the axon, the growth cone, is guided. We first describe the biochemistry of the growth cone.

3.1   The biochemistry of the growth cone

First identified by Ramón y Cajal (1893) the growth cone is a structure which develops at the tip of the neurite to guide the growing axon to its target (see Fig. 4.6). It has two major regions, the central and the peripheral zones.

In the central zone there is rapid directed transport of organelles, mainly neurosecretory granules and mitochondria. The cytoplasm in the central zone (axoplasm) has a high concentration of microtubules, polymerized proteins made up of tubulin dimers. Microtubules are important in giving structural support to the axon. The peripheral regions are dominated by filopodia and lamellipodia, the membrane stretched between filopodia. In contrast to the central zone, the cytoplasm in the peripheral regions (kinetoplasm) has a very low organelle density and a high concentration of F-actin polymer. The region of the growth cone comprising the central/peripheral interface is referred to as the transition zone (Forscher and Smith, 1988; Mitchison and Kirschner, 1988).

(a) THE GROWTH CONE

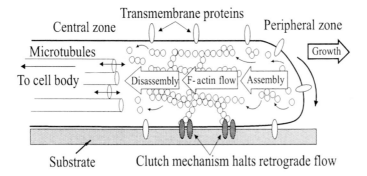

(b) LATERAL VIEW OF GROWTH CONE

FIG. 4.6. Diagrammatic representation of growth cone. (a) The major regions of the growth cone. (b) Schematic of the stages of growth cone movement (Hely, 1999).

F-actin

F-actin seems to play a vital role in maintaining motility of the growth cone and also in controlling the spatial distribution of microtubules. The peripheral zone has a high concentration of F-actin in both the monomer and polymer state. Actin monomers are polarized molecules that assemble into polarized filaments (F-actin) that have so-called 'barbed' (+) and 'pointed' (−) ends (see Fig. 4.6). Filament assembly is more rapid at the barbed end (Forscher, 1988). Monomeric actin normally polymerizes into F-actin at the leading edge of the growth cone and then flows rearward towards the central zone at a rate of 3–6 μm/min (Forscher and Smith, 1988). Rearward flow of F-actin seems to cause forward movement of the growth cone, analogous to the action of caterpillar tracks.

Microtubules

Microtubules are cytoplasmic filaments that are important structural elements of the axon and also play a role in the transport of organelles. They are primarily concentrated in the central domain of the axon and can extend far out into the peripheral zone, although they are not found in filopodia. Microtubules are the polymerized form of the tubulin dimer (made up of α and β subunit monomers). They are helical proteins, with 13 tubulin dimers per helical revolution. One end of the microtubule, the minus $(-)$ end, is usually stabilized in the neurite shaft. However the plus $(+)$ end of the microtubule is free to 'explore' the growth cone by the addition or subtraction of tubulin dimers in a process which is called dynamic instability (Mitchison and Kirschner, 1984).

The dynamically unstable microtubules found in the growth cone and the tip of the neurite shaft exist in either a growing or shrinking state. This gives them a unique role in the developing neurite. Conditions in which microtubule polymerization is favourable lead to the rapid extension of microtubules from the central zone of the neurite shaft into the leading edge of the growth cone. Much of the structural support for newly generated axon in the developing neurite comes from the invasion of microtubules from the central domain into the periphery of the growth cone.

Filopodia

At the leading edge of the growth cone membrane, filopodia appear as long thin spikes of membrane and act as sensory antennae. These convert directional signals from the extracellular space into an internal signal that is used by the growth cone to direct its movement.

Growth cone dynamics

The forward movement of the developing axon and growth cone is characterised by three stages: (i) exploration, (ii) orientation, and (iii) consolidation. In the exploration phase, the growth cone filopodia sample the extracellular space for directional signals. In the orientation phase, a single filopodium may establish the future direction of growth leading to invasion of this branch of the growth cone by large numbers of axonal microtubules. Finally, in the consolidation phase, a new growth cone forms at the tip of the leading filopodia. Over a period of about 20 minutes the old growth cone loses its adhesiveness to the substrate and is converted into new axon (Tanaka and Sabry, 1995). When a growth cone reaches its correct target, it halts, and remodels itself to form a synapse (Broadie *et al.*, 1993).

During the consolidation phase, any pathfinding decisions will be transient as long as both F-actin and microtubules are in their dynamic state. To make any forward advance of the growth cone permanent, the kinetoplasm of the peripheral region of the growth cone must be converted into the axoplasm of the central zone. During this phase, both F-actin and microtubules are stabilized to some extent. The F-actin which is stabilized in the direction of the target continues to flow rearward. This exerts a lateral force on splayed microtubules in the growth cone and may assist in the process of bundling the microtubules together into the densely packed array typical of axoplasm. During the bundling process microtubule associated proteins (MAPs), e.g. MAP2 in dendrites and tau in the axon, also play a large role in stabilizing the microtubules against shrinkage (Maccioni and Cambiazo, 1995). Finally the old growth cone loses its adhesiveness for the substratum. A new segment of axon has formed and a new growth cone will develop at the tip of the leading filopodia (Mitchison and Kirschner, 1988).

3.2 Mechanisms for Axonal Guidance

Classification of possible mechanisms
The process of outgrowth of axons to a specific target requires a way of guiding axonal trajectories and a way of stopping axonal outgrowth at the target. The mechanisms for both developmental tasks can use information from a variety of sources.

   All mechanisms that have been proposed for guidance and stopping are some combination of the following three basic types of mechanism which are classified according to the type of information they require.

1. No specific information is supplied to the axons during outgrowth.
2. The set of instructions for navigation is intrinsic to the cell itself.
3. The axons acquire information from the environment through which they grow, including the target structure itself.

1. No specific information—random outgrowth
One possibility is that axons grow out at random. As a mechanism on its own this is inadequate as axons do eventually connect to specific targets and so such a mechanism must be supplemented by one that selects out connections after contact with the target structure. Moreover, the tissue through which axons grow has numerous physical constraints (such as its edges) and, for most neurons, there will be directions that their axons simply cannot take. In the strictest sense, axonal outgrowth cannot be random. Most axons form part of a nerve bundle; the issue of axonal ordering within the bundle, or the lack of it, is important with regards to mechanisms of map formation and is discussed in more detail in Chapter 5.

2. Ballistic mechanism
Another possibility is that cells contain complete information as to how to get to their target. This information would be in the form of a set of instructions for pointing the axon in the right direction and for specifying the amount of growth. Given the inherent imprecision in the size and shape of neural structures and in the speed of developmental processes, any mechanism that sends axons off in a specific direction to travel for a specific time in a heterogeneous environment is likely to be too unreliable to operate alone.

3. Interactions with the environment
There is a rich set of possibilities. It is difficult to draw firm boundaries between many of them and it is likely that more than one operate in most developing

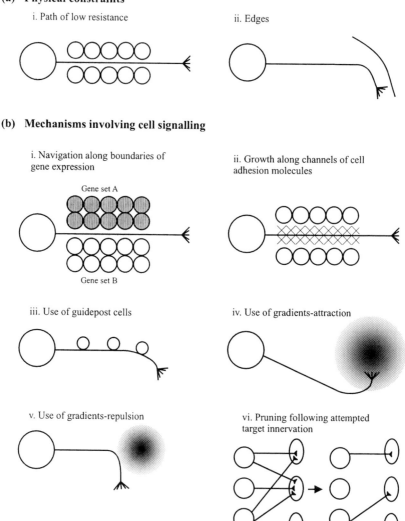

FIG. 4.7. Summary diagram of various possible mechanisms underlying axonal guidance.

pathways. Some of these possibilities are summarized in Fig. 4.7:

(a) Axons may be guided by physical constraints; for example, they may follow paths of least resistance. This mechanism requires contact between the growth cone and the environmental feature, but does not necessarily require

Table 4.2 Molecules implicated in axon guidance (diagrams are shown in Fig. 4.8).

Cell adhesion molecules (CAMs)

Many members can mediate homophilic adhesion, functioning as both a ligand on one cell and a receptor on another. Some also function as heterophilic ligands or receptors for cell surface or extracellular matrix molecules. Many CAMs have signalling functions, although only a few have protein tyrosine kinase or protein tyrosine phosphatase domains (Tessier-Lavigne and Goodman, 1996; Brummendorf *et al.*, 1998; Jessell, 1988; Edelman and Crossin, 1991).

Netrins and their receptors

Netrins are a small family of guidance molecules that can attract some axons and repel others. The attractive and repulsive effects may be mediated by different receptors (e.g. DCC and UNC5 respectively). They are proteins (about 600 amino acids) related to the much larger laminins (Table 3.3) and are diffusible (Tessier-Lavigne and Goodman, 1996; Kennedy *et al.*, 1994; Colamarino and Tessier-Lavigne, 1995). They have been shown to have attractive effects on cortical axons (Metin *et al.*, 1997) and, more recently, on thalamocortical axons.

Receptor protein tyrosine kinases (RPTKs)

These include the receptors for many neurotrophic factors (such as the neurotrophins and fibroblast growth factors, Table 6.2). The neurotrophic factors have major roles in the regulation of cell survival, and are discussed in more detail in Chapter 6; they do, however, have roles in other developmental processes, as discussed at appropriate points throughout the text. The largest group of RPTKs in vertebrates is the Eph family. Their ligands are membrane-anchored and several have been implicated in contact-guidance to the target (Drescher *et al.*, 1995; Cheng *et al.*, 1995; Nakamoto *et al.*, 1996; O'Leary *et al.*, 1999).

Semaphorins

A large family (> 20 members) of cell surface and secreted proteins that may function mainly as chemorepellants or inhibitors or growth, although there is some evidence that they may play attractive roles (Bagnard *et al.*, 1998). Members have extracellular semaphorin domains of about 500 amino acids that are conserved. The vertebrate semaphorins can be divided into at least four distinct classes. Recent work has suggested that members of the semaphorin family (Semaphorins A,D,E) have roles in the development of cerebral cortical connections (Bagnard *et al.*, 1998; Skaliora *et al.*, 1998; Giger *et al.*, 1996; Chedotal *et al.*, 1998; Polleux *et al.*, 1998). Their effects are mediated by neuropilins (Kolodkin *et al.*, 1997).

Extracellular matrix molecules (ECMs)

Many ECMs can promote or inhibit axon growth. Receptors for ECM molecules are predominantly integrins, immunoglobulin superfamily receptors, and proteoglycans. ECMs are described in Table 3.3.

Neurotransmitters

Neurotransmitters have been shown to influence growth cone turning *in vitro* (Zheng *et al.*, 1994, 1996).

that the contact induces intracellular signalling via secondary messenger systems within the growing cell.

(b) There may be communication either through contact or at a distance via specific molecules that activate cell surface receptors and intracellular secondary

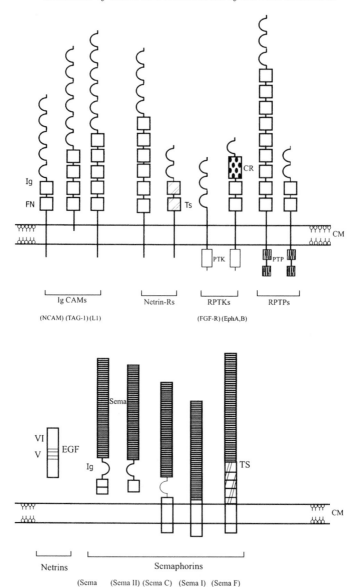

F I G .   4 . 8 . Schematic representations of the structures of some of the molecules implicated in guiding growing axons in various parts of the nervous system, including the cerebral cortex and its connections (e.g. Metin *et al.*, 1997; Bagnard *et al.*, 1998; Polleux *et al.*, 1998). The cell membrane (CM) is represented by horizontal lines. Abbreviations: CR, cysteine-rich region; EGF, epidermal growth factor domain; FN, fibronectin domain; Ig, immunoglobulin domain; PTK, protein tyrosine kinase; PTP, protein tyrosine

messenger systems. This mechanism requires a greater degree of participation in the guidance process by the axon than mechanism (a). The axon not only has to grow but it has to transduce extracellular cues and make decisions about the direction of its growth. Some of the molecules that may guide axons in this way are shown in Fig. 4.8 and listed in Table 4.2.

(c) Communication occurs through electrical signalling.

Physical constraints

Growing axons may follow discontinuities between layers of cells to get from their origin to their target. This is sometimes referred to as stereotropism (Harrison, 1914) or contact guidance (Weiss, 1958). A channel is a region of the tissue that offers reduced resistance to penetration by growth cones, perhaps because it is relatively cell-free. A possible example of this is in the pathway of the tibial Ti1 pioneer neuron in the grasshopper, which has been fully mapped (O'Connor and Bentley, 1993). In this pathway, the growth cones migrate along a gap between the cells of the basal lamina and the basal surfaces of the epithelial cells. As a result of cell death in the mouse optic stalk, spaces appear through which axons from retinal ganglion cells subsequently navigate. In the mutant ON^J, such spaces never appear and retinal fibres never enter the optic stalk (Silver and Robb, 1979).

These ideas have been embodied in the blueprint hypothesis (Singer *et al.*, 1979). This hypothesis is based on work on newt spinal cord showing that axons grow in channels of extracellular matrix which have been formed in advance of the growing axons, a finding which mirrored similar phenomena previously observed in studies on regeneration (Egar and Singer, 1972; Nordlander and Singer, 1978). According to this hypothesis, the pattern of future primary neuronal pathways (expressed in neurogenesis as channels or gaps between the processes of the epithelial cells) is inherent in the primitive neuroepithelium and its derived cells. The mechanism of guidance of axons along such channels could be mechanical. However, given that it is now known that many extracellular molecules induce intracellular responses, guidance through such channels may involve chemicals in them signalling to the growth cone.

---

phosphatase domain; Sema, semaphorin domain; TS, thrombospondin domain; V and VI, regions with similarity to the amino-terminal domains V and VI of laminin. The molecules illustrated in the *top* diagram are members of the immunoglobulin superfamily that are implicated in axon guidance as ligands, receptors, or both. They are cell adhesion molecules (CAMs), of which three examples are given (neural cell adhesion molecule or NCAM, TAG-1, and L1) (Brummendorf *et al.*, 1998), netrin receptors (netrin-Rs), receptor protein tyrosine kinases (RPTKs), which include the fibroblast growth factor receptors (FGF-R) and Eph receptors, and receptor protein tyrosine phosphatases (RPTPs). The molecules illustrated in the *bottom* diagram belong to the netrin and semaphorin families of axon guidance molecules. All of these molecules are highly conserved among vertebrates and invertebrates (Tessier-Lavigne and Goodman, 1996). Details of molecules are in Table 4.2.

Contact guidance that may involve signalling mechanisms

It is difficult to distinguish between a guidance mechanism that relies entirely on physical contraints and one that also involves signalling. An essential feature of the blueprint hypothesis retained in later variations is that it postulates the laying-down of guidance cues in the tissue prior to the growth of axons into that region. One variant on the blueprint hypothesis is that the boundaries demarcated by the expression of certain regulatory genes define the courses taken by early axonal pathways. This hypothesis is based on the correlations between axonal pathways and the expression domains of regulatory genes in the zebrafish brain, the vertebrate hindbrain, and the floor plate. The genes Pax-6 and Otx-2 (see Chapter 3) are examples of genes encoding transcription factors that have been implicated in the regulation of axonal growth in the developing forebrain (Ba-Charvet *et al.*, 1998; Mastick *et al.*, 1997). There are several possible ways in which the blueprint could be formed. For example, pathways for growing axons may be dictated by adhesive differences between adjacent domains. These differences could arise due to the region-specific expression of the transcription factors. Alternatively, the genes may establish certain orientating gradients in the neuroepithelium (Wilson *et al.*, 1993).

Directional guidance through relatively large channels and grooves by an adhesive gradient is known as haptotaxis. If the extracellular matrix is broad and allows the axon to grow in several directions an adhesive gradient would make one direction preferred over the others. One extracellular matrix (ECM) adhesion molecule is laminin. It has been shown *in vivo* that laminin provides a pathway through which trigeminal sensory axons grow to reach their peripheral targets (Letourneau *et al.*, 1988). Laminin has also been shown to influence the branching properties of hippocampal neurites *in vitro* (Lein *et al.*, 1992).

Guide posts and pioneer axons

In some cases the route of the extending axon is marked by guidepost cells— pre-axonogenesis neurons which are derived from epithelial cells. This represents another way in which cues embedded in the environment between the origin of axons and their targets can guide axons. Guidepost cells were first identified in embryonic grasshoppers. When certain identified cells in the limb bud were removed, it was found that pioneer neurons failed to navigate (Bentley and Caudy, 1983). Observations have been made on the navigation of the first growth cones in the grasshopper embryo which are navigating in an axonless environment. It was suggested that there is very selective filopodial adhesion to specific landmark cells and these may play an important role in the guidance of pioneer growth cones (Taghert *et al.*, 1982). On encountering a guidepost cell (Tr1 in the trochanter), the tibial axons in the grasshopper limb bud take a 90° degree right-hand turn and grow along a channel of the adhesive molecule fasciclin IV (this is a founder member of the semaphorin family; Pini, 1994). The axons continue to grow along this channel by preferential adhesion and may also be inhibited from forming new branches until they leave the channel following contact with guidepost cell Cx1 in the coxa.

In these studies, the guideposts are intended only to guide the pioneers so that there must be a subsidiary mechanism for guiding the axons which arrive later. Harrison (1910) suggested that in early development, when the axons have to navigate over fairly small distances, it might be sensible to think in terms of pioneers using a different mechanism from the later developing axons. It is possible that axons coming later follow the correct pioneers by recognizing and responding to molecules expressed by specific pioneer pathways (Goodman and Shatz, 1992).

Chemical gradients

The environment between the origin of axons and their targets may be filled with secreted factors produced by the target. Growth cones can be guided to a target by gradients of diffusible chemicals that are secreted by certain cells within the target region. This is known as chemotropism and was first suggested by Ramón y Cajal (1893) when studying embryonic chick neurons (as cited in Kandel *et al.*, 1991, p. 911). More generally, chemotropism can be used to describe the attraction of axons by distal structures in the absence of direct contact with them but by means of long-range interactions mediated through transportable molecules. One simple picture is that the concentration of the molecule varies monotonically along the intended route of the axon and the growth cone is able to move along its gradient.

The first compelling example that growth cones (from sensory neurons) can respond to a gradient of a soluble molecule was reported by Gundersen and Barrett (1979). In this case the soluble molecule was nerve growth factor (NGF) which was first purified by Cohen in 1960. A family of similar molecules has since been isolated (Lewin and Barde, 1996) (see Chapter 6) although there is little evidence that they have chemotropic roles. The first diffusible chemotropic factors described in the vertebrate central nervous system (CNS) are members of the netrin family, netrin-1 and netrin-2, which are related to the ECM molecule laminin (Kennedy *et al.*, 1994). Many of these growth factors may act in concert to guide the incoming axons to their correct target area. For example, in addition to the guidepost cells and adhesion channels marking the pathway of Ti1 pioneer neurons there are also at least three distal–proximal chemical gradients (Norbeck and Denburg, 1992).

There is evidence that tissues secrete diffusible chemoattractants at appropriate times during development. This evidence has been obtained mainly from *in vitro* experiments. However, there is little evidence as to the exact contribution that chemical gradients make to the guidance of axons in a developing embryo. It is likely that there are numerous overlapping, partially overlapping, synergistic, or antagonistic gradients of chemotropic and chemorepulsive (see next section) molecules. Chemoattractants probably act in combination with other cues, such as the scaffolds provided by earlier developing axons and contact-guidance molecules.

Chemorepulsion

Recent research has suggested that, in addition to chemoattractive signals drawing axons towards a target, chemorepulsive signals may be widely used to steer axons away from inappropriate regions (Fitzgerald *et al.*, 1993; Keynes and Cook,

1995; Pini, 1993; Serafini *et al.*, 1996). Such chemorepulsive signals may act when cellular processes make contact (contact-repulsion) or may be diffusible and act at a distance. The fact that contact-repulsion can occur has been demonstrated by studying interactions between (i) peripheral sensory axons and retinal ganglion cells in culture (Kapfhammer and Raper, 1987; Luo *et al.*, 1993), (ii) spinal nerves and the anterior or posterior halves of the somites (Davies *et al.*, 1990), and (iii) retinal axons and the developing optic chiasm or tectum (Walter *et al.*, 1987; Wizenmann *et al.*, 1993). Molecules implicated in contact-repulsion include the ephrins, which are membrane anchored ligands that act on receptor tyrosine kinases (Eph receptors). There are eight known ephrins, divided into the ephrin-A (A1–A5) and ephrin-B (B1–B3) subfamilies (O'Leary *et al.*, 1999). The molecules ephrin A5 and ephrin A2 are expressed as gradients in the chick optic tectum and the family of receptors to which they bind are expressed on retinal growth cones (Drescher *et al.*, 1995; Cheng *et al.*, 1995; Nakamoto *et al.*, 1996).

Whether contact-repulsion occurs during the development of the cerebral cortex or its afferents has not been clearly demonstrated, although it has been suggested as a mechanism by which growing thalamocortical axons might be held in an ordered bundle (Blakemore and Molnar, 1990; Molnar, 1998). With regards to chemorepulsion by secreted factors, many of the molecules that have been implicated as diffusible chemorepulsants in other parts of the nervous system are expressed in the cerebral cortex. For example, members of the semaphorin gene family are expressed in the cortex (see below). Semaphorin III has been shown to repel dorsal root ganglion axons and may help pattern sensory projections in the spinal cord (Messersmith *et al.*, 1995). Several other candidates for chemorepulsive molecules have been identified elsewhere in the nervous system, notably, collapsin, which induces growth cone collapse (Luo *et al.*, 1993), and netrin-1. The latter is expressed by floorplate cells of the developing spinal cord and has the interesting property of attracting spinal commissural axons (Kennedy *et al.*, 1994) but repelling trochlear motor axons (Colamarino and Tessier-Lavigne, 1995). Research implicating these molecules in the development of corticofugal connections is discussed below.

Utility of chemical gradients

In order for guidance of axons by chemical signals to be effective, the growth cones must be able to sense local changes in concentrations of chemicals; i.e. they need to be able to sense concentration gradients.

In developing systems where there is evidence for chemotropism, the target is less than 500 microns away from the growing axons (Lumsden and Davies, 1983, 1986; Tessier-Lavigne *et al.*, 1988; Heffner *et al.*, 1990). Chemotropic guidance in culture also requires that distances between the source of axons and their target be less than 500 microns. Recent theoretical work by Goodhill (1997) and Goodhill and Baier (1998) suggested that this limit can be explained in terms of the mathematics of diffusion of chemical factors. In these models, it is assumed from experimental evidence that there must be at least a 1–2% change in the concentration of the factor across the growth cone for detection of a gradient (Goodhill, 1997). The models consider the case of diffusion of a factor from a point source, which is unrealistic, and do not take into account many complicating conditions such as tissue heterogeneity and the nature of the extracellular matrix, with which diffusible factors might interact *in vivo*. Nevertheless, they have predicted that guidance by stable gradients should occur over distances of around 500–1000 microns, a prediction that fits well with experimental evidence. Interestingly, the models predict that guidance over distances up to several millimetres may be possible as gradients are forming. Gradients would form quickly for small molecules, but may take several days to form if the factors are large (such as the netrins). These models have provided an important first step in defining the constraints on chemotropic guidance and the conditions under which it can operate. They are likely to become more refined as knowledge of the biology of chemotropism progresses.

Electrical gradients

Electric fields have been observed in developing embryos (Hotary and Robinson, 1990) and it has been proposed that electric gradients act to define an invisible coordinate system for the establishment of the embryonic pattern (Shi and Borgens, 1995). Disruption of the natural electric fields may lead to developmental abnormalities such as skeletal and neural defects (Hotary and Robinson, 1994). These results suggest that electric gradients may induce the growth of functionally distinct regions in the early development of the embryo.

Electrical gradients can also be used to influence the direction of neurite outgrowth (McCaig and Rajnicek, 1991; Bedlack *et al.*, 1992). The mechanism for this appears to involve the redistribution of integral membrane proteins within the growth cone which migrate towards the negative cathode. This leads to an increase in the number of receptors, including the acetylcholine receptor, at the membrane facing the cathode. This results in increased numbers of growth cone filopodia and subsequently turning of the neurite (Stewart *et al.*, 1995).

Direct communication with the target

In addition to being the source of long-range signals, targets can supply information by direct contact with the growing axons. Information conveyed by direct contact can be used to:

(a) Instruct the axons to stop growing.

(b) Instruct the formation of synaptic structures.

(c) Remove some of the projecting neurons or prune off axonal branches.

Targets may play different roles at different stages of development.

The amount of information that is required to be supplied in this target-derived signal will depend on the use to which this information is to be put and on how much information has been acquired on the way to the target. One likely use of communication with the target is to signal to the growing axons when they have reached their destination. Cells may generate positive signals, marking them as targets, or there may be negative repulsive signals from surrounding cells. Newly arrived axons have the potential to influence their target structure. They may alter the morphology of that structure, or drive its differentiation; or a more subtle influence may stimulate a feedback of information that could strengthen the recognition of the target structure by the axons.

The development of motoneurons is one example of how interactions with the targets can influence some aspects of axonal growth and not others. Between embryonic days E5 and E12 in chick, around 40–50% of the original neurons in the lateral motor column are lost (Hamburger, 1975). The survival of the remaining neurons is target-dependent, as demonstrated by experiments showing that (i) removal of early limb buds increases the amount of cell death in the ventral horn (Hamburger, 1958; Oppenheim *et al.*, 1978); (ii) increasing the size of the target (by, for example, grafting in an additional limb bud) decreases the amount of cell death (Hollyday and Hamburger, 1976). These issues of resculpting of connections are discussed again in Chapters 5 and 6. At a later stage of development during axonal outgrowth, most motorneurons are guided precisely to the muscles that they innervate (Landmesser, 1984). Motor nerves can be guided to their muscle when forced to take abnormal routes (Lance-Jones and Landmesser, 1981; Hollyday, 1981) whereas in other cases nerves innervating rotated limb buds are guided to the inappropriate muscles (Stirling and Summerbell, 1979; Summerbell and Stirling, 1981). The most parsimonious explanation is that environmental cues can correct short-range but not long-range errors of guidance (Summerbell and Stirling 1981; Landmesser, 1984). This suggests that particular muscles are not marked as the targets for particular sets of motorneurons, but that motorneurons are guided by cues in the environment between the developing spinal cord and the muscles. Since these cues produce appropriate innervation, the expression of target-specific signals would be redundant.

4   GENETIC ANALYSIS OF AXONAL GUIDANCE IN NON-MAMMALIAN SPECIES

One approach to studying axon guidance has been to identify the genes involved by studying the abnormal patterns of guidance established in mutants. As has been described earlier, the two methods that have been used are the screening of large populations of mutants produced by for example X-irradiation or investigating the effects of knocking-out already cloned genes.

Genetic screens of the nematode *C. elegans* have revealed genes causing uncoordinated movements, the so-called unc genes. The gene products of unc-5 and unc-6 seem to be involved in axon guidance along the dorsal–ventral axis (Ishii *et al.*, 1992; Hamelin *et al.*, 1993). In the fruit fly *Drosophila melanogaster*, mutations in the gene commissureless results in flies without commissures; mutations in dreadlocks causes axons from photoreceptors to make pathfinding errors

(Seeger *et al.*, 1993; Garrity *et al.*, 1996). More recently, the retinotectal system in the zebrafish *Danio rerio* has been employed in large scale genetic screening (Baier *et al.*, 1996; Trowe *et al.*, 1996; Karlstrom *et al.*, 1996). The relative simplicity of the direct projection of retina onto contralateral tectum and the ease of viewing axonal pathways coupled with advances in screening techniques have made this a viable exercise.

Over 100 000 zebrafish embryos were screened for defects in axon guidance between eye and brain. This was assessed using the lipophilic tracers DiI and DiO, which were each injected into a small area of retina thus labelling a circumscribed population of axons. Over 100 mutant lines were identified in which pathfinding differed from that found in the wild-type, and these mutants were classified according to whether the abnormalities were in axonal guidance, ordered retinotectal maps, or development of the brain. Most mutants also showed other developmental defects.

The largest population of mutants showed altered ability of axons to cross the midline of the brain. In most cases the midline structures were abnormal but the retinotectal projection itself (now assembled on ipsilateral tectum) was not affected. In other cases the ability of axons to reach the tectum was affected once they had crossed the midline; and in other cases axons travelled in the wrong brachium yet still innervated the correct part of the tectum. Mutations that affect the retinotectal map itself are described briefly in the next chapter.

These studies suggest that that axonal navigation is likely to be controlled by a number of genes. The facts that the genes isolated affect more than one type of developmental event and the precision of assessment is fairly low makes it difficult to infer what the precise action of any particular pathfinding gene is. However, the results suggest that pathfinding mechanisms act somewhat independently of those controlling other properties, such as map formation (Trowe *et al.*, 1996). Now that pathfinding genes have been isolated, it should be possible to examine their roles more closely.

5 MECHANISMS OF AXONAL GUIDANCE IN THE CORTEX

Many or all of the mechanisms outlined above may play important roles in the guidance of cortical connections; so far, the development of these connections has been less well studied than that of other pathways, particularly those in non-mammalian species. In the following section we consider how these types of mechanism could apply to the development of neocortex.

The mechanisms of cortical axon guidance are likely to be similar in different species of mammal. This is a reasonable assumption since the main features of the cellular processes themselves are very similar in different species (Molnar, 1998). However, there could be important differences. As yet, there is no strong evidence for such differences, but this is hardly surprising given our lack of knowledge of the mechanisms that regulate the development of cortical connections. One of the most obvious differences between the brains of different species is their size. Size may be very important in a system whose regulation involves chemotropism. Diffusion gradients of morphogens are thought to operate over relatively short distances (Section 3.2) and the development of cortical connections in large brains may rely on the presence of more gradients or on the combination of chemotropism with a larger number of other mechanisms. While it might be thought that, to compensate for their size, larger brains might develop cortical connections relatively early, while they are still small, this does not seem to be the case. The age at which axons from the LGN reach the visual cortex may actually be relatively *earlier* in rodents than in cats; certainly it is no later (see above). Thus, the process of geniculocortical development from LGN formation to cortical innervation may occur earlier and may occupy a relatively shorter proportion of gestation in smaller species.

5.1   Trajectories of axonal growth in cortex

Two main questions can be asked regarding the trajectories followed by developing cortical connections. (i) What determines the initial direction of growth of the axons in the developing neural pathways? (ii) What maintains or alters that direction of growth as the axons navigate towards their target? There is strong evidence that chemotropism may operate in some of the pathways; there are indications that contact guidance, chemorepulsion, and neuroepithelial channels may play roles (Section 3.2). Recent work has shown that the development of groups of cells that guide thalamocortical axons is dependent on expression of specific regulatory genes (Chapter 3) (Tuttle *et al.*, 1999). In some pathways, specific projections may arise through initially undirected growth (as discussed above and in Chapter 5 on map formation) followed by selective withdrawal of connections.

So far, the best evidence for chemotropism in the development of cortical connections comes from studies of the influence of subcortical structures on the growth of deep layer corticofugal projections. During the first stages of their growth, corticofugal axons travel ventrally towards the basal telencephalon. There is evidence that the ganglionic eminence of the basal telencephalon (Fig. 2.5) is an intermediate target for these axons (Metin and Godement, 1996). As development continues, these axons form a tight bundle in the region of the ganglionic eminence, called the internal capsule (Fig. 2.5). Having exited from the internal capsule, axons make changes in their trajectories: layer 6 axons deviate into the thalamus, whereas layer 5 axons continue to grow caudally towards midbrain, hindbrain, and spinal cord (Fig. 4.1). Recent culture work has indicated that the ganglionic eminence has a chemoattractive effect on growing corticofugal axons and that netrin-1, first identified as a chemoattractant for subsets of neurons in the spinal cord (Serafini *et al.*, 1994; Kennedy *et al.*, 1994), may mediate this attraction (Metin *et al.*, 1997; Richards *et al.*, 1997).

Other authors have suggested that the thalamus might secrete diffusible chemoattractants for corticofugal axons (Bolz *et al.*, 1990; Novak and Bolz, 1993). If such attractants exist, they might draw specifically layer 6 axons towards the thalamus from the bundle of corticofugal axons that is leaving the internal capsule. However, although the embryonic thalamus does appear to secrete molecules that promote the growth of cortical axons, as yet there is very little evidence that such factors can act as attractants (Lotto and Price, 1996; Lotto *et al.*, 1999). It has been observed in co-cultures of the cortex and thalamus that corticothalamic axons form specifically from layer 6, irrespective of the position of the thalamus relative to the cortex, and this has been interpreted as resulting from specific chemoattraction of layer 6 axons by the thalamus (Bolz *et al.*, 1990; Novak and Bolz, 1993). However, this result, which is obtained even under conditions that are not conducive to the establishment of diffusion gradients (Yamamoto *et al.*, 1989, 1992), might be explained by selection of specifically layer 6 axons by the thalamus after contact (Tuttle and O'Leary, 1993; Lotto *et al.*, 1999).

There is better evidence that chemotropic influences direct the development of layer 5 axons as they grow caudally to the midbrain, hindbrain, and spinal cord. Not only can structures in these regions stimulate the growth of axons from the embryonic cortex (Lotto and Price, 1996), but *in vitro* studies have shown that the basilar pons, which is a target for cortical layer 5 neurons (Fig. 4.5), can attract cortical axons at a distance (Heffner *et al.*, 1990). The molecules that mediate this attraction are not known but it is thought that, *in vivo*, they operate over short-range to cause the formation of collaterals from caudally directed axons travelling towards the spinal cord (Fig. 4.5) (Heffner *et al.*, 1990; O'Leary and Terashima, 1988).

Chemoattraction of the axons of deep layer cortical neurons towards the ganglionic eminence may not be the only mechanism guiding corticofugal fibres. Recent reports have described how the initial trajectory of cortical efferents towards the underlying white matter may be influenced by diffusible chemorepulsive signals from the cortical marginal zone (Polleux *et al.*, 1998). Such signals may force growing cortical axons away from the marginal zone, and hence into the white matter. The evidence is that semaphorins (Fig. 4.8; Table 4.2), which are expressed in the embryonic cortical plate and marginal zone (Skaliora *et al.*, 1998; Giger *et al.*, 1996; Chedotal *et al.*, 1998; Polleux *et al.*, 1998), mediate this interaction via the neuropilin-1 receptor (Polleux *et al.*, 1998). Other work has shown that the responses of cortical axons to the semaphorins depends on the type of semaphorin and on its concentration profile (Bagnard *et al.*, 1998). Semaphorin D has chemorepellant actions, and is expressed in the proliferative zones of the cortex. Semaphorin E is inhibitory to cortical axonal growth when it is at uniform concentration, but when cortical growth cones encounter it in a gradient of increasing concentration it attracts them. Semaphorin E mRNA is expressed by cells of the subventricular zone, and it is proposed that a gradient of protein with its source in this zone attracts cortical axons towards it and away from the cortical plate. Semaphorin D is expressed in the proliferative zones, where it may block the entry of cortical axons. In this way, corticofugal axons may become confined to the upper edge of the proliferative zones, where they contribute to the axonal pathways of the emerging intermediate zone (Bagnard *et al.*, 1998).

Another consideration is that the axons of different neurons are likely to respond differently to the various extracellular guidance cues. For example, many layer 5 neurons project subcortically but others in the same layer send their axons to the contralateral hemisphere (Fig. 4.1). The two sets of axons might be guided selectively due to their differing responses to molecules produced subcortically (e.g. netrin-1) or at the midline. Members of the Wnt and BMP families are produced at the midline (Furuta *et al.*, 1997; Grove *et al.*, 1998; Lako *et al.*, 1998), which was the lateral part of the neural plate prior to neural tube closure (a region which is known to express diffusible morphogens, Fig. 3.6). Although these molecules are candidates for such a role, as yet there is no strong evidence of their involvement.

With regards the development of cortical afferents, *in vitro* studies have indicated that the cortex releases diffusible molecules that can stimulate the growth of thalamic axons (Molnar and Blakemore, 1991; Molnar, 1994; Lotto and Price, 1994, 1995; Rennie *et al.*, 1994; Price *et al.*, 1995). It has been suggested that these might attract thalamocortical axons (Molnar and Blakemore, 1991, 1995b). However, unequivocal evidence that these molecules influence the direction of thalamic axonal growth is lacking (Lotto and Price, 1994, 1995; Rennie *et al.*, 1994; Price *et al.*, 1995) and, so far, the best evidence that chemotropism operates in the development of cortical connections comes from studies of the development of corticofugal axons.

Contact guidance has also been implicated in the development of reciprocal connections between the cortex and subcortical structures. As thalamocortical axons emerge from the internal capsule, they grow through the subplate towards their cortical targets, suggesting that this structure may act as a guide to the growth cones. The subplate is known to express a variety of cell adhesion molecules, including L1, fibronectin, chondroitin sulphate core proteins, and glycosaminoglycans (Godfraind *et al.*, 1988; Chung *et al.*, 1991; Stewart and Pearlman, 1987; Chun and Shatz, 1988; Sheppard *et al.*, 1991; Derer and Nakanishi, 1983; Fukuda *et al.*, 1997; Miller *et al.*, 1995; Bicknese *et al.*, 1994; Henke-Fahle *et al.*, 1996; Kinnunen *et al.*, 1999). Specific carbohydrate moieties (Henke-Fahle *et al.*, 1996), glycosaminoglycans, chondroitin sulphate core proteins, and specific peanut agglutinin lectin binding (Gotz *et al.*, 1992) are all expressed selectively in the subplate. Functional *in vitro* assays have suggested that at least some of these molecules can influence patterns of afferent and efferent cortical axonal growth (Henke-Fahle *et al.*, 1996). In addition, the membrane associated protein LAMP has been suggested to have a role in the guidance of limbic and non-limbic thalamocortical projections (Mann *et al.*, 1998).

Another suggestion is that thalamic axons may fasciculate on their subplate counterparts, providing them with a pathway to follow to their cortical targets (Blakemore and Molnar, 1990; Molnar, 1998). This has been termed the handshake hypothesis, since it proposes that the two sets of axons meet in the internal capsule and then grow over each other, retaining their order as they do so. This may contribute to the generation of an orderly map of the thalamus in the cortex (Chapter 5). Although attractive, the idea remains controversial. First, subplate axons may not be the first axons to reach the internal capsule and contact the thalamocortical afferents; rather, layer 5 neurons may pioneer the efferent pathway (Clasca *et al.*,

1994, 1995). There is now considerable evidence that, whereas the thalamocortical afferents do indeed grow through the subplate, efferents from the cortical plate itself (which would include the pioneering layer 5 neurons) follow a different, deeper route (De Carlos and O'Leary, 1992; Bicknese *et al.*, 1994; Henke-Fahle *et al.*, 1996). Thus, while there may be an important role for an initial handshake between cortical afferents and efferents in the internal capsule, it may involve axons from the cortical plate. These axons may not be followed subsequently by the thalamocortical axons. Rather, it is possible that thalamocortical axons switch to follow subplate axons, i.e. perhaps an initial 'handshake' with one set of fibres is followed by a prolonged relationship with another. Secondly, *in vitro* experiments have suggested that axons growing from cortical neurons do not fasciculate with axons from thalamic neurons, but collapse after contact with them (Bolz *et al.*, 1995). It will be important to discover whether this is true for cells from all layers of the developing cortex; for the handshake hypothesis to work in its present form, one would expect cells from the layers that make initial contacts to be able to fasciculate with their thalamic counterparts.

In summary, there is growing evidence that chemoattractive, chemorepulsive, and contact-guidance mechanisms combine to guide the growth of thalamocortical and corticofugal pathways. Much work remains to demonstrate the exact mode of action of the factors that have been identified and the mechanisms that have been postulated.

5.2   Interactions with targets. I. The subplate

In mammals, the initial target of the thalamocortical axons is the subplate. Thalamocortical axons grow through the subplate, as we have discussed in the previous section, but they must also stop at appropriate points within it. The subplate is a transient structure (Chapter 2) and the thalamocortical axons form temporary synapses on cells in this region. Experimental evidence indicates that the subplate plays a role in the guidance of thalamocortical axons to appropriate cortical regions. Therefore, the subplate may have several overlapping functions, acting as a channel through which thalamocortical axons can grow, providing signals to stop these axons at appropriate points and providing temporary targets for them. Ghosh and Shatz (1992a) and Ghosh *et al.* (1990) lesioned the subplate before the arrival of afferents and found that these axons continued to grow beyond the lesioned area to innervate distant sites. This implies that the growing axons themselves do not contain the information necessary to make them stop in correct regions. Since the lesions were very localized, it is also unlikely that the axons acquire information on where to stop in the subplate before their arrival in an appropriate zone. It is most likely that the subplate contains information that instructs the ingrowing axons where they should stop.

Although target recognition occurs in the subplate, it is not any group of subplate cells that will terminate the growth of any thalamocortical axon; it must be an appropriate group. Two questions arise. On what scale does target recognition operate in the subplate? How do ingrowing axons stop among correct groups of subplate cells?

Currently, there is no direct evidence to answer the first question. However, since thalamocortical axons eventually enter the cortical plate with a cruder organization than they will eventually attain we can assume that the precision of the projection from thalamus to subplate is similarly crude.

There is a spectrum of possible answers to the second question. At one end of the spectrum, the subplate may contain molecular markers that are specific to each region and that interact only with the incoming axon carrying the complementary markers. Essentially, this follows Sperry's hypothesis of chemoaffinity (Sperry, 1943, 1951, 1963, 1965) (Section 3.2, Chapter 5) but applied at a fairly coarse scale. At the other extreme, subplate cells may contain no specific information allowing their positive identification and thalamocortical axons may terminate in the subplate because of chemical and/or physical spatiotemporal constraints on their growth. At the age at which the subplate is first innervated from the thalamus, there is evidence that the overlying cortical plate is not permissive for axonal ingrowth (Tuttle *et al.*, 1995; Gotz *et al.*, 1992; Henke-Fahle *et al.*, 1996). Thalamocortical axons growing through the subplate, which is permissive for their growth, are therefore constrained by their chemical environment. Further, it has been suggested that thalamocortical axons preserve an ordered arrangement as they approach the cortex and terminate in the subplate (Molnar and Blakemore, 1995a,b; Molnar, 1998). The notion that the subplate is devoid of any information instructing the incoming axons where to stop is hard to reconcile with the lesion experiments of Ghosh *et al.* (1990); but while some positive recognition process does seem likely, it is not known how complex it has to be. Intuitively, the chemoaffinity hypothesis is unattractive because of the amount of specification that it would require; an array of different molecules, or the same molecules at different concentrations, would need to be deployed in the subplate, to interact with a complimentary deployment of receptors in an appropriate manner among the afferents. A more plausible hypothesis might be to suppose (Sperry, 1963) that only a small number of molecules, perhaps one for each dimension of variation, are deployed in the subplate in a spatiotemporal gradient such that specificity is achieved by interactions between only those axons that have newly expressed a particular receptor (or receptors) and those subplate cells that have newly expressed a particular ligand (or ligands). Temporal gradients of development are known to exist in the cortex, but whether they could explain the recognition of specific regions of the subplate has not been explored. The general question of using gradients to set up maps of connections is discussed in Chapter 5.

5.3   Interactions with targets. II. Cortical plate

Some time after innervation of the subplate (the time depending on the species) thalamocortical axons enter the overlying cortical plate. The majority of these axons terminate in layer 4, although there is also a significant innervation of layers 1 and 6. Evidence suggests that this is due to the up-regulation of growth-promoting molecules in the cortical plate (Tuttle *et al.*, 1995; Gotz *et al.*, 1992; Henke-Fahle *et al.*, 1996).

Several experiments are pertinent to the question of how the ingrowing thalamic axons stop in specific layers, particularly layer 4. Some have been done *in vivo* and involved the lesioning of afferents to other cortical layers to discover whether the thalamocortical axons would take over the vacated layers (Price, 1995). They did not, indicating that appropriate laminar innervation is not achieved by preventing afferents innervating other layers because those other layers are already occupied, i.e. through some sort of hierarchy of occupancy. Other *in vitro* experiments have assessed the stopping of thalamocortical axons under various culture conditions (Molnar and Blakemore, 1991). The results of these *in vitro* experiments have argued against the suggestion that axons stop in layer 4 because of an inhibitory effect of the layers above layer 4. As in the case of the subplate, it is more likely that layer 4 expresses a positively identified signal. The nature of this signal is unclear.

5.4 Interactions with targets. III. Thalamus and reticular nucleus

The guidance of axons to their target zones in the thalamus may follow similar principles to those that underlie the development of thalamocortical axons. It has been suggested that cells in the reticular nucleus of the thalamus might act as guidepost cells for the various types of corticofugal projections that pass through them (Mitrofanis and Guillery, 1993). It is possible that this structure acts as a temporary target for corticofugal axons, which has prompted comparisons between it and the subplate (Mitrofanis and Guillery, 1993; Molnar, 1998). The way in which the internal capsule and thalamus sort out the various types of axon that pass through them is not known. There is evidence from culture experiments that the thalamus has the ability to distinguish between appropriate and inappropriate axons that contact it (Lotto *et al.*, 1999), but the molecules that mediate this interaction and its role *in vivo* are not clear.

5

Map formation

1   INTRODUCTION

In everyday usage, the term 'map' is taken to indicate a flat representation of the
earth's surface, or a part of it, showing physical features, cities, and so on. This term
has a more general meaning, namely a diagram showing the layout of the component parts of a complex structure. In mathematics, mapping involves associating
elements of one set with those of a second set according to the given relationship
between the two sets. According to the mathematical definition, all neurons in the
mature nervous system are mapped onto the neurons to which they connect and
therefore understanding how neural mappings are achieved could be considered
synonymous with understanding how every aspect of the connectivity of the nervous system is established. However, in line with neurobiological convention, we
take map formation to mean the generation of ordered connections between two
discrete neural structures e.g. connections between the thalamus (or its component
nuclei) and the cortex (or its component areas).

A striking feature of many of the connection patterns between collections of
nerve cells is that they are highly ordered. Evidence for this comes mainly from
two types of experiment. First, in electrophysiological experiments it is often found
that stimulation of adjacent regions in one structure, such as a sensory surface or a
nucleus, leads to activation of adjacent regions in its target (Talbot and Marshall,

1941; Apter, 1945; Woolsey, 1952; Gaze, 1958; Rose and Mountcastle, 1959). As the stimulus is moved systematically across the structure, the region of the target that responds often shifts in a corresponding fashion. Secondly, a correspondence between points in a target and its structure is often observed in anatomical experiments using axonal tracers (molecules that can be injected at discrete points to label axons running to and from those points). Tracer placed at one point in one structure often label a small, circumscribed area in the target, the spatial layout of points of administration (in different animals) being reflected in the layout of points to which the tracers go in the target (Mesulam, 1982; Cook and Rankin, 1984). Such ordered anatomical layouts of connections provide the substrates for the ordering observed in electrophysiological experiments.

Many maps can be thought of as mapping the elements of one two-dimensional surface onto another. For example, axons from each small cluster of ganglion cells in the mammalian retina project (via the LGN) onto a small area of visual cortex with the result that a map of the retina is spread over the surface of its target structure (Fig. 5.1a). In amphibia and fish the retina projects directly to optic tectum where, once again, an orderly map of the retina is found (Gaze, 1958) (Fig. 5.1d). A second example is in the somatosensory system in rodents (Rose and Mountcastle, 1959). The two-dimensional array of whiskers on the snout projects in a very precise way via midbrain nuclei to form a somatotopic map in the cortex, the barrel field (named after the cytoarchitectonics of this part of cortex), in which the order of whiskers on the snout is preserved (Fig. 5.1b). Other ordered maps are one-dimensional, such as the tonotopic map of frequency in auditory cortex (Rose, Galambos and Hughes, 1959) (Fig. 5.1c). Where axonal projections are through intermediate structures, the intermediate maps are themselves well-ordered. Ordered projections are the rule, although there are a few apparently disordered projections such as that of visual space onto the pyramidal cells of mammalian hippocampus, which in rats respond to specific locations in the animal's environment ('place cells'; O'Keefe and Nadel, 1978), and in the direct projection between cortex and striatum (Kincaid *et al.*, 1998).

The mapping of the elements in one structure onto another may be studied at the coarse-grained level, as in the case of the mapping of thalamic nuclei onto the cortex; or at a fine-grained level, as in the case of the mapping of cells within a particular thalamic nucleus onto a particular cortical region. Such maps are readily understood on the basis of zone-to-zone or point-to-point connections between the structures, mediated either by bundles of axons (in the case of coarse-grained mapping) or by individual axons (in the case of fine-grained mapping).

The fundamental type of map, that of one surface onto another (a topographic map), is well displayed in the mammalian visual cortex by a result of experiments from Tootell *et al.* (1982), shown in Fig. 5.1a. This figure shows the projection on macaque monkey striate cortex of a visual stimulus in the form of a half-circle and illustrates that firstly there is an ordered projection of retina onto cortex and secondly the projection may be distorted, different small regions of retina being represented on the cortex to a different extent.

(a)   (b)

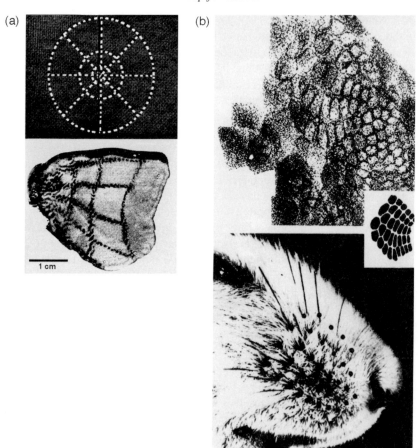

FIG. 5.1. (a) Showing the ordered projection of the retina onto the visual cortex of monkey. The animal was exposed to the image (*top* photograph) and activity in the visual cortex was revealed by processing for deoxyglucose uptake (*bottom* photograph). Note ordered projection and non-linearities. Reproduced from Tootell *et al.* (1982) with permission; ©1982 American Association for the Advancement of Science. (b) The pattern of whiskers on the adult rodent snout (*lower* photograph) and the pattern of barrels in somatosensory cortex (*upper* photograph, schematised in inset) to which the whiskers project in a one-to-one fashion. The pattern of whiskers is almost invariant from one animal to another. (Copyright acknowledged to Woolsey and van der Loos, 1970.) (c) The one-dimensional map of frequency in auditory cortex. (AI and AII: primary and secondary auditory cortex; EP: posterior ectosylvian gyrus; I: insula; T: temporal field; numbers 0.13–100: kHz). There is a regular tonotopic representation in cat but a distortion of this regularity in bat by a large representation of 61–62 kHz, the frequency of its echolocating signal (based on Shepherd, 1994, and Suga, 1978). (d) The ordered projection from retina to contralateral tectum in adult *Xenopus laevis*. The numbers indicate where in the visual field a small point stimulus evoked maximal response at the correspondingly numbered tectal position. Reproduced from Jacobson (1967) with permission; ©1967 American Association for the Advancement of Science.

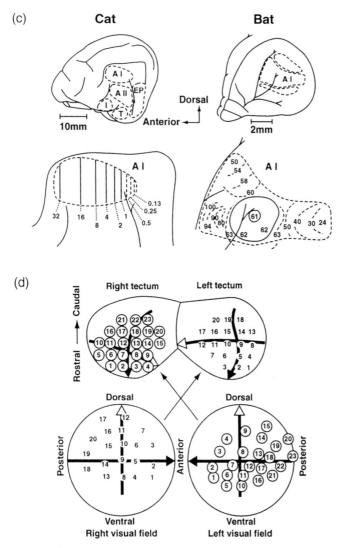

(c) Cat Bat

Dorsal

Anterior

10mm

2mm

A I

A I

0.13
0.25
0.5

32 16 4 1
8 2

50
54
58
60
100
90 80
94
53 62
61
62 63
50
40 30 24

(d) Right tectum Left tectum

Caudal

Rostral

21 22 23
16 17 18 19 20
10 11 12 13 14 15
5 6 7 8 9
1 2 3 4

20 19 18
17 16 15 14 13
12 11 10 9 8
7 6 5 4
3 2 1

Dorsal Dorsal

Posterior Anterior Posterior

17 12
16 11 7
20 15 10 6 3
19 9 5
14 2
18 13 8 4 1

15
9 14
4 20
3 8 13 19
2 7 12 17 22 23
1 6 11 16 21
5 10

Ventral Ventral
Right visual field Left visual field

FIG. 5.1. (*Continued*)

    In a complex structure such as the cerebral cortex, more complex properties of the afferent system are also encoded in the map. For example, in certain areas of the visual system, cells are found that are sensitive to the orientation of a stimulus or its direction of movement as well as its position in the visual field. Such attributes of the external environment can be detected by means of the neural circuitry and the connectivity of the CNS ensures that they are often represented in an ordered fashion. In the cortex, the nature of the stimulus required to produce

maximal excitation in each small area varies over its surface, defining feature maps
(Fig. 5.2a).

The ability to detect features of the environment, such as oriented lines, depends
on convergence of inputs from multiple afferent axons onto each postsynaptic

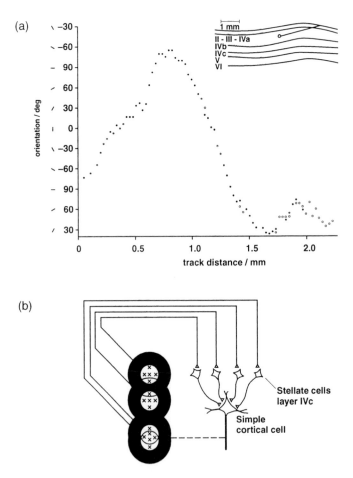

F I G .   5 . 2 . (a) A map of orientation specificity over mammalian visual cortex. The
diagram shows the variation in orientation preference of cells along a 2 mm electrode track
running obliquely through the visual cortex (inset).The orientation of the bar stimulus which
gives maximal excitation at each point varies smoothly over the surface of the cortex.
Cortical layers II–VI are marked on the inset. (b) Illustrates a hypothesis devised by Hubel
and Wiesel (1962, 1965) to explain how simple receptive fields (Chapter 7), displaying
orientation specificity, are formed in the cortex by a convergence of inputs from lower-
order neurons. The convergence of LGN cells with concentric fields that are arranged in a
straight line on the retina may generate oriented receptive fields in cortical cells.

neuron (Fig. 5.2b). Thus, the construction of feature maps within an overall geographical map of the innervating structure on the target is a complex achievement.

In theory, a faithful representation of one surface on another could be achieved by mapping each point on one surface to a unique point in the other, with preservation of order in the layout of connected points. In some cases, such a simple mapping of one surface onto another could be achieved by a set of connections that preserve their relative positions as they run between the two regions, without any crossing over (Fig. 5.3a); in other cases, the geometrical constraints make it impossible to achieve a map of connections arranged with the desired polarity without a wholesale crossing over of connections occurring (Fig. 5.3b). However, a system that can detect an array of features within a small region of a sensory surface, such as many possible orientations of a line presented on a small region of the retina, cannot be connected up in such a straightforward point-to-point way. At the level of individual axons there is considerable convergence and divergence of projections that does not violate the overall geographical mapping and sufficient to generate the circuitry required for the detection of an array of features presented to a given region of a sensory surface and the generation of feature maps (Fig. 5.2).

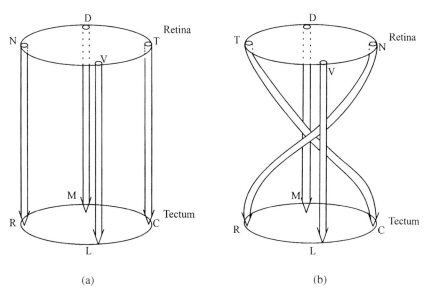

(a)　　　　　　　　　　　　(b)

FIG. 5.3. (a) Showing how an ordered map between retina and tectum could be attained by axons travelling directly from one structure to the other whilst maintaining their relative positions. (b) Maps with certain polarities cannot be achieved in this way; in the case shown, the required pattern of interconnections is attained only at the expense of a massive crossing over of fibres. N: nasal; T: temporal; D: dorsal; V: ventral; R: rostral; C: caudal; M: medial; L: lateral.

As a rule, we know more about the development of geographical (or topographic) maps of innervating structures over the surface of targets than about the development of feature maps. One particular example where the development of a more complex arrangement of inputs has been well-studied is found in binocular visual cortex (Figs. 5.14c,d; 5.15a) (LeVay *et al.*, 1975). Visual cortical cells receive innervation from both eyes, but with differences in the strength of the innervation from each eye that vary systematically across the surface of the cortex. These systematic variations in ocular dominance are superimposed on the basic retinotopic map (Hubel and Wiesel, 1977).

In the previous chapter we considered the mechanisms that may guide bundles of axons to their correct target structures. In this chapter we consider how the ordering of connections in these pathways generate various types of map in the target. There is considerable overlap between these topics; in some cases the same mechanisms that guide axons to correct targets may contribute to the development of orderly connections with the target. First we consider the generation of topographically ordered maps. We examine the various hypotheses that have been put forward for their generation and examine the evidence from non-cortical systems. We then consider various cortical systems where such maps of connections have been described. We go on to describe the different types of feature map and possible mechanisms for their generation. Finally we discuss different types of computer and mathematical models that have been proposed for map formation.

2   THE DEVELOPMENT OF TOPOGRAPHICALLY ORDERED MAPS OF CONNECTIONS

Most work has been carried out on the vertebrate visual system, either the projection from retina via the thalamus to cortex or, in amphibia and fish, the direct projection of retina onto optic tectum, the analogue of the superior colliculus in mammals. The first, crude maps were constructed from the results of axon degeneration studies (Attardi and Sperry, 1963) but the first maps with any precision were constructed by extracellular recording from the optic tecta of goldfish, and of the anura *Rana* and *Xenopus laevis* (Gaze, 1970; Sharma, 1972). The connections are not precise at the cell-to-cell level (as in invertebrates) but in *Xenopus laevis*, for example, at least 50 distinguishable recording positions are arranged in topographic order (Gaze, 1970). The other important attribute of such maps is that they always have a specific orientation. In all maps between retina and tectum, temporal retina projects to rostral tectum and dorsal retina to medial tectum (Fig. 5.1d).

The problem of understanding how maps are formed has often been formulated in terms of the establishment of a functional relationship between the cells in one set of cells with the members of a second set. More recently, with the advent of powerful methods for tracing patterns of connections, this problem has become that of the problem of specifying the connections themselves.

2.1   Hypotheses for map formation

Most of the main theories for the formation of topographic maps of connections were developed between the 1940s and the 1960s. Despite their age, they are still very much relevant today. It is worth noting that, ever since the studies of Langley (1895) (who carried out experiments on himself on the regeneration of peripheral nerve) most proposals for how maps of connections are *developed* were derived from *regeneration* studies. The main classes of theories are:

1. **The fibre ordering hypothesis** These are a collection of hypotheses which have the common feature that ordered maps are a result of the order of fibres within the pathway itself. One way (Attardi and Sperry, 1963) in which this could be done is through the guidance of axons by cues placed in the pathway- this is a variant of the cytodifferentiation hypothesis (Hypothesis **2**; see below). Alternatively, it has been suggested that the axons grow out in order and that maintaining this order is sufficient to determine the final pattern of connections (Horder and Martin, 1979; Rager and von Oeynhausen, 1979).

2. **The cytodifferentiation hypothesis** (Sperry, 1943, 1963; Meyer and Sperry, 1973). This states that there are preexisting sets of biochemical labels among both the presynaptic and the postsynaptic cells, that each label marks the position of that cell within the set and that the pattern of connections is generated by the matching together of the cells with complementary labels (Fig. 5.4a).

3. **Neighbour matching hypothesis** This derives from the idea that postsynaptic cells tend to accept or retain innervation from fibres having patterns of impulse firing in common with each other (Lettvin; cited in Chung, 1974). Under normal conditions, cells in the same structure with similar firing patterns will be close to one another. In this way neighbouring presynaptic cells will tend to develop connections with neighbouring postsynaptic cells. This hypothesis (Fig. 5.4b) can be extended to make use of any property of the system that has a spatial distribution (for example, freely moving molecules). This hypothesis uses information about relative position to impose relative order amongst the innervating fibres on the target structure and so is unable to specify the orientation of the final map of connections. Since all maps do have a predictable orientation, any mechanism for setting up the correct neighbourhood relations must be supplemented by one specifying map orientation.

4. **The induction of specificity by innervating cells** This hypothesis suggests that the postsynaptic cells acquire the ability to make contact with selected presynaptic cells through signals passed to them from the presynaptic cells (Willshaw and von der Malsburg, 1979; Ribchester and Barry, 1994).

5. **The timing hypothesis** This states that during neurogenesis the earliest fibres to reach their target make connections with the earliest differentiating

(a)

Presynaptic sheet

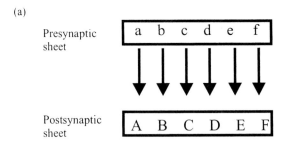

Postsynaptic sheet

(b)

Presynaptic sheet

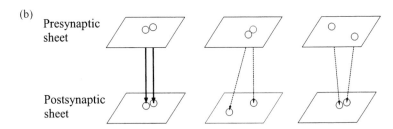

Postsynaptic sheet

FIG. 5.4. Various hypotheses for the formation of topographic maps. (a) The cyto-differentiation hypothesis. Axons of presynaptic cells carry labels reflecting their place of origin and they match to the postsynaptic cells carrying the complementary label. (b) Neighbourhood matching. If a mechanism operates that reinforces the contacts made by neighbouring axons from neighbouring cells of origin then an ordered mapping will result (*left hand* diagram, solid arrows). The two other diagrams show synaptic configurations that will not be reinforced.

postsynaptic sites (Gaze, 1960; Jacobson, 1960). This requires an underlying mechanism that converts positional information into temporal information.

6. **The retrograde modulation hypothesis** (Weiss, 1937a,b) Growing nerve fibres are assumed to make contact at random. The postsynaptic elements are attuned to respond to their proper signal only, which indicates the region of origin amongst the presynaptic cells. In this way specificity between presynaptic and postsynaptic elements is attained by functional means instead of through specific anatomical connections. Since connections are regarded as being made at random, there is no anatomical map formed and therefore no explanation of ordered patterns of connections. This is not discussed further.

We now examine the evidence for the first five hypotheses in turn, dealing first with non-cortical systems, mainly the retinotectal projection in lower vertebrates, and then with cortical ones.

3 THE DEVELOPMENT OF TOPOGRAPHIC MAPS IN NON-CORTICAL SYSTEMS—EXPERIMENTAL EVIDENCE

3.1 The role of fibre ordering in map making

In the construction of topographic maps, the mapping problem may already have been solved if the nerve fibres grow out towards their target structure in order. If this order is preserved to the point of synaptogenesis, a map of the first structure will be imposed on the second structure without there being any need for knowledge of what inputs each of the regions of the second structure should receive. At a gross level this seems to be true for the thalamocortical projection, where there is an ordered projection from the individual nuclei themselves onto neocortex (Section 4.1).

A more striking, long known example of a pathway in which nerve fibre order is preserved to a much higher level of detail is the projection of retina onto contralateral optic tectum in fish.

The retinotectal projection in fish
Various experimental models have been used to examine the hypothesis that nerve fibres are guided to their sites of termination through interaction between axons that are neighbours in the pathway. In the simplest possible case, fibres could grow out alongside those from their neighbouring cells of origin and maintain this ordering all the way to the target.

At first sight, this could be tested by looking for order in the mature pathway. One vertebrate that displays remarkably precise ordering of axons within the optic nerve is the *Cichlid* fish (Anders and Hibbard, 1974; Scholes, 1979; Rusoff, 1984; Presson *et al.*, 1985). In this animal, the axons of the retinal ganglion cells pass into the optic nerve in order. The cross-section of the nerve just behind the eye resembles a long folded up ribbon (Fig. 5.5). There is a polar coordinate representation of retinal position within the nerve cross-section, with the radial dimension of the retina represented along the long axis of the ribbon and the circumferential dimension along the short axis. The retina grows in rings, and as it does so, the axons from each annulus of newly formed cells add on as a band of unmyelinated fibres at one end of the ribbon. It is inferred that newly growing fibres travel over the substrate laid down by the older fibres. This order is maintained towards the optic chiasma as gradually the ribbon becomes shorter and fatter. The folds coagulate until finally the cross-section becomes roughly circular without any of the elaborate pattern of foldings seen in the optic nerve.

Despite this evidence of a high degree of order within the optic pathway, as an explanation of how the ordered retinotectal map is formed it is unsatisfactory for four reasons.

(a) 200–300 μm after the optic chiasma, the fibres change their position within the optic pathway very abruptly, each group of fibres of the same age (i.e. from the same annulus of retina) seeming to stay together. The fibres split up into

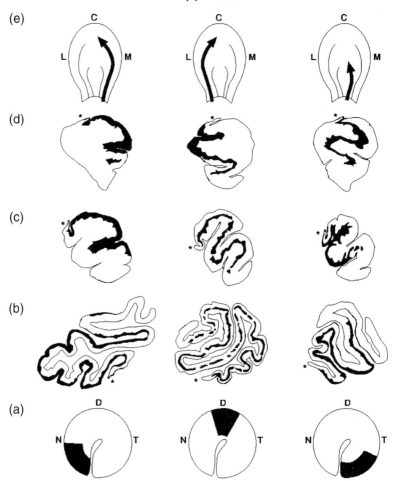

FIG. 5.5. The arrangement of fibres in the optic nerve of the *Cichlid* fish. Shows the patterns of osmiophilic degeneration of fibres in the optic pathway after selective lesioning the nasal retina (*lefthand* column), dorsal retina (*middle* column) or temporal retina (*right-hand* column). (a) The extent of the lesion. (b) Immediately behind the optic nerve head the optic nerve is, in cross-section, a very long and thin ribbon. There is an ordered representation of retina within the ribbon, the radius being represented along the long axis and the circumference along the short axis; i.e. a representation in polar coordinates. Unmyelinated, presumably newly arriving, axons are grouped at one end of the ribbon, shown by ∗. (c) A more posterior section of the optic nerve, showing that the ribbon has become shorter and wider yet the polar coordinate representation has remained. (d) Shortly before the optic tectum there has been rearrangement of fibre positions within the cross-sections, over a very small distance, which disturbs their neighbourhood relationships. (e) Illustrating the fibres being led onto the optic tectum. Reproduced from Scholes (1981) with permission. Labelling as in Fig. 5.3.

lateral and medial brachia and are led onto the tectum. It has not been possible to follow the course of these fibres as they change their positions.

(b) It is not known how optic fibres leave the two brachia to innervate the tectum. The situation may be complicated by the possibility that the fibres in the optic tract are destined for more than one area of termination; that is, two or more sets of innervating fibres are intermingled.

(c) It is doubtful whether *in principle* fibres could be led onto the optic tectum without grossly violating their relations with their neighbours when subject to the physical constraints imposed by the fibres already present. Imagine how a retinotectal map could be constructed by moving a disc (representing the retina) along the optic pathway, keeping it in the transverse plane of the nerve, eventually projecting it onto the surface of the optic tectum. Maps with certain polarities can be obtained by placing the retina onto the surface of the optic tectum and then rotating it (Fig. 5.3a); to produce the actual polarity of the map, the disc has to be flipped over, which would correspond to a violation of neighbourhood relations between fibres. The biological case is more complicated than this; the specific transformations that occur within the three-dimensional optic pathway have to be taken into account. In particular, retinal fibres undergo a centre-to-periphery inversion of order on leaving the retina. The importance of geometrical constraints could be investigated by constructing 3D geometrical computer models of the optic pathway.

(d) The tacit assumption is made that the ordering of fibres in the adult is a faithful historical record of developmental events. It is assumed that there is no reordering of fibres within the nerve during development; direct experimental evidence is needed.

The channel catfish (Dunn-Meynell and Sharma, 1986) has a different ordering of fibres in the optic nerve. In the first part of the nerve, the ganglion cell axons are arranged in 13 separate optic papillae. Close to the optic nerve head, the papillae are arranged in the cross-section in a U-shaped formation. Fibres of dorsal origin are at one tip of the U and ventral fibres at the other tip, with fibres of both nasal and temporal origin at the base of the U. At the level of the optic chiasma, the U-shape has flattened out whilst retaining the relative ordering of the papillae. In the optic tract, a substantial re-ordering of fibres takes place.

These studies illustrate that there are cases where fibres keep contact with their neighbours for much of the way along the pathway, which could contribute to the formation of a map but without being the whole story. The *Cichlid* fish seems to be an extreme case where there is a high degree of ordering in the optic pathway. There are signs that similar types of ordering exist in many other species of fish; but to a lesser extent or obscured by such factors as the pattern of fasciculation (Bunt, 1982).

3.2   The cytodifferentiation hypothesis

The simplest statement of this hypothesis is due to Roger Sperry, who proposed the doctrine of chemoaffinity. This is that both the presynaptic and the postsynaptic cells carry prespecified, distinguishing labels, probably cytochemical in origin, and the making of connections involves a matching up of each presynaptic cell with the postsynaptic cell carrying the matching label. In the original papers (Sperry, 1943, 1944, 1945) the cells were regarded as matching together in the way that a lock fits into a key. As it was inconceivable that each cell could carry a different label, later he proposed (Sperry, 1963) that the molecular labels were spread across the retina to form gradients of concentration, one type of molecule for each dimension of variation. Each gradient would be matched by a complementary gradient over the surface of the optic tectum. Each incoming axon would then find the tectal cell with the matching set of labels, to which it would make contact (Fig. 5.4a).

Sperry's hypothesis was formulated to account for the behavioural responses observed after nerve regeneration following cutting the optic nerve and rotating the eye in adult newt (Sperry, 1943, 1994, 1945). He found that the animal's response to visual stimulation after restoration of visual function was not adapted to the eye rotation. For example, after a 180 degrees eye rotation, the animal's response to visual stimulation of nasal retina was appropriate to the effect of stimulation of temporal retina in normal animals, and vice versa. The conclusion was that regenerating retinal axons from the rotated eye had found their old partners on the tectum.

Much experimental and theoretical work has been carried out on the development of the ordered retinotectal mapping of retina onto optic tectum in lower vertebrates to test this hypothesis. The prime experimental issues have been (i) whether connections are as rigid as the hypothesis suggests and (ii) how the retina and tectum acquire their labels and what the labels might be.

Plasticity of connections

Sperry's proposal was intended to account for various experimental findings involving the regeneration of connections following surgical removal of parts of retina or tectum from adult goldfish. Degeneration staining indicated that the optic fibres from a surgically diminished half-retina regenerated to the appropriate half of the tectum (Attardi and Sperry, 1963). However, later experiments found that in this experiment retinal fibres eventually moved to form an ordered map over the entire tectum (Horder, 1971; Yoon, 1972; Schmidt *et al.*, 1978). Complementary experiments revealed that after removal of half the tectum from goldfish, the projection from the entire retina eventually becomes compressed, in order, on to the surviving half-tectum (Gaze and Sharma, 1970; Cook and Horder, 1974; Yoon, 1971). These results exemplify the typical finding in the mismatch experiments: that the retina and the tectum match together as a system (Gaze and Keating, 1972), regardless of the actual sizes of both structures, which might have been reduced in the surgery. There is therefore much more plasticity in the patterns of connections made than envisaged in the doctrine of neuronal specificity (Fig. 5.6). Similar findings were found in developmental studies. In *Xenopus laevis*, the retina and tectum grow in different ways (Straznicky and Gaze, 1971, 1972). New cells are added on as rings of cells to the outside of the retina whereas tectal growth is along the rostro-caudal axis, most new cells being added to caudal tectum. None the less, there is an ordered projection of retina onto tectum from a very early stage. This implies a gradual shifting of connections. For example, central retina projects to central tectum, the position of which moves progressively backwards as more tectal cells are added. These inferences were confirmed by extracellular recording (Gaze *et al.*, 1974) and by electron microscopy studies demonstrating the degeneration of synapses during development (Gaze *et al.*, 1979a). In *Rana pipiens* tadpoles, Reh and Constantine-Paton (1983) labelled small groups of retinal ganglion cell terminals with HRP and investigated their tectal projection sites with reference to [³H]thymidine labelled tectal cells, at various stages of development. They found that the retinal terminals move from a position rostral to the labelled tectal cells to a position caudal to these cells, travelling a distance of 1.4 mm during early developmental stages. Separate electrophysiological and electron microscopy studies established that the retinal ganglion cell terminals had made functional synaptic contact and therefore were continually changing their tectal partners during development.

A second set of related experiments are those involving the projection from *Xenopus* compound eyes onto the optic tectum (Gaze *et al.*, 1963). Compound eyes are made at tailbud stage by replacing one-half of an eye rudiment by a

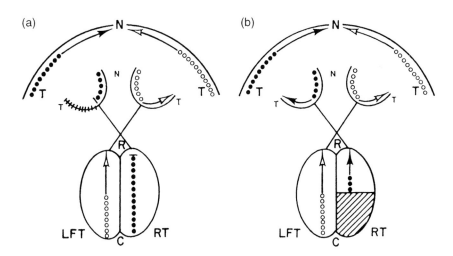

FIG. 5.6. The mismatch experiments. (a) Following removal of half the left retina from adult goldfish and optic nerve cut, the remaining half retina expands its projection, in order, to cover the entire right tectum. (b) Conversely, a whole left retina forms a compressed and ordered projection onto a right half tectum. Circles are used to represent nasal retinae (N); arrows are used to represent temporal retinae (T). R: rostral; C: caudal. (After Edds, 1979)

half from another eye. For example, replacing a temporal-half eye rudiment with a nasal-half yields a double nasal (NN) compound eye. Double temporal (TT) and double ventral (VV) compound eyes are also possible. These eyes develop apparently normally and develop a single optic nerve which projects to contralateral optic tectum, as in normal animals. Electrophysiological recording reveals that the retinotectal projection is ordered but two spatially separated receptive fields are found to drive each tectal position. Each half eye projects in order across the *entire* optic tectum rather than to the half predicted from neuronal specificity, to form a double projection (Fig. 5.7) (Gaze *et al.*, 1963).

Acquisition and identification of labels

At some stage in development, different parts of the retina and the tectum must acquire their own identity. The issue of how and when this occurs has been hotly debated in terms of how the axes of the retina and the tectum are specified. When does the retina become polarized; i.e. provided with the information that will enable nasal retina to develop connections with caudal tectum, temporal retina to rostral tectum, and similarly for dorsal and ventral retina? Following rotation of an eye rudiment of *Xenopus laevis* prior to embryonic stage 28, the retinotectal map measured in the adult was normal; that is, that part of the retina that came to occupy the nasal pole in the eye orbit projected to caudal tectum, as it does in normal animals; similarly for the cells from temporal, dorsal, and ventral poles. In contrast, following rotation of the eye rudiment at stage 32, the map in the adult was found to have been rotated by the same amount (Jacobson, 1967; Gaze *et al.*, 1979b). The interpretation was that the retinal axes were laid down between these two stages. Further experiments suggested that (i) the naso-temporal and dorsoventral axes of the eye are specified independently, one after another (Jacobson, 1967) (which mirrored similar inferences about the specification of the axis of the limb) and (ii) the axis of one of the two half eye rudiments put together in the same orbit to form a compound eye could be reprogrammed after the time of axial polarisation by the presence of the other half eye (Hunt and Frank, 1975). These latter findings were, and remain, controversial. However, some of them have been resolved by the use of albino tissue as an indicator of retinal origin. The results of these experiments suggested that in some of the controversial cases eye rudiments that had been rotated experimentally had then died to be replaced by regenerating tissue with the normal orientation.

Work has also been done on specification of optic tectum. Rotation of tectal precursors at very early stages can potentially furnish evidence about when the optic tectum is polarized. Chung and Cooke (1975, 1978) rotated portions of *Xenopus* pretectal tissue. In the cases where the tissue that gives rise to diencephalon, normally immediately anterior to tectum, had been rotated as well, the retinotectal map was rotated. In cases where there was no rotation of the diencephalon, a normal map resulted. Based on a relatively small number of experiments, the inference was that presumptive diencephalon contains an organizer (a 'beacon') that determines the polarity of tectal tissue.

(a)

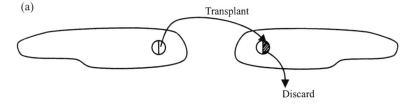

(b)

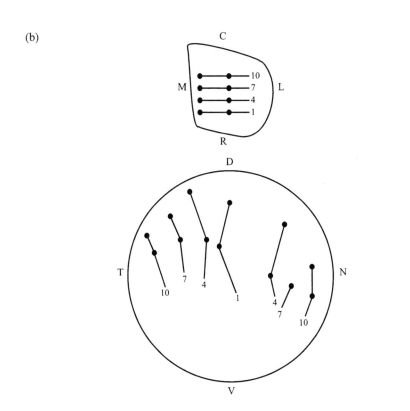

FIG. 5.7. Projections from *Xenopus* compound eyes. (a) Compound eyes are made in larval animals by replacing a half eye rudiment by a different half from another animal. This shows the construction of a double nasal (NN) compound eye. (b) The map formed by a NN eye, recorded electrophysiologically, in an adult *Xenopus*. Tectum is drawn above with recording positions marked; the visual field is drawn below. Each half of visual space corresponding to one half of the compound eye projects in order across the entire tectum, rather than being restricted to one half of the tectum From Gate and Straznicky (1980). Reproduced with permission of Company of Biologists Ltd. Labelling as in Fig. 5.3.

Genetic determinants

A different way of reversing the tectal axis has been attempted at the genetic level. Itasaki and Nakamura (1992) transplanted mesencephalic alar plate into the diencephalon of chick embryos. They found that this tissue reverses the normal rostro-caudal gradient of expression of the gene engrailed in optic tectum. Engrailed is a homeobox gene (Chapter 3), originally discovered in *Drosophila* (Morata and Lawrence, 1975; Kornberg, 1981) and now known to have homologues in many vertebrates (Patel *et al.*, 1989). It has a gradient of expression along the rostro-caudal axis of chick optic tectum, with a high level in caudal tectum, to which nasal fibres normally project, and a low level in rostral tectum, innervated by temporal fibres (Itasaki and Nakamura, 1996). It may control the ligands of the Ephrin class of receptors (see below).

The effect of reversing the rostrocaudal axis of expression of engrailed is that nasal fibres come to innervate rostral tectum; conversely temporal fibres innervate caudal tectum rather than rostral tectum. Several authors have used a retroviral gene transfer technique to produce animals with high levels of engrailed expression at specific regions throughout chick tectum (Itasaki and Nakamura, 1996; Friedman and O'Leary, 1996). They found that nasal fibres preferentially innervate the areas of high expression of engrailed whereas temporal fibres do not. This suggests that there is a causal link between the expression of engrailed and the establishment of retinotectal maps.

Recent experiments attempting to identify the genetic basis of axonal path finding and map making have examined the retinotectal projection of the zebrafish, which has an arrangement similar to that found in *Cichlids* but with a lower degree of order.

Use of large scale screening of zebrafish mutants has found a number of genes that affect the ordered mapping of retina onto contralateral tectum. Mutations in some genes are related to abnormal mapping of connections along the dorsoventral axis and in other genes to similar abnormalities along the anterior–posterior (rostral–caudal) axis. In some cases the arrangement of optic fibres within the optic pathway is normal; in other cases it is abnormal (see Section 4, Chapter 4). It is tempting to view these results as providing evidence for genes that control the establishment of gradients of guidance cues arranged along these axes (Trowe *et al.*, 1996). However, the precision of the retinotectal projection so far assessed in the mutant studies is too low to allow any firm conclusions.

Evidence for gradients of molecules

At the time the idea of neuronal chemoaffinity was proposed the essential molecular labels were considered as hypothetical objects and evidence for their existence depended on what seemed to be necessary to account for the connection patterns obtained under normal and experimental circumstances. Since the 1970s many molecules have been considered as candidates for Sperry's chemical labels. Initial work was carried out *in vitro*. To explore the possibility that the chemoaffinity labels could be adhesion molecules, it was investigated whether there were preferential adhesions between retinal cells and tectal cells. Cells prepared from central chick neural retina adhere preferentially to medial tectum and cells from dorsal retina adhere to lateral tectum (Roth and Marchase, 1976; Gottlieb *et al.*, 1976). Similar results were obtained using axonal tips instead of entire neurons (Halfter *et al.*,

1981). More recent experiments have tested the growth responses on retinal axons. Walter *et al.* (1987) allowed retinal cells to extend axons onto a membrane made up of alternating stripes derived from rostral and caudal tectum respectively. Ganglion cells from nasal retina innervated each type of stripe equally. However, cells from temporal retina extended axons onto stripes of rostral origin. The effect seemed to be one involving repulsion of cells of temporal origin by caudal cells. This was shown in experiments where after contact of tectal cell membranes by a growth cone of temporal origin, the growth cone filopodia withdrew, leading to the collapse and retraction of the growth cone (Cox *et al.*, 1990).

This evidence is suggestive of the existence of molecular labels but does not indicate the identity of the labels. A number of candidate molecules have been proposed such as TOP (Trisler and Schneider, 1981) and RGM (repulsive guidance molecule) (Stahl *et al.*, 1990). Most recently, interest has focused around the Eph receptors, the largest known subfamily of receptor tyrosine kinases, and their associated ligands, now known as ephrins (Flanagan and Vanderhaeghen, 1998). The existence of the Eph receptors has been known for some years and originally they were identified on the basis of their molecular structure alone. More recently it has been found that these receptors are expressed in the developing and adult nervous system (Tuzi and Gullick, 1994) and the family of associated ligands has recently been cloned (Flanagan and Vanderhaeghen, 1998). The ligand ELF-1, discovered in mouse optic tectum (Cheng and Flanagan, 1994), becomes bound to the receptor Mek-4 found in retinal ganglion cells. These molecules seem to fulfil the requirements for the labels required for chemospecificity. In chick there is a gradient of Mek-4 receptor density across the nasotemporal axis of the retina whereas there is a complementary gradient of ELF-1 across the rostro-caudal axis of optic tectum (Cheng *et al.*, 1995). ELF-1 is now known as ephrin-A2 and Mek-4 is known (confusingly) as EphA3. The evidence for these molecules being involved in map formation is:

(a) They are produced at the time when retinal axons travel into the tectum to make their connections (Cheng *et al.*, 1995).
(b) Incoming axons destined for the low end of the ephrin-A2 gradient avoided this region in cases where ephrin-A2 was overexpressed in this region (Itasaki and Nakamura, 1996).
(c) Axons that normally innervate high ephrin-A2 regions of the tectum were unperturbed by the overexpression.

From these experiments it was inferred that connections are made because axons are repelled by ephrin-A2 in the following way (Nakamoto *et al.*, 1996). The ligand ephrin-A2 is distributed over the optic tectum, a gradient being built up from rostral to caudal tectum. Axons of temporal origin normally project to rostral tectum. They have large numbers of EphA3 receptors on their surfaces, making them highly sensitive to ephrin-A2. These axons enter rostrally and grow until they meet increasing amounts of ephrin-A2 and stop. By contrast, axons of nasal origin normally map to the back of the tectum where ephrin-A2 levels are high. These axons have few EphA3 receptors, rendering them nearly oblivious to the ligand and allowing them to pass through increasing concentrations of it as they cross the tectum.

Other ligands have been found. Ephrin-A5, originally cloned as a ligand for the receptor EphA5 (Winslow *et al.*, 1995) is distributed in a graded fashion within the posterior part of the tectum (Drescher *et al.*, 1995). This too seems to have a repellent effect on both temporal and nasal cells. It may be that the role of ephrin-A5 (previously called RAGS) is to stop retinal axons from leaving the tectum. On the other hand, it could be that both ligands cooperate in generating the overall map of connections, in the rostro-caudal dimension at least.

Nakamoto *et al.* (1996) have proposed an informal model for topographic mapping to account for the findings that ephrins and their receptors are arranged in counter gradients; that is, axons from the high end of the retinal gradient normally project to the parts of the tectum at the low end of the tectal gradient and vice versa; and that the interaction of receptors and ligands causes repulsion. According to their model, all axons have an equal tendency to grow towards posterior tectum. In the final stable state, once the mapping has been set up, this tendency is counter balanced by an equivalent amount of negative signal. The amount of negative signal is determined by the number of receptors bound by ligand. In the simplest case, if the axon has an amount R of receptor which binds to an amount L of ligand, the strength of negative signal would be the product of $R \times L$. The same amount of signal would result from either high receptor and low ligand, low receptor and high ligand, or a medium amount of both quantities. This would account for the necessity of having counter gradients.

Certainly this is an interesting possibility but immediately several problems with it come to mind. First, this model specifies only how order can be arranged along one dimension and cannot be generalized in a straightforward fashion to two dimensions. As retinal axons enter the tectum at the rostral pole and then progress caudally it is natural to envision that molecular gradients can pull them in this direction. However, they cannot by the same mechanism be made to grow along in the mediolateral direction. Two possible solutions to this problem are that ordering of axons along the second axis is controlled by a separate set of gradients: or there is an entirely different mechanism for exploiting the information supplied from molecular gradients; see Section 7.1 for such a proposal. The second problem is that this model is only concerned with how to generate matching gradients in retina and in tectum. Like all models employing fixed labels, it will not account for the variety of results from both experimental and normal situations that demonstrate plasticity of connections in the system (Gaze and Keating, 1972). Finally, the model has one of the fundamental weaknesses of Sperry's proposal itself, which is that there is a lack of information concerning how, in early development, matching gradients could be set up in two disparate structures. Goodhill and Richards (1999) review models for map-making based on the recent findings about ephrins and their receptors, relating these to the theoretical models discussed in section 6.

3.3 Neighbour matching hypothesis; activity-independent versus activity-dependent mechanisms

A hypothesis that is completely different from that put forward by Sperry is that the nature of the contacts made by any given axon depends on which contacts are formed by its *neighbours* (Fig. 5.4b). This gives rise to a very different type of relation between retinal and tectal cells, particularly that there is no fixed relation between them.

The general idea is there is a mechanism that ensures that axons with different cells of origin which are close together on the retina tend to make connections on nearby tectal cells. This could be because cells in the retina are spontaneously active and axons from neighbouring cells have strongly correlated patterns of activity enabling activity-dependent synaptic modification (Lettvin: cited in Chung, 1974); or because there is a set of labels assigned to the retinal cells with a graded spatial distribution and cells of nearby retinal origin carry similar labels and therefore establish contact on the same part of the tectum on the basis of their carrying similar labels (Willshaw and von der Malsburg, 1979). This distinction gives rise to the issue of the evidence for *activity-dependent* against *activity-independent* mechanisms for map formation.

Evidence for activity-independent mechanisms
The positive evidence for this is provided by findings, discussed in section 3.2, for complementary gradients of labels, possibly the ephrin ligands and their associated receptors, of the type implied by Sperry's doctrine of chemospecificity (Sperry, 1943, 1963). Further evidence comes from work showing that maps of connections can develop in the absence of neural activity or where the normal activity patterns have been disturbed.

The Californian newt *Taricha torosa* manufactures tetrodotoxin (TTX) which when applied to nerve cells is a blocker of voltage-sensitive sodium channels and therefore prevents the propagation of nerve impulses. The nervous system of this newt itself is insensitive to TTX. Harris (1980) grafted eye rudiments to this newt from an axolotl which is tetrodotoxin-sensitive. The eye developed as normal and formed a normal optic nerve which innervated the optic tectum apparently normally. In this eye all action potentials were blocked yet neuroanatomical techniques revealed that a retinotopic map formed. However, only a low degree of order could be demonstrated due to the particular anatomical techniques employed. The transplanted silent eye could maintain an optic projection even in the presence of competition from the electrically active normal eye.

It may be that activity-independent mechanisms act to arrange fibres in the optic tract as they approach the tectum. Stuermer (1990) demonstrated that an initial ingrowth of optic fibres into the tectum of zebrafish is not affected by blocking activity with TTX. Cook and Becker (1988) investigated the regeneration of an orderly projection from retina to tectum in goldfish following optic nerve cut. In normal animals, axons from ventral retina travel in the medial brachium of the optic tract and axons from dorsal retina in the lateral brachium. After regeneration, both ventral and dorsal retina are represented in both brachia. Optic nerve fibres reach the optic tectum some three weeks after optic nerve cut. Three weeks later, the number of inappropriately directed fibres have decreased, due probably to elimination of external collaterals rather than cell death. Cook and Becker (1988) found that this so-called brachial refinement was not affected either by intraocular injection of TTX or by subjecting the animals to continuous stroboscopic illumination (which in previous experiments had been found to impair the refinement of the map itself).

Evidence for activity-dependent mechanisms

In vertebrates such as fish and frog, it is difficult to investigate the effects of activity on the development of maps directly. In *Rana*, blocking NMDA receptors disrupts the retinotopic organization (Cline and Constantine-Paton, 1989). Other evidence comes either from surgically created situations or by arguing from findings from the regeneration of projections. Reh and Constantine-Paton (1985) used the three-eye preparation. This had been developed by Constantine-Paton and Law (1978), who implanted an extra eye rudiment into the frog *Rana pipiens* at early embryonic stage. In many cases one of the two optic tecta developed a projection from two eyes rather than one and so it was possible to investigate how the two projections would compete with each other to innervate their common target. Typically the innervation from each of the two eyes formed a pattern of stripes over the optic tectum, a somewhat simplified version of the pattern of zebra stripes seen in binocular innervated mammalian cortex (Fig. 5.15a) (LeVay *et al.*, 1975). Two weeks after crushing both of the normal optic nerves in these three eyed tadpoles, the projection from the supernumerary eye covered the tectum in a continuous fashion. After four weeks the host optic fibres had reached the tectum and six to seven weeks after nerve crush the pattern of stripes had been re-formed. In other experiments (Reh and Constantine-Paton, 1985), during the last three weeks of this process, activity in the optic nerve was abolished with TTX and in this case segregation of the projection into stripes did not occur. Blocking nervous activity with TTX without optic nerve crush also showed continous, overlapping projections after three weeks of continuous TTX blockade. These experiments taken together indicated that activity is essential for both the development and maintenance of striped projections in binocularly innervated structures.

Other authors have investigated the effect of neural activity on map formation in the regeneration of adult projections. Meyer (1983) and Schmidt and Edwards (1983) made repeated injections of TTX into the goldfish eye following optic nerve crush. It was found that the maps regenerated in the presence of TTX were ordered to some degree but not with the same amount of detail found after regeneration without application of TTX. To counteract the possible criticism that the TTX had other unknown metabolic effects, Cook and Rankin (1986) investigated the refinement of the regenerated goldfish optic projection under conditions of abnormal electrical stimulation, produced by keeping the animals under stroboscopic illumination. They made a careful quantitative study where retrograde transport of HRP from a standard tectal injection site was employed to measure the precision of the mapping. They calculated the mean squared distance of each labelled retinal cell to its nearest neighbour and expressed this as a proportion of the area of the retina. Early in regeneration, without exposure to stroboscopic illumination, labelled retinal cells were very widely dispersed and over the next two or three months, precision was improved until the normal figure of 1% was reached. After three months of exposure to strobe light, the precision of the mapping was still very diffuse and corresponded to that seen one month after regeneration in connections in normal lighting conditions.

These various sets of experimental results suggest that both activity-independent and activity-dependent effects are essential for the establishment of ordered nerve connections. One popular view is that activity-independent effects direct the nerve fibres onto the tectum and are responsible for producing an initial coarsely-grained map and that the refinement of connections into the precision seen in the adult is driven by activity. One possible type of activity used for the setting up of maps is that of correlated activity. Strongly correlated spontaneous activity has been demonstrated amongst ganglion cells in the adult at least (Arnett, 1978; Rodieck, 1967). This makes spontaneous activity a plausible basis for the formation of ordered maps.

3.4   The induction of specificity hypothesis

The experimental basis for this originates in work carried out on the retinotectal system in goldfish, which can be seen as an attempt to introduce a different hypothesis for how cells make connections on the basis of the labels that they carry.

A surgically constructed half retina regenerates an ordered projection to the entire optic tectum, rather than innervating that half of the tectum that it would innervate if part of a normal eye. This could be because either the retinal labels had been changed by the surgery, or the tectal labels had been changed, or both. Schmidt (1978) carried out a set of experiments in adult goldfish. By forcing a surgically diminished half retina to innervate the optic tectum together with a normal retina he was able to use the projection made by the normal retina to calibrate the putative labels carried by the tectum and by the experimental retina. In a first set of experiments he removed one-half of the retina from an adult goldfish and allowed the remaining half retina to regenerate its connections to the entire contralateral tectum. He then diverted this projection to ipsilateral tectum, which carried a projection from a normal retina, and showed that it innervated, in order, only its 'appropriate' half (Fig 5.8a). This established that the half retina was still a half retina in terms of the labels that it was assumed to carry. In a complementary set of experiments he diverted the projection from a whole retina onto the ipsilateral tectum carrying an expanded projection from a half retina. In this case, only the half of the retina which had matching origin with the experimental half retina

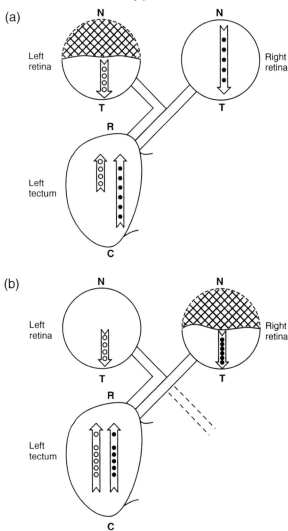

FIG. 5.8. Evidence for induction of markers in the retinotectal system of goldfish (Schmidt, 1978). (a) A left half retina that had previously regenerated an expanded projection on the contralateral optic tectum (not shown) is forced to innervate the ipsilateral tectum holding a projection from a normal eye. (b) An intact left retina is forced to innervate the ipsilateral tectum, which is already holding an expanded projection from a half retina. (After Edds, 1979)

established an ordered projection on the ipsilateral tectum, showing that tectum itself carried a half set of labels (Fig. 5.8b). These results demonstrated that in a surgically constructed half eye which made an expanded projection on the optic tectum the retinal labels did not change but the tectum acquired a half set of labels;

they must have been induced from the retina. Later on in this chapter we describe a model for marker induction developed prior to this experimental work (von der Malsburg and Willshaw, 1977; Willshaw and von der Malsburg, 1979).

3.5 The timing hypothesis

There is some evidence in invertebrates (Lopresti *et al.*, 1973) that connections are made on the basis of the time of arrival of axons at their target structure. Rager and von Oeynhausen (1979) proposed that, in chick, axons arriving at one area of tectum (such as the rostral edge) make contacts there and occupy the space, preventing later arriving fibres from innervating this region and forcing them to contact regions nearby. In this way, a temporal pattern is converted into a spatial pattern. It is fairly simple to imagine how such a mechanism could specify the ordering of optic fibre terminals along the direction of ingrowth of optic fibres but not along the direction perpendicular to it. The basic problem is that timing provides for variation along one dimension only whereas most maps are at least two-dimensional. Moreover, timing is inherently unstable and on this hypothesis disruption of timing relations would result in disruption in the map. This is contrary to the experimental findings. Maps are not affected by delaying the arrival of optic fibres by diverting optic fibres to take a different route (Beazley, 1975; Beazley, 1977). In surgical constructed *Xenopus* eyes made up of two halves of different ages, the normal temporal pattern of axonal outgrowth is reversed but the initial pattern of innervation is normal (Holt, 1984).

4 THE DEVELOPMENT OF TOPOGRAPHIC MAPS IN CORTICAL SYSTEMS

We now examine the ways in which maps form between subcortical and cortical structures and between cortical areas. We review the mechanisms discussed above in a series of cortical systems at both coarse-grained level (i.e. the projection from the entire thalamus to the entire cortex) and a finer-grained level (i.e. projections to individual cortical areas).

In cortical systems there has not been such a systematic examination of possible mechanisms as there has been in lower vertebrates. Here we examine each system in turn.

4.1 The thalamo-cortical projection—is the cortical map specified prior to innervation?

Many adjacent neocortical areas receive projections from adjacent thalamic nuclei (Caviness and Frost, 1980; Crandall and Caviness, 1984b; Jones, 1985; Caviness, 1988; Molnar, 1998). As a general rule, in the adult, neighbouring thalamic neurons preserve their relative positions as they project to the cortex; the spatial order of the nuclei in the thalamus, and of the cells in each nucleus, is transformed with considerable accuracy onto the neocortical sheet. The thalamo-cortical map so produced is of a three-dimensional thalamus projecting onto the two-dimensional surface of the neocortex and so is of a higher degree of complexity than the map between retina and tectum.

In recent years there have been a number of studies of ordering within thalamo-cortical projections as they grow. This work has been made possible by the development of new methods for tracing axonal projections with different coloured dyes that diffuse in fixed embryonic tissue, the carbocyanine dyes (Honig and Hume, 1986; Godement *et al.*, 1987). The growth of thalamo-cortical projections has been studied using these dyes by several groups (Erzurumlu and Jhaveri, 1990; Catalano *et al.*, 1991; Erzurumlu and Jhaveri, 1992; Kageyama and Robertson, 1993; Miller *et al.*, 1993; Molnar, 1998). When dyes are placed into the embryonic thalamus, thalamic axons are seen to reach the internal capsule in an ordered fashion. When dyes are placed into the embryonic cortex, adjacent parts of the cortex are found to receive their projections from adjacent groups of thalamic cells and the axons connecting the cortical and thalamic regions are ordered, preserving neighbourhood relationships along their lengths (Fig. 5.9). These studies have provided evidence

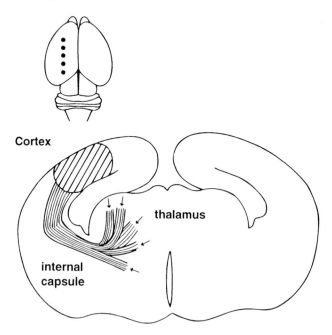

FIG. 5.9. Results of an experiment in which different coloured tracers were placed in a row in the cortex (five filled circles on the upper drawing, dorsal view of the brain) of a rat just before birth. The tracers diffused along the axons connected to each point. In coronal sections five distinct bundles were seen passing through the internal capsule without obvious mixing or crossing and running to different thalamic nuclei. (After Blakemore and Molnar, 1990; Molnar, 1998)

that, as thalamic fibres arrive in the subplate, they may already be organized with a degree of order approximating to the order of thalamic nuclei. This may form an important foundation on which to build the eventual cortical map of the thalamus. The refinement of the initial map probably involves the detailed sorting of afferents; evidence for this is that some thalamic axons send transient collaterals towards inappropriate regions of cortex as they grow towards their correct target area (Naegele *et al.*, 1988; Ghosh and Shatz, 1992a). The mechanisms that refine the initial projections and lead to the removal of the transient collaterals are not clear. It is possible that refinement is a result of interactions between the afferents, which impose patterns of neural activity and/or biochemical markers on the cortex that are broadly ordered and are read by the transient collaterals. On the other hand, the different regions of the cortex may possess some form of intrinsic knowledge concerning which thalamic nuclei should innervate them before the afferents arrive. Or both mechanisms may contribute.

For many developmental neurobiologists, the question of how much of the regionalization of the cortex is imposed on it by the order of its afferents and how much is specified before innervation has become a major preoccupation. Extreme views have been espoused, with some suggesting that the cortex is a naive sheet of cells whose identities are determined by the nature, the order and the detailed connectivity of the afferents that they receive; others have suggested that the cells of the cortex do have at least some regional identity before they become innervated (Rakic, 1988; O'Leary, 1989; Molnar and Blakemore, 1995b). As discussed in Chapter 2, there is some evidence for region-specific differences in proliferative rates and the expression of molecules in the cerebral cortex prior to innervation, and in some cases these molecular differences are not altered when expressing regions are transplanted to non-expressing sites, suggesting that some differences may be determined (i.e. irreversible) prior to innervation (Cohen-Tannoudji *et al.*, 1994; Barbe and Levitt, 1992; Levitt *et al.*, 1995). These results argue in favour of cortical cells having some positional identity without innervation, although how much is far from clear.

Others experiments have addressed this issue by studying the properties of different cortical regions either in culture or after transplantation. Molnar and Blakemore (1991) carried out a series of experiments with cultured explants of the cerebral cortex and thalamus to investigate the specificity of axons from different thalamic regions for different cortical areas. They found that axons from thalamic explants showed no preference for the area of neocortex with which they were cultured. They grew equally well on their normal target areas as on other non-target areas of the neocortex. Other experiments have involved the transplantation of regions of the developing cortex to abnormal sites (O'Leary and Koester, 1993). When transplants were done between neocortical regions, the donor tissue was found to develop attributes of the new host region rather than retaining its normal attributes. Thus, when pieces of visual cortex were grafted into motor cortex, they developed persistent projections to the spinal cord, as does normal motor cortex but unlike normal visual cortex; when pieces of motor cortex were grafted into the visual cortex, they developed persistent projections to the superior colliculus, as does normal visual cortex but unlike normal motor cortex. Sur *et al.* (1988) carried out a series of experiments on the regeneration of connections in ferrets where target structures of sensory fibres were ablated, leading to the fibres being diverted to other cortical structures. Ablation of lateral geniculate nucleus and visual cortex led to visual afferents innervating medial geniculate nucleus (the destination of auditory fibres), with the result that cells of the auditory cortex became responsive to visual stimuli and acquired the characteristics of classical simple and complex visual cortical cells (Chapter 7).

All of these experiments indicate that different regions of the embryonic and neonatal neocortex have a low level of commitment to their specific regional fates. Although it is widely accepted that the fates of embryonic cortical regions are not determined by birth (i.e. they are not irreversible), the degree to which they are specified remains controversial. The results of the experimental challenges described above suggest that it is easy to deflect developing neocortical regions from their normal developmental pathways. However, recent transplant experiments similar to those outlined above have come up with opposite results with no clear explanation for the difference (Roger, 1998). Furthermore, it may be harder to alter the fates of embryonic tissue transplanted between the neocortex and other cortical areas, such as the limbic cortex. Pieces of embryonic limbic cortex transplanted into neocortex retain their normal pattern of thalamic innervation provided they are old enough to express limbic system-associated protein (Barbe and Levitt, 1992; Mann *et al.*, 1998).

In summary, it is likely that both specification prior to innervation and the influence of cortical afferents contribute to cortical regionalization. The development of a cortical map of the thalamus is probably due to both the preservation of order in the bundle of growing thalamo-cortical axons and to the removal of transient collaterals through interactions with an increasingly elaborate array of cortical cells. Whether the transient collaterals have a specific function or whether they are a consequence of there being a degree of error in the detailed ordering of growing thalamo-cortical axons is not known. Examples of more specific pathways in which the sorting of initially disordered projections to form an orderly map is readily apparent include the geniculocortical projection from the visual thalamus to the visual cortex (in which initially overlapping maps of the two retinae later segregate) and the callosal and ipsilateral corticocortical projections (in which initially widespread projections are later narrowed); these pathways are discussed later in this chapter.

4.2   Mapping to specific cortical areas

Barrel formation—ordered maps in rodent somatosensory cortex
The most detailed evidence for the existence of precise maps of connections in cortex is found in the somatosensory cortex. Muride rodents, such as the terrestial rat and mouse, make much more extensive use of tactile information than visual information. Correspondingly, their somatosensory cortex is relatively large whereas

their visual cortex is relatively small and simple. A large area of primary somatosensory cortex is occupied by the barrel field which is an ordered representation of the facial whisker pad (Woolsey and van der Loos, 1970) (Fig. 5.1b). Layer IV of this part of cortex is made up of groups of cells surrounded by cells of different sizes, defining a series of barrel-shaped regions. There is an intimate relationship between the arrangement of whiskers and the arrangement of barrels: where the muzzle contains an extra whisker, there is an extra barrel in the topologically equivalent place and vice versa (van der Loos and Dorfl, 1978). Neurophysiological recordings have established that activation of an individual whisker excites the cells in the corresponding barrel. There is also a topological representation of the whiskers in the nuclei of the brain stem trigeminal complex (subnuclei principalis, interpolis, and caudalis—the barrelettes) and the ventrobasal thalamus (barreloids). The mapping pattern is not preserved throughout the length of the pathway from sensorium to cortex but rather is recreated at each individual relay station.

The pattern of vibrissal follicles is laid down seven days before birth; barrelettes form before barreloids which themselves form before the barrels; barrels form three days after birth. Deoxyglucose studies demonstrate that this sequence is mirrored in the development of functional properties (Killackey *et al.*, 1995; Melzer *et al.*, 1994).

Barrel formation—information from developmental and regeneration studies
In the adult, the representation of a single whisker in the thalamus is mirrored exactly in the cortex. At birth the thalamo-cortical projection is precise, but it is not precise enough to account for the adult projection. About 70% of the thalamocortical axons are at a position equivalent to being within 1.3 presumptive barrel diameters of their topologically precise target whereas to account for the of mapping seen in the adult, at this stage of development 100% of the axons would have to be within 0.4 barrel diameters (Agmon *et al.*, 1995).

There is much evidence for plasticity in the whisker-to-barrel pathway in rodents. An intact sensory periphery is required during a certain critical period of development for the normal map to develop. When rows of follicles are injured at birth, before barrels form, the corresponding row of barrels is not present in the adult, and is replaced by a small barrelless territory (Melzer *et al.*, 1993). Barrels develop in the first postnatal week and their morphology can be manipulated by the selective lesioning of the whisker follicles. The earlier the follicles are removed, the more extensive the resulting morphological aberration. Lesions within the first two days after birth leads to the development of enlarged barrels with partially disrupted borders surrounding a disorganised zone in place of the barrels that would have represented the removed follicles (Melzer *et al.*, 1993). Seven days after lesions of all probisci except one row, the cortical representation of the spared row increases in width by 60% (Fig. 5.10) (Jablonska *et al.*, 1995).

Most evidence in this system points to the instructive role of afferents in establishing this pathway. There are many suggestions that use of whiskers or, at least,

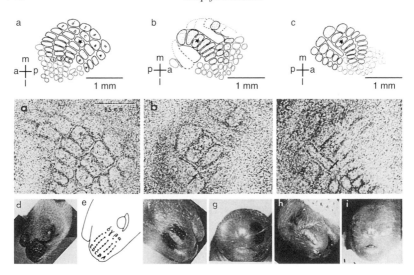

FIG. 5.10. a–c: Top row shows reconstructions from serial sections through layer 4 of adult mouse barrel field. a: anterior, p: posterior, m: medial, l: lateral. The matching sections are shown in the lower panels, the asterisks in the corresponding pictures indicating matching barrels. d–i: show muzzles. d, e: normal muzzle of a 6 day old mouse, with barrel rows and columns labelled. f, g: muzzle of a newborn mouse in which all papillae except β and the C row were ablated (major injury). h, i: muzzle of a newborn mouse in which only the β papilla and those in the C row were ablated (minor injury). a: control barrel field. b: barrel field that results after the major injury. c: barrel field that results after the minor injury. Reproduced from van der Loos and Woolsey (1973) with permission; ©1973 American Association for the Advancement of Science.

activity in the sensory neurons contributes to the formation of the map. For example, there is a high correlation between the length of the whisker (signalling perhaps its use) and the area of the corresponding cortical field. Some of this evidence is only suggestive for developmental processes as it comes from studies in the adult.

Several lines of evidence imply a crucial role for the thalamic afferents in the development of barrels. The pattern of probiscal follicles is laid down seven days before birth, preceding the pattern of barrels which is established three days after birth. Thalamo-cortical afferents are the first barrel components to have a periphery-related pattern. The patterning observed is transiently present in the deep cortical layers prior to the emergence of layer IV, the layer in which barrels later develop (Schlagger and O'Leary, 1994). In newborn mice, no whisker-related patterns are found in either the cortex or thalamus. Consequently, the thalamo-cortical projection at birth is a topological mapping of the thalamus onto the cortical sheet, as yet unrelated to the periphery (Agmon *et al.*, 1995). Around postnatal day 2, thalamic barreloids are formed and thereby cells in the ventrobasal thalamus (Agmon *et al.*, 1995) acquire a whisker-specific identity. The presumptive thalamic barreloids are already connected up to the presumptive cortical barrels, which relates the whole system back to the whiskers.

The evidence cited above concerning the degree of order in the thalamo-cortical projection suggests that the whisker maps formed are not as a result of the preservation of order amongst axons. In addition, there is evidence that fibre tracers placed close together in the newborn somatosensory cortex label fibres which are unsegregated along the thalamo-cortical tract. Furthermore, at this age fibres from some barreloids course directly through other barreloids. These results should be interpreted with caution as although the tracts are relatively immature, at this stage the axons within them are not actually in the process of navigating to their targets. Given the very rapid changes in the dimensions and geometry of the brain that are occurring at this time, it is dangerous to draw strong conclusions about the mechanisms by which a system developed on the basis of its organization once that stage of development is complete.

Overall, it seems unlikely that axons from neighbouring whiskers remain together and thereby innervate neighbouring subcortical and cortical areas. One possibility is that there is early widespread growth of connections followed by refinement of connections. Agmon *et al.* (1995) suggested that rather than there being a maintenance of fibre order in a developing thalamo-cortical tract, once the axons reach the deep cortical layers an active process of resegregation occurs which results ultimately in the appropriate connections being made. However, they found that developing thalamo-cortical axons arborize only locally within layer 4 with a horizontal extent never wider than a single barrel. In addition, there is negligibly little overlap between incipient terminal arborization in adjacent (presumptive) barrels. The other possibility is that there is long-range guidance of axons to specific targets by signals derived from the target, perhaps under peripheral control. This would have to be activity-independent as the whisker-related map develops normally in the face of neonatal blockade of sensory evoked electrical activity in the barrel cortex.

In summary, despite the existence of highly ordered maps of the whisker fields in all the intermediate nuclei and the cortex itself, the evidence points to instruction by the innervating fibres guiding barrel formation, and sorting of thalamic afferents at the target rather than a mechanism of fibre ordering in the growing tract.

Visual cortex—afferent pathways in albinos
A number of mammalian species have mutant strains in which reduced pigmentation is associated with congenital abnormalities of the visual pathways. These mutants include the Siamese cat, the albino rat and ferret, the white tiger, and the pearl mink (Guillery, 1974). In all these strains, there is an impaired projection of axons from the retina to the LGN. Mutations of genes coding for enzymes that catalyse reactions in the synthesis of the dark pigment, melanin, appear to be responsible for the abnormalities of the projections from the retina. There is a layer of melanin-producing cells in the pigment epithelium underlying the retina, although it is not clear how the absence of melanin from these cells produces abnormalities in the specification of the direction taken by ganglion cell axons in the retinogeniculate pathway (Guillery, 1974; Stent, 1981).

In the normal cat, fibres from ganglion cells in the temporal retina project ipsi-laterally to lamina A1 of the LGN; cells in the nasal retina cross in the optic chiasm to innervate the A lamina of the contralateral LGN. In each layer of the LGN there is a retinotopic map representing the contralateral visual field and these maps are in register. In other words, adjacent points on the retina are represented at adjacent points in each layer of the LGN, and each point on the retina is represented in columns of cells that run perpendicular to and traversing all layers. Afferents from both geniculate laminae converge onto visual cortical neurons to generate a single topographic, binocular representation of the contralateral visual field. Figure 5.11 shows the retinogeniculocortical pathways of the Siamese cat. Axons of some of the ganglion cells in the temporal retina, that normally project ipsilaterally to the LGN, cross at the optic chiasm to innervate layer A1 of the contralateral LGN. Thus, the contralateral input to the A layers remains normal, but the A1 layers receive afferents from both ipsilateral and contralateral retinae. In the region of the A1 laminae receiving abnormal crossed projections, the retinotopic map is reversed and is clearly out of register with the map in the overlying A layers.

One consequence of these abnormalities of the retinogeniculate pathway is to alter the development of the geniculocortical afferents. The reorganization of the projection from the LGN to the cortex occurs in one of two ways. In some Siamese cats (called Boston cats), the order of the geniculocortical axons from the abnor-mally innervated region of the A1 layer is reversed as they traverse the white matter (Fig. 5.11b). The rest of the fibres from the LGN maintain their order and they project to an adjacent portion of the visual cortex. As is seen from Fig. 5.11b, the result of this is to generate a normal sequence of visual field representations, but with much less binocularity than normal (Hubel and Wiesel, 1971; Guillery, 1974; Shatz, 1977a). In other Siamese cats (Midwestern cats), the anatomical appearance of the geniculocortical projections is normal, at least as far as can be discerned with the methods used. However, the inputs from the abnormally innervated portion of the A1 layers are functionally suppressed (Kaas and Guillery, 1973; Guillery, 1974, see Fig. 5.11a). Thus, in both reorganizations of the geniculocortical pro-jections, the result is that cortical neurons do not receive conflicting inputs from two separate regions of the visual field.

The anatomy of the callosal projections is abnormal in Boston Siamese cats (Shatz, 1977b). Whereas in normal cats only the borders of areas 17 and 18 are interconnected, in the Boston Siamese cat callosal cells are found well within the body of areas 17 and 18, at points to which the representation of the vertical merid-ian is displaced. Thus, cortical sites representing similar receptive field coordinates in each hemisphere remain appropriately interconnected via the corpus callosum in the mutant.

Similar observations to those on Siamese cats have been made in albinos of other species. Moreover, it has been reported that an albino-like alteration of the geniculocortical pathway can be experimentally induced in normal pigmented cats by sectioning one optic tract at birth, thereby stabilizing initially exuberant con-tralateral retinogeniculate projections (Schall *et al.*, 1988). All these findings are of

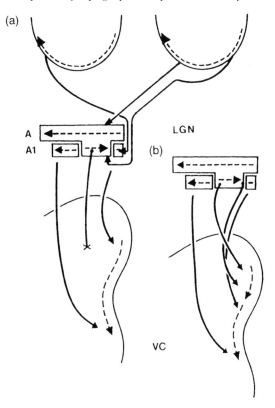

FIG. 5.11. Diagram illustrating the abnormalities of the visual pathways in the Siamese cat. The nasal retina of the right eye and the temporal retina of the left eye normally project to layers A and A1 of the left LGN. respectively. The opposite is true for the projection to the right LGN. (not shown here). The retinotopic maps (indicated by broken lines) in layers A and A1 are normally in register. In the Siamese cat, there is an abnormal crossed projection from the temporal retina to layer A1. Thus, regions of the A1 laminae have retinotopic maps that are out of register with those in the A laminae. Normally, the projection from the A1 laminae to the visual cortex (VC) is superimposed on that from the A laminae, generating a single coherent binocular retinotopic cortical map. In the Siamese cat, the inputs from the abnormal part of layer A1 are either (a) suppressed (in Midwestern cats) or (b) reversed and rerouted to an adjacent cortical zone (in Boston cats). Both reorganizations achieve a similar result, i.e. the avoidance of the functional ambiguity that would occur if information from different parts of the visual field were to converge onto the same cortical sites. (Based on Guillery, 1974)

considerable relevance to a discussion of the mechanisms of afferent development in the visual cortex. It is clear from the rerouting of axons that occurs in the Boston Siamese cat that the topographic nature of the afferents to the visual cortex is not determined exclusively by the positions of the cell bodies of the axons in the LGN. Moreover, these observations make it unlikely that topography in the geniculo-cortical pathway is generated by a system in which each region of the cortex is preprogramed to accept only specific axons. The evidence seems to point towards a mechanism in which there is an overriding necessity for afferents ending on the same cortical target to represent the same point in the visual field and to have similar functional properties. Discrepancies between the functional characteristics of the inputs are avoided. However, a hypothesis that seeks to explain the normal development of the major characteristics of the geniculocortical afferents on the basis of a comparison of functional properties alone seems insufficient, not least because of the general similarities of the final system in different individuals of a species. There must presumably be additional, probably genetically specified, mechanisms that form a framework within which activity-dependent processes can operate to enrich and refine the pathways. Within the framework there could be enough plasticity to allow modification by afferent activity, and this may occur in albinos.

4.3   Development of callosal and ipsilateral corticocortical projections

The cortical areas of the right and left hemispheres are reciprocally interconnected by axons that run through the corpus callosum. These projections link mirror-image points on the two sides of the brain and many are concentrated around the areal borders where the vertical meridian of the visual field is represented (e.g. Berlucchi 1972; Sanides 1978). Within each hemisphere, the different areas of visual cortex are linked reciprocally by ipsilateral corticocortical axons. The organization of corticocortical projections has been examined in considerable detail in the visual system in cats and primates. In adults of these species, corticocortical cells that interconnect pairs of areas originate and terminate in patches or bands that run tangentially, mainly through the superficial layers of the visual cortex (Ferrer *et al.*, 1988; Zeki and Shipp, 1988; Price and Zumbroich, 1989). In the monkey, there is a correlation between the function of the cells of origin in the patches or bands and the function of the extrastriate area to which they project. In other species, the functions of the corticocortical pathways and the significance of the patchy organization of connections are not clear, which is unfortunate since many studies of corticocortical development have been carried out in the cat, where assessment of function is difficult.

The problems that confront the developing callosal and corticocortical fibres are essentially the same as those that must be overcome by the developing geniculocortical projection. Axons must grow through the white matter towards other regions of the visual cortex, they must penetrate the cortex, and they must form topographic connections in the correct target laminae with the appropriate tangential distribution (i.e. patchy in the case of the corticocortical axons, and mainly confined to the areal borders for the callosal projection).

The development of the callosal and corticocortical afferents to visual cortex has been studied in a number of species using anterogradely and retrogradely transported tract-tracers, such as tritiated proline or HRP. Although the distributions of callosal and corticocortical terminals are quite different in the adult animal, there are striking similarities in the ways in which the two pathways develop.

There is now a large body of evidence demonstrating that, although many visual cortical neurons generate immature projections that grow towards other regions of the ipsilateral and contralateral visual cortex early in development, only some of these cells are successful in producing persistent callosal or corticocortical connections. There are initially highly exuberant projections, with many axons travelling both from and towards inappropriate regions of the cortex. Later, some of these early projections are somehow validated and form persistent connections, while others disappear. Much of this evidence has come from studies on the development of the callosal pathway in the cat (Innocenti *et al.*, 1977; Innocenti, 1981; Innocenti and Clarke, 1984b), and work on these projections in other species has confirmed the major findings (Olavaria and Van Sluyters, 1985). The information on the development of corticocortical connections is derived mainly from studies on the cat (Dehay *et al.*, 1984, 1988a; Innocenti and Clarke, 1984a; Price and Blakemore, 1985a,b; Innocenti *et al.*, 1988; Price and Zumbroich, 1989).

Development of callosal afferents
In the adult cat the callosal projection from areas 17 and 18 originates from and projects to narrow regions around the border between these areas; in the newborn kitten, injections of retrograde tracers into visual cortex and white matter of one hemisphere label neuronal cell bodies not only in the vicinity of the contralateral areal boundaries but also throughout the rest of the areas (Innocenti *et al.*, 1977). Experiments with long-lasting retrograde tracers have demonstrated that many of the cells scattered throughout the immature visual cortex that initially send projections into the corpus callosum survive, and that narrowing of the pathway is achieved by their losing callosally projecting axons without dying (Innocenti *et al.*, 1977; O'Leary *et al.*, 1981). At least some of these transiently projecting neurons form persistent connections with ipsilateral area 18 after eliminating their callosal axon (Innocenti *et al.*, 1986). In the monkey, much of the development of callosal projections in the visual cortex occurs prenatally. Although area 17 remains acallosal throughout development, the projection from area 18 may be more widespread early in gestation, and may later narrow to produce an adult-like pattern by the time of birth (Dehay *et al.*, 1986, 1988b; Chalupa *et al.*, 1989). However, further quantitative studies are required to demonstrate how far the processes of callosal development from area 18 in the monkey mirror those already described in the cat (Vercelli, 1992; Ozaki and Wahlsten, 1992; Meissirel *et al.*, 1991; Weisskopf and Innocenti, 1991; Schwartz *et al.*, 1991; Norris and Kalil, 1991; Haukin and Silver, 1988).

As fibres emerge from the callosum and traverse the white matter of the contralateral hemisphere, they fan out widely. Many grow towards regions of the visual cortex that receive no callosal afferents in the adult animal (Fig. 5.12). This non-specific growth has been observed using anterograde tract-tracers in the cat (Innocenti and Clarke, 1984b) and in the rodent (Olavaria and Van Sluyters, 1985). However, it is principally those axons that grow to the zones that are innervated by callosal projections in the adult (e.g. the area 17/18 border) that are able to

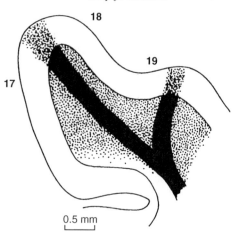

F I G . 5 . 12 . Diagram illustrating the distribution of callosal terminals in the right visual cortex of a kitten within the first postnatal week, revealed by anterogradely transported horseradish peroxidase injected into the left visual cortex. Many axons are arranged in bundles projecting to the border between areas 17 and 18 and to the lateral part of area 19 (filled areas). However, a large number grow in a more non-specific fashion throughout the entire white matter, although they barely enter the overlying cortex (stippled areas). It is only in those regions destined to receive callosal innervation in the adult that fibres penetrate the full extent of the grey matter and eventually form persistent connections. (Based on Innocenti, 1981)

penetrate far into the grey matter and form persistent connections. The remainder grow to the grey matter/white matter border underneath areas that are not destined to receive callosal afferents, but most go no further and appear to be withdrawn later (Innocenti and Clarke, 1984b).

In newborn kittens, injections of retrograde tracers into the area 17/18 border without any involvement of the underlying white matter label neurons only at the area 17/18 border in the contralateral hemisphere, and not the entire exuberant population of callosal neurones (Innocenti and Clarke, 1984b). These results demonstrate that it is only those axons that originate around the area 17/18 border and grow to the contralateral area 17/18 border that can penetrate significant distances into, and form persistent connections with, the cortex. It is possible that the initial population of axons traversing the callosum grows entirely non-specifically, whether it originates from the areal boundaries or not, and only those fibres that come from and attempt to penetrate appropriate regions of cortex persist.

Corticocortical projections—mature organization
The factors controlling the development of ipsilateral corticocortical connections remain relatively obscure. Much work on this subject has concerned the development of connections in the visual cortex of the cat. The areas of the visual cortex are interconnected by a highly organized and complex system of corticocortical pathways. Previous studies on intrinsic and corticocortical connections in the cat

have suggested that these projections connect groups of cells with similar preferred orientations (Gilbert and Wiesel, 1989). This observation has led to the generally accepted view that these long-range horizontal connections are excitatory, despite some evidence to the contrary (Matsubara *et al.*, 1987). Nevertheless, the way in which these projections contribute to receptive field organization is not clear, since the majority of cells in extrastriate cortex continue to respond and maintain qualitatively similar properties after inactivation of area 17 (Dreher and Cottee, 1975; Sherk, 1978). It is probable that the inability to discover the role of the corticocortical connections in cat is because, despite the density and precise organization of the corticocortical inputs, their contribution is to enhance or add more subtle aspects of receptive field organization than have so far been examined.

In an attempt to obtain a clearer idea of the function of these projections, we carried out a series of anatomical and neurophysiological experiments. We have shown that there is considerable convergence and divergence of the projection from area 17 to area 18 (Ferrer *et al.*, 1988, 1992), and that the degrees of anatomical divergence and convergence are rather precisely related to the retinotopic organization, receptive field size, and scatter within the two visual areas (Price *et al.*, 1994a). Injection of tracer into area 18 labels a group of clusters in area 17 that extends over a region of cortex that is wider than the injection site by an amount that is consistently related to the magnification factor. In terms of retinotopic coordinates, the territory in area 17 extends over a wider area of visual field than the uptake site in area 18, by a similar distance in visual field representation in all directions.

The receptive fields of cells (defined in Chapter 7) in area 18 are, on average, larger than those of cells in area 17. Our results indicate that it is *possible* for convergence and divergence in the association pathway to compensate for this difference by providing cells in area 18 with input from cells in area 17 whose receptive fields cover the same extent of visual space. This contrasts with intrinsic corticocortical connections within area 17, which are sufficiently widespread that they can provide input from regions of visual field outside the classical receptive fields of the receiving neurones (Ts'o *et al.*, 1986). Although this may still be the case for interareal association connections, our results demonstrate that it is not *necessarily* so.

Thus, it remains possible that the input from area 17 to any cell in area 18 provides subunits within the extrastriate cell's receptive field, each subunit being smaller than the overall receptive field and presumably all having roughly the same preferred orientation. This remains to be tested. The overall picture is that long-range ipsilateral corticocortical connections, both intrinsic to one visual area or interareal, are excitatory, have similar preferred orientations, and may increase receptive field complexity either by generating subunits within them or by influencing them from beyond their edges. They may be responsible for establishing phase-locking between neuronal assemblies with oscillatory activity in the cat, even over large distances (Eckhorn *et al.*, 1988; Engel *et al.*, 1991).

However, none of this answers the question of why the corticocortical connections are clustered. We have demonstrated with large injections of retrograde tracers in a number of extrastriate areas that these patches are not just artefacts of making small injections, but represent a truly discontinuous sampling of the activity of area 17 (Ferrer *et al.*, 1988, 1992). We have sought to correlate these association clusters with periodically distributed features of visual cortical functional architecture. We have concentrated primarily on ocular dominance and orientation columns, although other columnar organization may be present and worthy of study (e.g. spatial frequency columns, Tootell *et al.*, 1981). We found a strong tendency for area 17 to 18 cells to be clustered over regions of area 17 with a strongly binocular input from the LGN (Price *et al.*, 1994b). It is possible that association pathways to other extrastriate areas are also clustered over strongly binocular regions, since the injection of multiple extrastriate regions with different retrograde tracers labels patches in area 17 that partially overlap and avoid particular regions (Ferrer *et al.*, 1992; Bullier *et al.*, 1984). Whether these regions are strongly monocular remains to be tested.

It is not clear whether the coincidence of areas of binocularity and patches of association cells in area 17 is because it is the binocularity itself that is important or because some property that is related to binocularity, such as disparity selectivity (Price *et al.*, 1994a), is conveyed by these connections. The coincidence does suggest that experimental manipulations involving input in one or both eyes may influence the development not only of ocular dominance columns but also of the association cells (Price *et al.*, 1994b); see below for further discussion.

Development of corticocortical connections

Like the development of callosal connections in the cat, the development of ipsilateral corticocortical connections is a good example of a process in which initially widespread connections are later narrowed to give a greater degree of precision in the mapping. Just as many callosal fibres do not grow directly to the borders between contralateral visual areas, many corticocortical fibres do not grow through white matter in an ordered, topographic fashion to their targets. Experiment with the anterograde tracer [^{3}H] proline suggested that, in newborn kittens, cells in each small region of area 17 send axons through a broad expanse of white matter in only the general direction of other ipsilateral visual areas (Price and Zumbroich, 1989). These developing axons fan out until they reach the subplate, immediately below layer 6, or penetrate the deep cortical layers (Fig. 5.13). More recently, studies with the carbocyanine dyes DiI and DiA have indicated that, despite their widespread projection, there is a tendency for axons growing from each point in area 17 to be bundled in tracts projecting towards topographically appropriate target zones (Caric and Price, 1996). Order in the corticocortical projections had not been seen previously since the earliest we had studied corticocortical axons with anterograde tracing was about four days postnatal, at which age there is a massive outgrowth of connections and any order in the tract is largely obscured. Fibres that end up under appropriate cortical regions penetrate the overlying cortex itself, generating at least a rough topographic order. Most corticocortical axons that terminate under topographically incorrect regions of visual cortex appear to be eliminated (Fig. 5.13a,b) (Price and Zumbroich, 1989). Thus, specificity of connections in these afferent pathways may be established by processes that are quite similar to those involved in the development of callosal projections. Despite the possibility that there is considerable guidance of, or constraints on, axonal growth through the white matter at very early stages, there is still considerable imprecision in the early corticocortical connections.

Recent experiments on the development of corticocortical connections in the rodent's visual system have demonstrated that axons arrive at their cortical targets in the same order in which their cell bodies are generated (Coogan and Burkhalter, 1988). Thus, connections from the deep layers of the striate cortex reach their targets before those from the superficial layers arrive; a similar sequence may occur prenatally in other species such as the cat, where the projections at birth arise from both superficial and deep layers (Price and Blakemore, 1985a,b).

In the kitten, corticocortical fibres from area 17 to extrastriate visual cortex are clustered as they penetrate topographically related regions of extrastriate visual areas and start growing to their target laminae shortly after birth (Price and Zumbroich, 1989). The tangential periodicity of these dense patches of developing terminals is similar to that in the adult. Thus, the specificity with which these projections actually invade the cortex is quite striking. Corticocortical afferents from area 17 probably do not wait until the migration of neurons into their major target sites in layers 2 and 3 is complete before they penetrate extrastriate visual cortex. Corticocortical axons from area 17 first enter area 18 before postnatal day 4 and penetrate area 19 and the lateral suprasylvian cortex only slightly later, around postnatal day 12 (Price and Zumbroich, 1989). Yet the migration of cells into layers 2 and 3 (their targets) is not complete until the end of the third postnatal week in the cat (Chapter 4). In this respect, the development of these projections is different from that of the geniculocortical pathway.

After the corticocortical axons have penetrated the cortex, they grow rapidly from the deep cortical layers to reach targets mainly in layers 2 and 3. In the cat this occurs during the first three postnatal months. The density of terminals in the deep cortical layers decreases in relation to that in the superficial layers; relatively few terminals persist in layer 4 of areas 17 and 18, the main recipient layer of geniculocortical afferents in these areas (Price and Zumbroich, 1989). It is conceivable that developing corticocortical fibres form persistent connections with target cells that are in the process of migrating to their final positions in the superficial layers, although there is no evidence for this.

At the same time as corticocortical afferents from area 17 are growing to increasingly superficial layers in area 18 in the newborn kitten's visual cortex, the distribution of the cell bodies of these invading fibres is undergoing major changes. Retrograde tract-tracers have been used to demonstrate that there is a topographic relationship between the position of the cell bodies in area 17 and of the penetrating fibres in area 18, particularly when only the superficial layers of

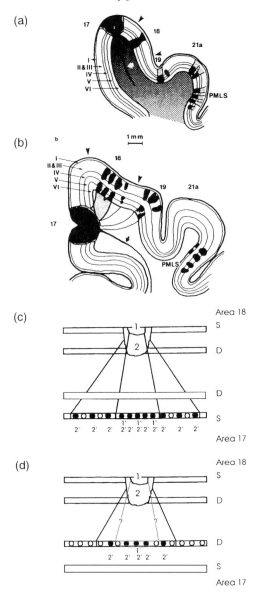

FIG. 5.13. The development of corticocortical connections. Camera lucida drawings of coronal sections through the right visual cortex of (a) a 12-day-old kitten and (b) an adult cat. Injections of tritiated proline were made into area 17 (filled areas) and the degree of shading is proportional to the density of anterograde label. The arrows indicate label in corticogeniculate axons. (a) At 12 days there is extensive labelling of the white matter and all of the visual cortical areas lateral to area 17 contain dense, patchy label whose location is topographically related to the position of the injection site in area 17. In area 18, this label is densely distributed across layers 2–6, but in more lateral areas it is still mainly in deep

area 18 are injected (Fig 5.13c,d). But until postnatal day 10 the cell bodies are distributed continuously in two tangential bands throughout both superficial and deep cortical layers. After postnatal day 10 these cells become distributed in patches, mainly in superficial layers 2 and 3 (Price and Blakemore, 1985a,b). The use of long-lasting retrograde tracers has demonstrated that the emergence of patches of association cells from an initially continuous distribution is due largely to axonal retraction, although it has been suggested that the loss of deep layer connections is achieved by cell death (Price and Blakemore, 1985b). These regressive phenomena may occur after the overall topography of the corticocortical projections has been established by selective invasion of the cortex (Price and Zumbroich, 1989).

Studies with two different retrograde tracers in each of a series of young kittens have suggested that the incidence of bifurcation among corticocortical connections from area 17 is as low as in adult cats (Price and Ferrer, 1993). Thus, most of the axonal elimination that refines the early exuberant projections from area 17 to each extrastriate area may leave many of these neurons with no association connection at all. It remains possible that such cells regrow an association axon to another extrastriate area after removal of the first projection; alternatively, there may be a large number of truly transient corticocortical cells that, after axon elimination has occurred, become neurons with connections exclusively intrinsic to area 17 (Gilbert and Wiesel, 1983; Price, 1986; Callaway and Katz, 1990; Luhmann *et al.*, 1990).

When retrogradely transported tracers (such as diamidino yellow or fast blue) are injected into visual cortical areas in adult cats, the labelled regions of other visual areas are considerably wider than the injected regions, indicating a considerable

---

laminae. (b) In adult cats, there is dense patchy label in several extrastriate areas: the label in the white matter is confined to the fibre tracts leading from the injection site direct to the terminal zones. Arrowheads indicate areal boundaries. (c,d) Schematic representations of projections from area 17 to area 18 in kittens aged three to four days: (c) represents the pattern of projections from the superficial layers of area 17; (d) represents that from the deep layers of area 17. In both (c) and (d), the horizontal elongated parallel lines represent the superficial layers (S: cortical plate and layer 1) and deep layers (D: layers 5 and 6). The results of injections involving different layers in area 18 are illustrated by considering two injections, numbered 1 and 2: 1 involves only the cortical plate and layer 1; 2 involves all the cortical layers. (c) Injections of only the superficial layers in area 18 (injection 1) label cells in a relatively narrow region of the superficial layers in area 17 (labelled cells are represented as filled circles with 1' written beneath them). Injections of all layers in area 18 (injection 2) label cells over a much wider region of the superficial layers in area 17 (filled circles with 2' written beneath them). (d) Injections of only the superficial layers in area 18 (injection 1) labelled very few cells in the deep layers of area 17 (indicated by question marks). Injections of all layers in area 18 (injection 2) labelled a region in the deep layers in area 17 that was narrower than the region labelled in the superficial layers in area 17 by similar injections (conventions as in c). In (c) and (d), the lines linking the representations of areas 17 and 18 illustrate that the amount of convergence from area 17 onto area 18 was less for projections to the superficial layers of area 18 than for projections to the deep layers. Based on Price and Zumbroich (1989), Price (1991) and Caric and Price (1996).

degree of convergence of inputs from one area to another. The degree of convergence and divergence in the corticocortical pathways is a measure of the precision of the topographical mapping. In kittens, the degree of convergence and densities of corticocortical projections are very large at the time of birth but rapidly decrease during the first two postnatal months to reach adult values (Price *et al.*, 1994b; Kato *et al.*, 1991b; Batardiere *et al.*, 1998). Current evidence is that many of the exuberant corticocortical connections produce a very widespread innervation of layers 5 and 6 although there is a much more focused penetration of the superficial layers (Fig. 5.13c,d). Thus, it appears that, as in callosal development, only those corticocortical connections that are in an appropriate retinotopic location penetrate deep into the grey matter. The rest remain in layers 5 and 6.

Although the hypothesis that interactions around the white matter/grey matter border are important in eliminating inappropriate connections seems reasonable for the developing callosal projections and corticocortical connections from striate to extrastriate cortex, the situation is more controversial for the transient projections that arise from non-visual cortex and grow towards ipsilateral areas 17 and 18 in the newborn kitten (Dehay *et al.*, 1984, 1988a; Clarke and Innocenti, 1986; Innocenti *et al.*, 1988). Some reports have suggested that the majority of these early projections grow only as far as the deep part of layer 6 before being eliminated (Clarke and Innocenti, 1986) whereas others have found evidence for deep penetration of the grey matter by considerable numbers of such transient axons (Dehay *et al.*, 1984, 1988a). On balance, it seems intuitively more likely that the numbers of penetrating fibres were underestimated in some experiments than the reverse. At present, then, it appears that interactions at the white matter layer 6 border may be less important for the transient projections from non-visual areas to visual cortex than in the development of the other afferent pathways discussed above. However, further work in this area is important, and it is as well to concede that current conclusions about the extent of grey matter penetration, that hinge crucially on the sensitivity of tract-tracing methods in young animals, may have to be modified for pathways other than just transient non-visual to visual cortex projections.

Similar events to those occurring during the development of inter-areal corticocortical connections are observed during the formation of horizontal or vertical connections intrinsic to a single cortical area (Katz, 1991). Axons from a small region within each visual area initially grow towards retinotopically inappropriate zones of the same cortical area, and many of these projections may later be lost (Price and Zumbroich, 1989). As for as the corticocortical connections, the cell bodies of intrinsic projections are initially continuously distributed, and later become patchy (Price, 1986; Callaway and Katz, 1990, 1991, 1992; Katz and Callaway, 1992; Lubke and Albus, 1992; Luhmann *et al.*, 1990).

Development of corticocortical connections—effects of lesions and deprivation studies

A classic way of challenging the developing system (used to great effect in the retinotectal system of adult lower vertebrates; Section 3) is to carry out controlled surgical or chemical ablation of tissue or sensory deprivation and investigate the response of the system. We have tried to modify corticocortical connections in several ways.

(a) Lesioning area 18 in developing kitten brains prevented patchiness of projections from area 17 to area 18 from emerging normally (Kato *et al.*, 1993). Thus, the destruction of one region of the visual cortex appeared to prevent the emergence of a clustered distribution of corticocortical projecting cells. Why this should have occurred is not clear. One hypothesis is that by removing one set of connections within the cortex, the competition of other sets of connections for trophic support from the deafferented regions was diminished.

(b) In normal kittens, the overall number of axons projecting from area 17 to area 18 increases after birth and then decreases again to adult values. Following monocular deprivation, the second phase, the decrease, does not occur and the density of projections from the superficial layers is abnormally high (Price *et al.*, 1994b); following binocular deprivation, the density of projections is abnormally low. The explanation for this may be dependent on the overall level of activity in the cortex. Since monocular deprivation may release neurons from the inhibitory effects of disparity selectivity, monocular deprivation should increase the activity of the visual cortex (Price *et al.*, 1994b). Binocular deprivation on the other hand will decrease it.

(c) The embryonic LGN was destroyed with ibotenic acid, an excitotoxin used to kill cells that have glutamate as their neurotransmitter. As assessed with the anterograde tracer, DiI, the normal localized ingrowth of axons into the superficial layers of area 18 did not occur. There was a relatively widespread penetration of even the most superficial layers and clustering did not emerge properly. It appears that under these experimental conditions the cells that form the corticocortical projections are not committed to making a particular pattern of projections. This suggests that geniculate growth factors and/or activity may be used at this point in developmental time to help mould the developing pathways (Caric and Price, 1999).

4.4 Summary

Mechanisms that involve the maintenance of fibre order in growing cortical connections or that guide specific subsets of cortical axons may be essential for establishing coarse-grained cortical maps and their polarity. However, it seems that an early overproduction of connections combined with later withdrawal of those that are somehow deemed inappropriate is also a widely used strategy in the development of cortical maps. Axonal retraction can either involve the removal of very long fibres, as occurs in the callosal and corticocortical pathways, or the short branches of initially exuberant terminal arbors, as occurs in the formation of ocular dominance columns in the geniculocortical pathway (see below). Thus, elimination of axons and/or axonal branches can operate at different levels, either ensuring the matching of appropriate growth cones and target areas, or, within a target area, the matching of inputs to appropriate cells. The complexity of the cortex makes it difficult to draw conclusions about the way in which specific connections are formed at the level of individual cells. It is possible that each individual developing axon is not destined to contact a specific target cell, but only to reach a population of cells in a particular target region. Within that zone, potential target cells may be multipotent and may have specific functions conferred on them as a result of the contacts they receive.

5   THE DEVELOPMENT OF FEATURE MAPS IN THE VISUAL SYSTEM

In addition to the topographically ordered maps of connections between two sets of cells, there are other more complex maps in which some attribute or feature of the activity in the presynaptic structure is represented in the cells of the target. The order of connections from each thalamic nucleus to each cortical sensory area generates maps of the sensory surfaces of the body in the corresponding areas and convergence of inputs generates more complex functional properties of cortical cells that are laid out as feature maps (as defined in Section 5.1).

The visual cortex has been examined in numerous species of carnivores, primates and rodents (Gilbert and Wiesel, 1981; Graybiel and Berson, 1981; Van Essen and Maunsell, 1983; Zeki and Shipp, 1988). It is divided into a number of areas, each of which is retinotopically organized and contains an ordered representation, or map, of the visual field. The areas of the visual cortex differ in the precise details of their cytoarchitecture, connections, and functional properties.

Figure 5.14 illustrates the locations of the principal visual areas in the cat and monkey cortex. Each visual cortical area may be at least partially specialized for a particular visual task. In the monkey, for example, areas V1 and V2 appear to be involved in segregating information on the orientation, direction of movement, and wavelength of visual stimuli, while area V3 may be important for dynamic form analysis, area V4 for colour and static form analysis, and V5 for motion analysis (Zeki and Shipp, 1988, Fig. 5.14). In cat, segregation of function among the visual areas of cortex is less clearly defined, although there is evidence that the posterior lateral suprasylvian cortex (PMLS) is specialized for a role in the analysis of image motion (Zumbroich et al., 1988a).

The visual cortex receives input from the retina via the lateral geniculate nucleus (LGN) of the thalamus. In addition, extrageniculate thalamic nuclei, including the pulvinar and lateral posterior complex, project to the visual cortex (Raczkowski and Rosenquist, 1983). In the cat, the LGN and extrageniculate thalamic nuclei send many axons to both striate and extrastriate cortical areas. In the monkey, almost all of the neurons in the LGN project to V1 and very few project to prestriate visual areas (Kennedy and Bullier, 1985). Geniculocortical axons terminate mainly in

(a)

(b)

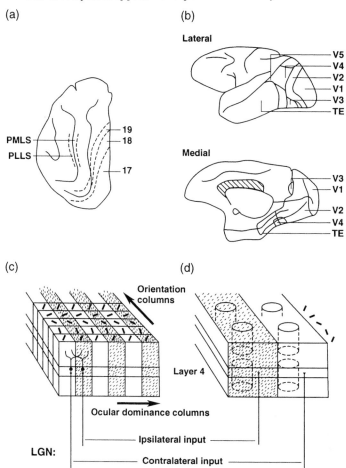

FIG. 5.14. (a) Dorsal view of the left hemisphere of the adult cat showing some of the major visual areas; areas 17, 18 and 19; PMLS, posteromedial lateral suprasylvian area; PLLS, posterolateral lateral suprasylvian area. (b) Some of the visual cortical areas in the macaque monkey: lateral (*top picture*) and medial (*bottom picture*) views. Visual areas V1 to V5 are shown; TE, temporal visual areas. (c) Diagram showing a model of the relationship between ocular dominance and orientation columns in the cat visual cortex. In this model, ocular dominance and orientation columns run at right angles to each other. (d) Diagram of the visual cortex of the monkey showing blobs and stripes. Based on Hubel and Wiesel (1962, 1974); Salin and Bullier (1995); Price (1991); Livingstone and Hubel (1983, 1984, 1987, 1988), and Livingstone (1996).

cortical layer 4, although there are also projections to layer 6, layer 1, deep layer 3, and superficial layer 5 (reviewed by Gilbert and Wiesel, 1981). The inputs from the two eyes are segregated tangentially (i.e. parallel to the surface of the brain); while the overall density of geniculocortical terminals is roughly constant throughout layer 4, the density of innervation from either eye fluctuates periodically, generating interdigitating ocular dominance columns (Fig. 5.14; Fig 5.15a).

Hubel and Wiesel (1962, 1963) discovered that cells in binocular visual cortex vary in their responsiveness to two eyes. Similar ocularity preferences extend down to layer IV, where cells in the LGN terminate, and thus the concept of ocular dominance columns arose. Subsequently existence of such columns was confirmed anatomically; the map of ocularity specificity across the entire surface of binocular cortex resembles a pattern of zebra stripes (Fig. 5.15a). Ocular dominance columns seem to emerge from an initially overlapping distribution of innervation of left and right eye origin. In cat and monkey, segregation begins at or around birth and is complete at about six weeks later.

Cells in certain visual areas are orientation selective; i.e. each cell is responsive to a small bar of light when presented in a particular orientation at a particular position in the visual field (Figs. 5.2, 5.14, 5.15b). The existence of orientation maps was established by extracellular recording and, more recently, the method of optical recording has been used to produce detailed orientation maps over the entire surface of the visual cortex (Blasdel and Salama, 1986; Bonhoeffer and Grinvald, 1991). The maps produced are quite complex and have a number of features such as periodically repeating patterns and more complicated features such as saddle points and singularities (points on the cortex around which orientation domains are clustered in a pinwheel fashion). This type of data (Fig. 5.15b) has provided an irresistible challenge to modellers.

The magnitude of the response elicited by a moving bar stimulus in a particular orientation may depend on the direction of movement (at right angles to the orientation of the bar). This makes it possible to construct a directionally selective map and the properties of this type of map have been investigated recently (DeAngelis *et al.*, 1995).

There are a number of relationships between the three types of maps produced. Effectively the ocularity map interrupts the retinotopic map; if all the pieces of cortex innervated by one of the eyes were removed and the remaining pieces, innervated by the other eye, pushed together, then a completely ordered retinotopic map would result. In monkey visual cortex, areas that are stained for cytochrome oxidase (CO) are located in the middle of ocular dominance stripes (Fig. 5.14d) and are very unselective to the orientation of the stimulus. In cat visual cortex, pinwheel centres are mainly located to the middle of ocular dominance columns (Hübener *et al.*, 1997). The other relationship between orientation and ocular dominance is that, according to recent optical recording experiments in cat, the orientation domains tend to intersect at right angles the borders of ocular dominance stripes (Hübener *et al.*, 1997). In the classic model of Hubel and Wiesel (1977), developed for the cat (Fig. 5.14c), iso-orientation columns run in straight lines at right angles to the interdigitating ocular dominance columns.

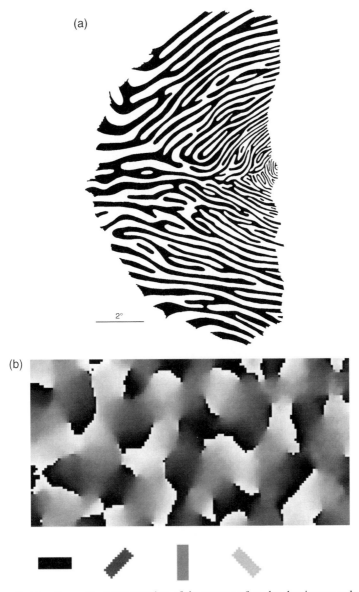

F I G . 5 . 15 . Computer reconstruction of the pattern of ocular dominance columns in layer 4c of area 17 of a macaque monkey, produced by reduced silver staining, translated into the visual field (Fig. 25 from Hubel and Wiesel, 1977. Reproduced with the permission of The Royal Society London.) (b) Orientation preference map for area 17 of the cat visual cortex, constructed by optical recording. The orientation at each point is indicated on a grey-scale. The key below shows how orientations are assigned on the scale. The length of the bars corresponds to 0.5 mm. This type of picture is best seen in colour (e.g. Hübener *et al.*, 1997). Reproduced with the permission of M. Hübener.

5.1   Development of geniculate projections to the visual cortex

The segregation of afferents according to eye input, generating ocular dominance columns in layer 4, begins during the first postnatal month in the cat (LeVay *et al.*, 1978) and prenatally in the monkey (Rakic, 1976a, 1977). For the geniculocortical inputs from each eye, an initially continuous distribution of terminals becomes patchy. In the newborn kitten or monkey, the arborizations of geniculocortical fibres ending in layer 4 overlap extensively (Rakic, 1977; LeVay *et al.*, 1978, 1980); individual fibres from the LGN initially spread over a wide area in layer 4 in area 17, continuously innervating a region large enough to contain several future ocular dominance columns (Wiesel, 1982). As these afferents mature, there is a selective loss of branches, so that each fibre innervates the ocular dominance columns of one eye and leaves gaps for the inputs from the other eye. The establishment of separate domains supplied exclusively by one eye or the other is completed during the first six weeks of the animal's life. There is evidence for ocular dominance columns in humans, of about 1 mm in width, but there is no evidence about their development (Hitchcock and Hickey, 1980).

Although much of the evidence obtained so far on the maturation of the geniculocortical afferents supports the idea that, after penetration of the cortex, there is a refinement of the inputs by a process of pruning of initially exuberant arbors, there is some work suggesting that this may not occur in all visual cortical areas. Friedlander and Martin (1989) used intracellular staining methods to study the postnatal development of the innervation of area 18 of the cat's visual cortex. These workers began their study at the relatively late postnatal age of four to five weeks, but their results seem to contrast with those from area 17 in that they describe an expansion of geniculocortical axonal arbors to innervate larger areas of cortex by adulthood. Indeed, these authors question whether there is any reduction of the early binocular mixing in area 18, as there is in area 17. Further studies comparing ocular dominance column development in these areas is required to help clarify the issues raised by this work.

5.2   Effects of neural activity, particularly relating to functional deprivation

It is well established that the lack of normal visual experience early in postnatal life prevents the normal development of the visual cortex. This would suggest that some of the information required to generate normal visual pathways is derived from the interactions of the developing system with the external environment. Clearly, many aspects of cortical development occur prenatally and are immune to the effects of postnatal functional deprivation. Innate mechanisms generate many of the most fundamental aspects of afferent organization. Studies in both cats and primates have shown that before the neonate has received any visual experience, geniculocortical fibres find their main target (layer 4), converge to generate immature orientation selective cells clustered into rudimentary orientation columns, form a retinotopic map and, at least in the primate, begin to segregate to form ocular dominance columns (Blakemore and Van Sluyters, 1975; Rakic, 1976a; LeVay *et al.*, 1978; Albus and Wolf, 1984; Blakemore and Price, 1987a).

Visual deprivation early in life, during the so-called critical period, does not abolish these features of early organization. The continued refinement of cortical connections is strongly influenced by patterned neural activity. Visual deprivation can have a devastating effect on the development of the detailed circuitry required for the normal functional properties of visual cortical neurones. For example, in areas 17 and 18 of the cat, the normal appearance of a large proportion of orientation selective cells is prevented by dark-rearing or by binocular eyelid suture (e.g. Blakemore and Van Sluyters, 1975; Blakemore and Price, 1987b). There is a variety of results showing how experimental interference can affect the development of ocular dominance columns. Most of these experiments involve the manipulation of conditions of activity by (i) monocular deprivation; (ii) rearing of animals in the dark; (iii) distorting the retinal input by artificially inducing strabismus, and (iv) removal of spontaneous retinal activity by administering tetrodotoxin (TTX). The results of most of these experiments indicate the important role of neural activity in the formation of ocular dominance columns.

Thus, deprivation prevents the emergence of the full richness of functional architecture and receptive field properties of the normal adult visual cortex.

The most striking effects of deprivation are found when vision through only one eye is impaired during the critical period (Wiesel and Hubel, 1965; Blakemore *et al.*, 1978; Wiesel, 1982) (Fig. 6.5a). This procedure results in expansion of the cortical territory of the projection serving the normal eye relative to that of the projection serving the deprived eye. Neuronal activity plays a crucial role in this organization, and it appears that monocular deprivation places the geniculocortical afferents from the deprived eye at a competitive disadvantage. The effects of monocular deprivation can be reversed by opening the deprived eye and closing the other before the end of the critical period (reverse suture) (Fig. 6.5b). These changes involve the sprouting and/or trimming of geniculocortical arbors (Wiesel, 1982). It appears that, as the developing geniculocortical fibres elaborate on their initial, innately predetermined framework of immature inputs, it is especially important that those projections serving one eye should be as active as those serving the other eye. A balance of activity is required to ensure that the growth of terminals from each eye is restricted within its own cortical territory. The deprivation of patterned visual experience by binocular eyelid suture and dark-rearing does not totally prevent the formation of ocular dominance columns in the visual cortex, but only depresses their full elaboration (Swindale, 1988). Stryker and Harris (1986) reported that, in kittens, continuous bilateral retinal impulse blockade from shortly after birth until six to eight weeks leads to a complete absence of ocular dominance columns. Stryker and Harris (1986) made repeated bilateral intravitreal injections of TTX in kittens from the age of 14 days onwards, and searched unsuccessfully for evidence of ocular dominance columns after four to six weeks with both electrophysiological and anatomical methods. By 14 days, ocular dominance columns are normally detectable in kittens, at least physiologically (Blakemore and Van Sluyters, 1975; Albus and Wolf, 1984; Blakemore and Price, 1987a). On the basis of this evidence, it appears that bilateral TTX injections produced a degeneration of the early ocular dominance columns. At least the maintenance, and possibly the initial appearance, of these rudimentary ocular dominance columns require retinal activity, although it need not be related to external stimuli. Whether this activity plays an instructive role in the segregation of the geniculocortical afferents or is merely permissive is not clear. This issue is discussed further in Chapter 7.

6 MODELS FOR MAP MAKING

Much of the experimental evidence already cited yields results that are suggestive of the action of general principles rather than confirmatory of the existence of specific mechanisms for map making. Amongst the general principles noted are those concerned with axonal guidance, competition, interactions between axon and target, cell death, refinement of connections, and the role of neural activity. It is quite possible that in any particular situation mechanisms based on a number of these principles may act in combination. One way of pinning down how any particular mechanism might operate is to build a formal model of it and examine its properties. We now discuss formal models in which the ideas of synaptic modification through (i) interactions between nerves and their targets and (ii) competition are developed. Axonal guidance was discussed at length in Chapter 4. We first discuss models for the development of topography, with special reference to the retinotectal system of lower vertebrates, for which they were devised.

7 MODELS FOR THE DEVELOPMENT OF TOPOGRAPHY

7.1 Models based on chemoaffinity

Sperry's basic model of neuronal specificity (Sperry, 1943, 1945, 1963) has already been described above, as applied to the retinotectal system of lower vertebrates (Fig. 5.4a and Section 3.2). Various issues about the labels that were proposed to exist were also discussed, together with various informal models.

Gierer (1983) proposed a model based on the idea that axons grow in the direction of the maximal slope of a growth parameter, or *potential*. The potential assigned to each axon is assumed to be a function of the coordinates of its retinal cell of origin and its current location on the tectum. The direction of growth of an axon is down the sleepest slope of its potential, thereby decreasing its value. The axon will continue to change its position until its potential cannot be diminished any further. The form of the potential function is such that at this point the axon will have found its correct location in the tectum. This model can be thought of as a more computationally plausible model than that due to Nakamoto *et al.* (1996) for how molecular gradients give rise to maps of connections (which Gierer's work predates considerably). As such, Gierer's model is a straightforward demonstration as to how gradients can provide guidance signals. However, there is no provision for plasticity of connections under conditions of mismatch.

Models providing for plasticity of connections

If (i) two sets of nerve cells interconnect to form an ordered map of connections on the basis of the labels carried by the participating cells, and (ii) after surgical diminution of retina or tectum the presynaptic cells project to positions that they would not have occupied if there had been no surgery (Gaze and Keating, 1972), then it would seem that surgery has changed the labels. Various proposals have been made, as follows.

Regulation

An important variant (Meyer and Sperry, 1973) presents an alternative to neuronal specificity. It is envisaged that labels are used but they can be modified under certain conditions, which thus provides for a plasticity of connections. In order to account for the finding that regeneration of ordered maps is still possible after surgical diminution of one or both structures, as in the mismatch experiments, (Section 3.2, Fig. 5.6), it was suggested that removal of cells triggers off a reorganization of labels in the surgically affected structure. Following retinal hemiablation, for example, the set of labels initially deployed over the remaining half retina would be rescaled such that the set of labels possessed by a normal retina would now be spread across the reduced retina (Fig. 5.16b). This would allow the entire, reduced, retina to come to project in order across the entire tectum. The mechanism was called regulation by analogy with similar findings in the field of morphogenesis where a complete structure can regenerate from a partial structure (Weiss, 1939). However, this is a *post-hoc* explanation and lacks predictive power (Gaze and Keating, 1972).

Plasticity through competition?

Gaze and Keating (1972) suggested that it may be possible for systems-matching to occur without the necessity for changes in labels. Retinal axons could compete for space and, if each retinal axon has the same amount of 'synaptic strength', the set of axons can expand or contract to fill the amount of tectal space available. Prestige and Willshaw (1975) formalized the notion of chemospecificity by distinguishing between two types of chemical matching schemes. According to schemes of their type I, each presynaptic cell has affinity for a small group of postsynaptic cells and less for other cells (i.e. chemospecificity). Cells that develop connections according to this scheme will make specific connections with no scope for flexibility. According to schemes of their type II, all axons have high affinity for making connections at one end of the postsynaptic sheet and progressively less to other cells; similarly postsynaptic cells have high affinity for axons from one pole of the retina

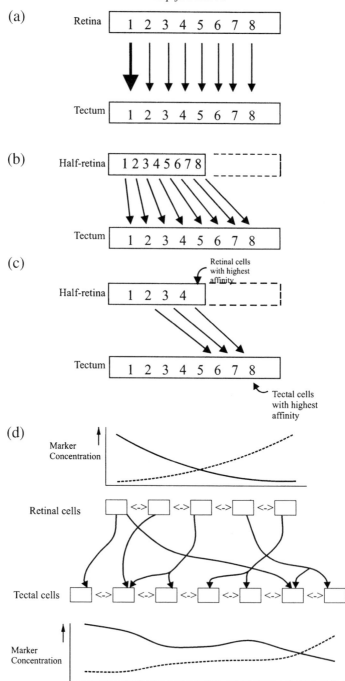

F I G .   5 . 16 . Legend opposite.

and less from others; there is *graded affinity* between the two sets of cells. Prestige and Willshaw (1975) explored models of the second type where the affinities were fixed. Simulations showed that ordered maps (albeit in one dimension only) can be formed if competition is introduced by limiting the number of contacts that each cell can make. This ensures an even spread of connections; without competition, the majority of the connections would be between the retinal and tectal cells of highest affinity. Whereas this competitive mechanism allows plasticity of connections, in order to produce plasticity when the two systems are of different sizes, the additional assumption had to be made that the number of connections made by each cell can be altered. This assumption is akin to introducing a form of regulation, even though the labels as such are not changed (Fig. 5.16c). Schemes of type II are formally similar to the model proposed by Nakamoto *et al.* (1996) (see page 136); both account for the formation of one-dimensional maps only.

Marker induction

Another possibility was developed by von der Malsburg and Willshaw (1977), who suggested that in all cases the presynaptic structure retains its labels and the postsynaptic structure's labels change. This was in the context of theoretical work (Willshaw and von der Malsburg, 1976, 1979; von der Malsburg and Willshaw, 1977) which explored the idea that a mechanism which ensures that each pair of neighbouring retinal cells projects to a pair of neighbouring tectal cells will give rise to an ordered map of connections.

This proposal contains features of both the *Neighbour matching* and *Induction of specificity* hypotheses of map making discussed in Sections 3.3 and 3.4. As remarked there, a neighbourhood mechanism on its own can only determine the relative order in axon terminals over the target surface. A neighbourhood mechanism that is suitable for map-making must have two components: the first one, requiring information of a very low order, establishes the map in the correct polarity; the second one ensures that retinal neighbours project to tectal neighbours. These authors argued that a crucial feature of the mechanism is how the neighbourhood information could be supplied and they suggested that it could involve either correlated neural activity (Willshaw and von der Malsburg, 1976) or specific labels, or markers, assigned to cells (von der Malsburg and Willshaw, 1977; Willshaw and von der Malsburg, 1979).

(a) One-dimensional illustration of the hypothesis of chemospecificity. (b) Illustration of the regulation hypothesis for the case of a half retina generating connections to a complete tectum. (c) The type II scheme of Prestige and Willshaw (1975) for the same case. (d) Illustration of marker induction scheme. Retinal cells acquire labels of two types in concentrations shown in the top graph. Tectal cells acquire markers from the retinal cells through the retinotectal synapses in proportion to synaptic strength and through intratectal exchange. Connections are continually refined according to the similarity between retinal and tectal markers. This leads to refinement in the tectal marker profile and refinement in the pattern of connections. The distribution of the two markers over the tectum during an intermediate stage of development is shown in the bottom graph.

The idea behind this marker induction model is that the retina is labelled by a set of markers continually generated at fixed locations within the retinal surface and subject to lateral transport and degradation. At steady state this sets up a fixed set of markers assigned to each retinal location, nearby retinal cells carrying similar sets of markers. As connections are formed, the markers are induced through the synapses already made into the tectum, which holds no markers initially. The rate of transfer of markers over a synapse is in proportion to the strength of the synapse. At each tectal site, markers from the various retinal cells that are innervating it become blended together with markers from adjacent tectal regions. By this means each tectal cell acquires a characteristic set of markers. Synapses are progressively strengthened in proportion to the similarity between the markers carried by the corresponding retinal and tectal cells. Hence each tectal cell becomes specific to the retinal cells carrying the markers most similar to its own set. This sets off a positive feedback mechanism, resulting in each tectal cell becoming more and more specific to particular retinal cells and thereby attracting more and more markers of this type (Fig. 5.16d). Because nearby retinal cells and nearby tectal cells carry similar sets of markers, retinal neighbours tend to project to tectal neighbours. Provided that the initial pattern of innervation is so biased to favour the desired orientation of the map, the result is that the set of retinal markers and a retinotopic map is induced onto the tectum in the desired orientation. Recently, the same idea has been applied to the problem of the elimination of superinnervation in developing muscle. This is the induced-fit hypothesis due to Ribchester and Barry (1994).

The marker induction model emphasizes the role of the presynaptic cells in establishing connections somewhat similar to the way the periphery is involved in the development of barrel fields in somatosensory cortex. This model solves the problem of how a sets of markers (or labels) in one structure could be reproduced in a second set in a way that is resistant to variations in the developmental program for the individual structures. It is able to account for the systems-matching sets of results (Gaze and Keating, 1972) at the same time as those on the reinnervation of optic tectum following graft translocation and rotation that suggest that in some, but not all, cases different parts of the optic tectum have acquired specificities for individual retinal fibres (Jacobson and Levine, 1975; Levine and Jacobson, 1974; Hope *et al.*, 1976; Yoon, 1971, 1980; Gaze and Hope, 1983). This model is consistent with the conclusions drawn by Schmidt (1978) in support of the induction of specificity hypothesis.

According to the marker induction model each half eye of a *Xenopus* compound eye contains a half set of labels even though it projects across the entire tectum (Willshaw and von der Malsburg, 1979). Evidence for this is discernible in the results from experiments by Straznicky and Tay (1982) on diverting compound eye projections in an analogous manner to that used by Schmidt (1978) in his regeneration experiments and from the fact that the position of retinal axons growing from compound eyes in the optic tract are characteristic of the position occupied by fibres from the appropriate half of a normal eye (Straznicky *et al.*, 1979). In addition, the non-linearities in the extracellularly recorded maps of compound eye projections during development (Straznicky *et al.*, 1981) are predicted directly from the marker induction model.

What militates against this model is firstly that Schmidt's experimental results (Schmidt, 1978) have never been confirmed. Secondly, a problem that is shared by all molecular-based mechanisms of this type is that the evidence for sets of complementary labels in retina and in tectum is slight (but see Section 3.2). Finally, currently there is much interest in activity-mediated mechanisms, to which we now turn.

7.2 Activity-based mechanisms

As originally formulated, the idea was that cells interconnect on the basis of the similarity in their patterns of activity (derived from Hubel and Wiesel, 1965; Wiesel and Hubel, 1965; Keating, 1968). This could form the basis of the formation of binocular connections in amphibian optic tectum, to bring together the connections from matching cells from ipsilateral and contralateral retinae; or as two neighbouring cells in a single retina would have more similar activity patterns than cells further apart, in principle neighbouring retinal cells could come to connect to neighbouring tectal cells.

Activity-based models originate in the model for the development of orientation specificity due to von der Malsburg (1973). He showed that when connections between two sets of cells are modified according to the amount of simultaneous pre- and postsynaptic activity present for each synapse (Hebb, 1949; Fig. 5.17a) retinal activity patterns in the form of straight lines of activated cells will cause the cortex to acquire orientation preferences. The pattern of orientation preferences in the orientation map so produced corresponds roughly to what is measured experimentally.

The first activity-based model for the development of retinotopy, called the neural activity model, is due to Willshaw and von der Malsburg (1976). This was the first of two proposals that they made for how neighbourhood mechanisms for the making of connections could be realized in the nervous system, the second being the marker induction model (von der Malsburg and Willshaw, 1977), discussed above. Conceptually the two models are very close.

Both models are based on the idea that ordered maps of connections will form if all pairs of neighbouring retinal cells connect with tectal cells that also are neighbours. They differ in that in one model, molecules are used to implement the neighbourhood mechanism, in the other neural activity is used.

Willshaw and von der Malsburg (1976) assumed that the retina is spontaneously active and that, through the action of short-range lateral interconnections, cells which are closer together are more likely to be spontaneously active concurrently than cells that are further apart. If initially connections are made between retina and tectum at random, spontaneously active retinal cells will come to excite cells at random positions on the tectal surface and the tectal cells which are closer together would be also more likely to fire in synchrony than cells further apart (due to lateral interconnections in the tectum). The synapses between presynaptic cells

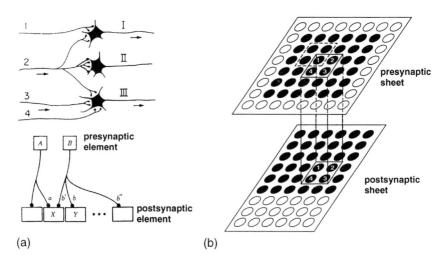

(a)   (b)

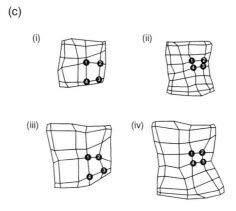

FIG. 5.17. (a) Illustrates the conditions under which Hebbian synaptic modification (Hebb, 1949) takes place. Activity in cells 1, 2 and 4 cause activity in cells I
and III. The synapses between the pairs of cells axons originating from (2,I),(2,III)
and (4,III) are modified as only for these synapses is there activity in the presynaptic
and postsynaptic cells simultaneously (diagram adapted from Brodal, 1992). (b,c) The
development of connections between 64 presynaptic cells arranged as a 8×8 square
and 54 postsynaptic cells arranged as a 9×6 rectangle, according to the neural activity
model (Willshaw and von der Malsburg, 1976). (b) Initial configuration of 36 presynaptic
and 36 postsynaptic cells indicated as filled circles. The 36×36 connections each
have random strength except that there are strong connections between the members
of each of the 4 numbered pairs of cells, to specify the orientation of the map. Open
circles indicate cells that are to be added; see below. (c) The configurations that
have developed, shown as a map of the geometrical means of the position of each
postsynaptic cell on the presynaptic surface, weighted by the strengths of connections
to it. The positions of adjacent postsynaptic cells are connected by a line, to form the
grid patterns shown. Diagram top left: the map developed between the original two sets of 36

and postsynaptic cells which are simultaneously active would then be strengthened, in a Hebbian fashion (Fig. 5.17a). They demonstrated by computer simulation how such a mechanism could lead to the formation of ordered neural mappings. To specify the polarity of the map, some of the retinal cells were assumed to be connected initially to the postsynaptic cells in the right orientation (but not necessarily in the right position). The simulation results illustrated the plasticity of connections that is allowed under such conditions which will account for the size-disparity experiments (Fig. 5.17c).

Amari and colleagues (Takeuchi and Amari, 1979; Amari, 1980) carried out a one-dimensional analysis of a continuous version of the neural activity model. They showed that when the width of the input stimuli is smaller than the extent of the lateral interactions in cortex then an ordered map results; when the width is greater, then on a large scale the map is ordered but on the small scale it breaks up into blocks. Later work (Amari, 1983) showed that the area of the postsynaptic sheet occupied by parts of the presynaptic sheet which are stimulated relatively frequently during development occupy proportionally more of the postsynaptic sheet; more recently this analysis has been extended to the case where the postsynaptic sheet is made up of excitatory and inhibitory cells (Da Silva Filho, 1992)

The predictions and assumptions made from the neural activity neighbourhood type of model require detailed verification, much of which is lacking. With reference to the assumption that the retina is spontaneously active and that the amount of correlated activity between two points is positively correlated with distance between them, there is some evidence for this (Rodieck, 1967; Arnett, 1978; Galli and Maffei, 1988). At the more general level, much careful work has been done to demonstrate the activity-dependent sharpening up of retinotectal projections in experimental paradigms (such as adult goldfish) where activity can be manipulated (see, for example, Schmidt and Edwards, 1983; Cook and Rankin, 1986; Cook, 1987, 1988; Rankin and Cook, 1986). Many people talk of activity-dependent 'refinement' of connections, implying that this may be a secondary mechanism that refines a map that has already formed. It is possible that the primary mechanism is limited to forming the initial crude map — that is, it is the mechanism for specifying the polarity of the map.

7.3 Related models

Several authors have argued that the mechanisms for map formation involve the simultaneous operation of several submechanisms which under different

---

cells. The other three diagrams shown how this map is reorganised after the addition of new cells to one or both structures, to mimic the different modes of growth in *Xenopus* retina and tectum (Straznicky and Gaze, 1971, 1972). Top right: add 18 cells to one end of the postsynaptic sheet; bottom left: add 28 cells around the circumference of the presynaptic sheet: bottom right: add these cells to both sheets simultaneously. Note that the positions of the 4 numbered cells vary from diagram to diagram, indicating that cells do not have absolute specificities.

circumstances can act together in different ways. We have already seen this in the cases of the marker induction model (Section 7.1) and the neural activity model (Section 7.2) for which, it is proposed, there is a mechanism for determining the polarity of the map and one for ensuring that neighbouring presynaptic cells connect to neighbouring postsynaptic cells.

Whitelaw and Cowan's model
Whitelaw and Cowan (1981) integrated mechanisms involving markers and activity by combining the idea of a gradient of adhesive selectivity proposed by Prestige and Willshaw (1975) with synaptic updating as in the neural activity model (Section 7.2). The formula for changing individual synaptic strengths follows the prescription of the neural activity model but then the raw changes in strength are multiplied by the degree of adhesion between the corresponding pre- and postsynaptic cells. In a recent modification to the model a postulated random depolarization which might occur due to spontaneous release of transmitter is added to account for the finding that a map will form in the absence of externally applied electrical activity (Cowan and Friedman, 1990). With this and other modifications the model accounts for a wide variety of experimental results.

Fraser's model
The approach adopted by Fraser (1981) was to introduce the idea of an 'adhesive free energy'. This is a number which can be calculated for every state on the system which describes how well the various constraints postulated by Fraser to control the development of the mapping have been satisfied. In order of increasing importance, the constraints relate to:

1. The degree of adhesion between retinal and tectal cells.
2. The degree of competition amongst retinal axons for tectal space (this constraint as well as constraint 1 is position-independent).
3. A tendency for axons which occupy nearby places on the tectum to stabilize their connections if their cells of origin are also neighbours.
4. A gradient of adhesive specificity along the dorsal-ventral axis of the retina together with a matching gradient on the tectum.
5. Similar gradients of specificity in the nasal-temporal axis of the retina (which matches to the rostrocaudal axis of the tectum).

Hope, Hammond and Gaze's arrow model
Another way of looking at map formation is due to Hope *et al.* (1976). The assumptions made in their arrow model are that each retinal fibre has to 'know' whether it is in the correct relative position with respect to the neighbouring fibres on the tectum. Fibres which are in the incorrect relative positions are assumed to be able to swap over their positions and the process of comparison of fibre positions is repeated. Starting from any initial pattern of connections, an ordered map of connections in the correct orientation will result and, provided that each axon is

additionally imbued with a certain degree of random exploratory behaviour, the set of retinal fibres will come to occupy, in order and in the correct orientation, the appropriate area of tectum available ('systems-matching'). This model has absolutely no fixed labels of the type suggested by Sperry (1943, 1944, 1963); all that each fibre is required to know is information about the desired polarity of the map.

Comments on related models
The problem inherent in all these three proposals is that the models are formulated in fairly abstract terms and little guidance is given as to how the particular mechanisms assumed are implemented in the nervous system. For example, the advantages of Fraser's hypothesised energy function are mathematical rather than biological. The arrow model is perhaps unique amongst models in that it is immediately falsifiable. It predicts that the maps produced by allowing optic nerve fibres to reinnervate the adult tectum after a portion of the tectum has been removed and then replaced after rotation will be a normal map with the small portion of the map identified with the rotated part of the tectum being rotated by a corresponding amount. However, since there is no information about absolute position on the tectum, if two parts of the tectum are interchanged without rotation (translocation), the arrow model will predict a normal map. A variety of experimental results have been obtained but the interpretation of the authors of the arrow model (who themselves have carried out translocation experiments) is that the maps obtained after the translocation experiments are not normal but contain matching translocated portions, which falsifies their own model (Hope *et al.*, 1976). The model due to Cowan and coworkers in its mature form (Cowan and Friedman, 1990) contains several different mechanisms acting together. As such it is comprehensive but lacks predictive power.

8   MODELS FOR THE DEVELOPMENT OF CORTICAL FEATURE MAPS

The aspects of visual cortical organization that are primarily of interest are the development of a continuous 'geographical' topographic mapping from the retina onto the cortex; the development of regions in the cortex that are specific to a particular eye (eye dominance stripes); the development of selectivity for a specific orientation of stimulus. The models for these phenomena are presented either as a set of mathematical equations or in terms of a simulation program. Most models embody roughly the same principles. Usually it is assumed that certain patterns of retinal activity drive the process; there are local interactions within the populations of cells; there is some sort of activity-based synaptic modification; and constraints on the values of the synaptic strengths ('weight normalization') ensures stability of the dynamic system. It is generally assumed that the same basic mechanism underlies all three types of cortical organisation mentioned, or at least there is a strong relationship between them, as the same type of model has been applied to all three situations. Currently the favourite idea is that neural activity drives the development of specific nerve connections.

Retinotopy

As already discussed in Section 5.7, most of the modelling work has concentrated on the development of retinotopy in the retinotectal systems of lower vertebrates. Retinotopic maps in mammals have the additional feature that they are non-linear (Fig. 5.1) and there has been work attempting to characterize the mathematical form of this non-linear transformation (Schwartz, 1977).

Ocular dominance

Early models of this phenomenon considered the development of ocularity specificity in isolation (von der Malsburg and Willshaw, 1976; Swindale, 1980) but it can be regarded as the additional phenomenon that results when the target structure is innervated retinotopically by two eyes rather than one eye. This is well illustrated by related results of Fawcett and Willshaw (1982), who examined the double projections made in *Xenopus* compound eyes. In these animals, each half of a surgically made compound eye projects in retinotopic order across the entire tectum. Staining one-half of the eye with HRP revealed that the tectal projection from each half eye is interdigitated with that from the other to form a pattern of stripes. As ocular dominance stripes are not formed normally in *Xenopus*, the patterns formed in this case must be entirely a byproduct of a mechanism used for another purposes. Striped projections are also formed in frogs into which a third eye has been transplanted at embryonic stages (Constantine-Paton and Law, 1978; Law and Constantine-Paton, 1981). The results from these experiments are more variable and difficult to interpret, probably because of the instability of the preparation. As there was no evidence for segregation of fibres in the tract in Fawcett and Willshaw's results, they concluded that ocular dominance specificities develop through interactions at the optic tectum and not in the pathway.

The basic question is: what discriminates between the fibres of the two eyes? If the underlying mechanisms are activity-based then it might be reasonable to suppose that each eye has its own distinctive pattern of activity, and various models have been built on this assumption (e.g. Miller *et al.*, 1989; Goodhill, 1993). However, this idea is difficult to reconcile with the results of Fawcett and Willshaw (1982); it is unlikely that each half of a compound eye has characteristically different and independent patterns of activity. The other possibility is that the differences between the two halves have a molecular origin — in this case obtained possibly because the two half eyes are of different origin and different molecules are expressed by the different genes in the two halves. However, double projections of the compound eye type can be produced from a single eye, by rounding up half-eye rudiments (Feldman, 1978; Straznicky *et al.*, 1980). Ide *et al.* (1983) showed that such double projections are striped. Most activity-based models for ocular dominance account for the size and shape of the striped patterns of ocular dominance within the limits of variation of the biological phenemona (Fig. 5.18a). Models such as Goodhill's, where the width of stripes is determined by the intraocular

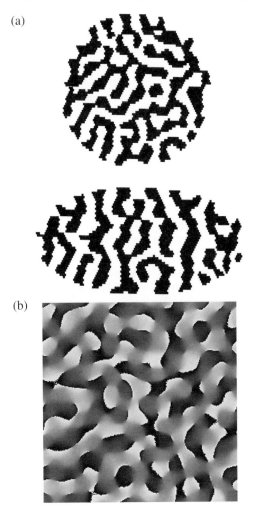

FIG. 5.18. (a) Results from a model showing simulated ocular dominance maps (Goodhill and Willshaw, 1994), derived from the elastic net algorithm (Section 8.1). The two figures illustrate that, on circular targets, the ocularity columns have no preferred orientation whereas on elliptical targets the orientation is parallel to the short axis of the ellipse. (b) A pattern of orientation preferences after the model due to Swindale (1996); reproduced with permission. Conventions as in Fig. 5.15b.

correlations in neural activity, can account for the effect of strabismus on stripe width whereas other models where stripe width is determined by the extent of the lateral interactions within cortex cannot (Goodhill and Löwel, 1995). Most models account successfully for the effects of monocular deprivation (Hubel *et al.*, 1977; Shatz and Stryker, 1978). However, none can account for the various effects of binocular deprivation seen in different areas of cat and monkey cortex (discussed in Swindale, 1996).

The ocularity stripes produced artificially on a three-eyed frog tectum and on *Xenopus* tectum carrying a compound eye projection do not change their width during development. It is not clear how this fact constrains the models for the generation of ocularity stripes but it does suggest that the width of stripes is laid down by an absolute rather than a relative value of some spatial parameter.

Orientation columns

Most models for this phenomenon involve neural activity and they divide into two classes: (i) those that require that the stimuli to which individual cortical cells are to develop a preference are presented explicitly to the system (von der Malsburg, 1973; Durbin and Mitchison, 1990; Obermayer *et al.*, 1990; Tanaka, 1990) and (ii) those that assume that no such patterns are required (Linsker, 1986; Miller, 1994). As there is some evidence that orientation specificity exists in visual cortex before the animals have opened their eyes, models of type (i) are not adequate on their own. For models of type (ii), the required specificity is assumed to derive from the underlying connections which are assumed either to be wired in from the outset or to be a result of the natural development of the system under the given rules for activity-based synaptic modification. For example, in the models due to Linsker (1986) and Miller (1994), radially symmetric patterns of spontaneous activity drive the production of oriented receptive fields through a process of symmetry breaking. The principal other differences between the models concern the assumed pattern of convergence of geniculate afferents and the nature of the intracortical interactions. Models of type (ii) might not involve neural activity at all but as yet no formal model of this type has been produced.

A large amount of detailed information is now available about the fine structure of the orientation maps. The maps produced by many of the models cannot be distinguished from the experimental data (see Swindale, 1996) (Figs. 5.15b,5.18b). Further experimental evidence is required to distinguish between the models. In addition, most models do not attempt to replicate the developmental process and a model that incorporates the three-dimensional geometry of the developing system is needed.

8.1 Abstract models

An alternative approach to modelling is to devise a principle that may underlie a particular developmental phenomenon and then construct a model in which this principle is implemented. Most models of this type are intended to optimize the amount of some physical quantity, e.g. the length of connections between cells, if the principle is to interconnect cells using the minimum amount of wiring. If a procedure can be devised that will alter the configuration slightly to make it more optimal then continued application of the procedure will result in the required configuration being reached. In the development of feature maps, there has been discussion on how to maximize the amount of information passing through the system (Linsker, 1989);

or the total amount of receptive field covered by individual feature-sensitive cortical cells (Swindale, 1991); or the degree of continuity in the map (Erwin *et al.*, 1995); or to minimize the total length of axons used (Cowey, 1979; Mitchison, 1991).

A different approach has been to apply the notion of dimension reduction. This is the notion that, for example, each point on the two-dimensional surface of the visual cortex has to represent the three coordinates of space, ocularity preference and a direction of orientation. Models for how such mappings can be produced have been devised. The elastic net (Durbin and Willshaw, 1987) is one such model, which had been devised to solve the Travelling Salesman Problem, the classic computer science problem of finding the shortest circuit around a given set of points (Lawler *et al.*, 1986). This problem can be thought of constructing a mapping from a two-dimensional space on to a one-dimensional space, whilst maintaining neighbourhood relationships. When applied to the feature map problems discussed here, a model based on the elastic net can account for the production of retinotopy, ocular dominance, and orientation simultaneously (Goodhill and Willshaw, 1990; Erwin *et al.*, 1995). The elastic net was not designed for biological plausibility and this is its drawback. It may be interesting to note that it was in fact developed from the marker induction model (Willshaw and von der Malsburg, 1979) from which many of the biological features of that model were removed. The marker induction model itself has not been applied successfully to all three types of map; von der Malsburg (1979) showed how it could account for retinotopy and ocularity by assuming that the development of retinotopy precedes that of ocularity.

6

Mechanisms controlling the development of cortical connections at the target

1   INTRODUCTION

In the preceding chapters, we have described how the embryonic anatomy of the early forebrain is established (Chapter 2) under the control of regulatory genes and extracellular signalling molecules (Chapter 3). Axons navigate through the developing forebrain to create its major afferent and efferent neural pathways (Chapter 4). Once this is achieved, there is considerable growth and refinement of connections between regions of the cortex to form specific patterns of connections (Chapter 5) and many of the afferent and efferent cortical pathways are resculpted into their adult form. These changes involve several cellular processes, in particular the elimination of connections by cell death, the development of very precise patterns of axonal connections through selective loss of axons, collaterals, or terminals without death of the cell and the further growth of specific axon terminals. Some of these processes involve changes in connectivity through modifying cell number (i.e. through cell death), others involve modifying the patterns of connections without cell death. In this chapter we describe these processes and the underlying mechanisms that operate at the cellular and subcellular levels. Amongst the key influences that we shall discuss are the role of neurotrophic factors and activity-dependent events.

2 MECHANISMS OF CELL DEATH

Of all the mechanisms involved in the formation and maintenance of neural connections, cell death is the best understood, especially at the level of how genetic
instructions can bring about cellular self-destruction. It has long been realized
that cell death can be a physiological as well as a pathological process, that it
requires protein synthesis, and that many cells die during normal brain development
(Hamburger and Oppenheim, 1982; Cowan *et al.*, 1984; Oppenheim, 1985).

As a general rule, during development neurons are produced in numbers that
are greater than those in the adult, only to be reduced in number shortly after
their production (Oppenheim, 1991; Henderson, 1996; Pettmann and Henderson,
1998). That so much cell death should occur during normal development is coun-
terintuitive and, if we are thinking anthropomorphically, it appears wasteful. It is
not clear why such a developmental process should have been selected during evolution. Indeed, when the process of normal neuronal death is blocked by making
transgenic mice with mutations of genes that regulate cell death, thereby increasing
the numbers of neurons, lifespan is not affected (Martinou *et al.*, 1994; Knudson
et al., 1995). None the less, cell death is a significant developmental process that
demands an explanation both in terms of its role in development and the molecular
mechanisms that control it. A widely accepted hypothesis is that neuronal death is
the way in which the numbers of neurons in one neural structure are adjusted (regulated) so that the targets of that structure receive the correct amount of innervation
(discussed in Section 4.3). One proposal is that neurons are thought to compete
for neurotrophic factors, which are taken to be survival factors in short supply.
However, there are many other possible roles for neuronal death, such as the creation of sex differences between neural structures (Breedlove and Arnold, 1983;
Cooke *et al.*, 1998; Bottjer and Arnold, 1997), the elimination of entire structures
that may act as transient scaffolds, such as the subplate (Chapter 2) or transient
branches of the tree of lineage, or the removal of erroneously routed projections
(Oppenheim, 1991; Burek and Oppenheim, 1998).

Although relatively little work has been done on the regulation of cell death in
the cortex, it is likely that the final biochemical pathways that result in cortical cell
death are the same as those that cause cell death elsewhere. Naturally-occurring
cell death is tightly regulated and involves the expression of specific cell death
genes that induce a process called apoptosis (Kerr *et al.*, 1972), in which the DNA
is cleaved at regular intervals and characteristic cellular changes such as chro-
matin condensation and DNA fragmentation occur. Apoptosis is distinguished
from necrosis, a pathological form of cell death that results from overwhelming
cellular injury, by criteria listed in Table 6.1. Although this distinction has proved
extremely useful for the study of cell death processes, it is not absolute (Clarke,
1998) and many stimuli that induce apoptosis can also induce necrosis under different conditions (e.g. chemicals at higher doses: Stewart, 1994; Bredesen, 1995).
The list of cell death genes that regulate apoptosis is long and is still increasing
(Hale *et al.*, 1996). Detailed reviews can be found elsewhere (e.g. Bredesen, 1995;

Table 6.1 Cellular changes in apoptosis and necrosis. Detailed accounts can be found in reviews such as Stewart (1994), Bredesen (1995), and Naruse and Keino (1995). Note that these criteria have general applicability, but may not hold in all situations. For example, internucleosomal fragmentation of DNA can occur in necrosis (Stewart, 1994).

	Apoptosis	**Necrosis**

Nucleus	Internucleosomal cleavage of DNA
	Early stage: >50 kb fragments
	Intermediate stage: 180–200 bp
	  fragments
	Late stage: soluble mono- or
	  oligonucleotides
	Chromatin condensation
		Degradation

Membrane integrity	Persists until late stage	Lost early
Mitochondria	Normal ultrastructural appearance	Swell and take up Ca^{2+}
Inflammatory changes in surrounding tissue?	No	Yes
Cell volume	Decreases	Increases early

Cell fragmentation	Plasma membrane forms blebs;
	  fragments of cell form
	  characteristic apoptotic bodies
		Lysis occurs

Steller, 1995; Vaux and Strasser, 1996; Raff, 1998): a simplified view of how apoptosis is brought about is shown in Fig. 6.1.

Numerous events can induce apoptosis, with different triggers having different degrees of importance in different tissues, and at different times in development. There are two ways in which neurons are caused to die. First, there is evidence that, in normal development of the nervous system, cells rely on a supply of one or more neurotrophic factors to block their own tendency to activate apoptotic molecules by default (Raff, 1998, 1992; Davies, 1997; Pettmann and Henderson, 1998; Bergeron and Yuan, 1998; Henderson, 1996). In other words, it appears that cells will commit suicide unless they are prevented from doing so by external factors (Fig. 6.1). This process of death by trophic deprivation has been the most intensively studied mechanism. The second possibility is that cells die because specific death-inducing receptors are triggered (Bergeron and Yuan, 1998; Pettmann and Henderson, 1998). So far, this ligand-mediated activation of death-signalling receptors, such as tumour necrosis factor receptor, has been better characterized in non-neuronal cells (Yuan, 1997). It is very likely that future research will demonstrate the importance of this mechanism in the developing nervous system. Paradoxically, the first discovered neuronal death receptor was the low-affinity receptor for nerve growth factor, called p75, which is a member

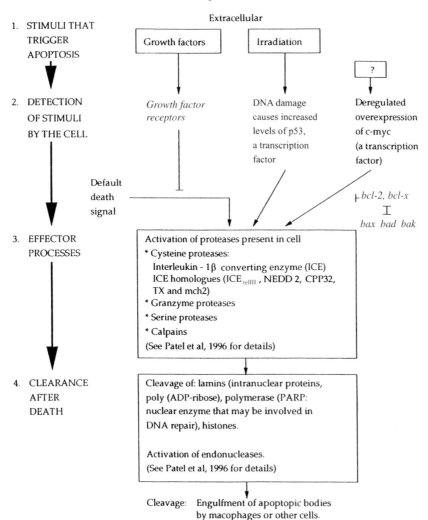

1. STIMULI THAT
   TRIGGER
   APOPTOSIS

Extracellular

| Growth factors | | Irradiation |

?

2. DETECTION
   OF STIMULI
   BY THE CELL

Growth factor receptors

DNA damage causes increased levels of p53, a transcription factor

Deregulated overexpression of c-myc (a transcription factor)

Default death signal

⊦ *bcl-2, bcl-x*

bax bad bak

3. EFFECTOR
   PROCESSES

Activation of proteases present in cell
* Cysteine proteases:
  Interleukin - 1β converting enzyme (ICE)
  ICE homologues (ICE$_{relIII}$, NEDD 2, CPP32, TX and mch2)
* Granzyme proteases
* Serine proteases
* Calpains
(See Patel et al, 1996 for details)

4. CLEARANCE
   AFTER
   DEATH

Cleavage of: lamins (intranuclear proteins, poly (ADP-ribose), polymerase (PARP: nuclear enzyme that may be involved in DNA repair), histones.

Activation of endonucleases.
(See Patel et al, 1996 for details)

Cleavage: Engulfment of apoptopic bodies by macophages or other cells.

FIG. 6.1. Some of the best characterized molecules regulating apoptosis in the context of the four stages of apoptosis (Stewart, 1994; Vaux and Strasser, 1996; Patel *et al.*, 1996). Lines ending in arrows indicate activation; lines blocked by a short perpendicular line indicate inhibition. For example, bcl-2 and bcl-x inhibit death, and bax, bad and bak have the opposite effect by inhibiting bcl-2 and bcl-x. Molecules having inhibitory roles are in italics.

of the tumour necrosis factor receptor family (Frade *et al.*, 1996; Dechant and Barde, 1997; Casaccia-Bonnefil *et al.*, 1996). Nerve growth factor (NGF) is one of the family of neurotrophins and normally it promotes cell survival by acting through a high affinity tyrosine kinase receptor, called TrkA, in association with the p75 receptor (described below). In early chick retina, nerve growth factor and the p75 receptor are expressed in the absence of TrkA. Blocking the action of nerve growth factor on the p75 receptor in these early retinal cells promotes their survival, suggesting that endogenous stimulation of the p75 receptor in the absence of TrkA receptors promotes apoptosis (Frade *et al.*, 1996). This experiment indicates that whether cells live or die is the result of a complex balance between the type and level of extracellular death-inducing or death-preventing molecules and the type, level, and intracellular signalling properties of the corresponding receptors on the cell surface. In addition, the state of activity of neurons affects whether or not they undergo cell death. Removal of afferents and blocking afferent activity *in vivo* can increase cell death in many developing systems including the cerebral cortex, where lesioning the posterior thalamus in hamsters at birth decreases the numbers of cells in layer 4 of the occipital cortex (Windrem and Finlay, 1991). In culture, there is evidence that the survival of several types of neuron, including those of the developing thalamus and cortex, is enhanced by their depolarization (Ghosh *et al.*, 1994; Meyer-Franke *et al.*, 1995; Magowan and Price, 1996). Depolarization may enhance survival by increasing the responsiveness of neurons to neurotrophic factors or by increasing the production of these factors. Understanding how the balance between all of these variables affects neuronal survival in different places and at different times in development is a major future challenge.

The numerous apoptotic stimuli, be they lack of neurotrophic support or presence of death-inducing ligands, lead to the post-translational activation of several proteases in a final common pathway (effector molecules). The products of other genes, such as bcl-2, bcl-x, bax, bad, and bak, can modulate these processes (Fig. 6.1). These genes comprise a family that in mammals corresponds to the single ced-9 gene that regulates developmental cell death in the nematode *Caenorhabditis elegans*. Although the *C. elegans* ced-9 gene encodes a negative regulator of developmental cell death, the mammalian family of related genes includes both inhibitors and promoters of apoptosis (Merry and Korsmeyer, 1997). The bcl-2 gene was the first to be detected, as a putative oncogene. Its oncogene-like role results from its ability to prolong the survival of non-cycling cells, and it cooperates with other oncogenes that have mitogenic effects rather than having an independent ability to induce proliferation (Hale *et al.*, 1996). It has been suggested that the ratio of apoptosis-inhibiting (such as Bcl-2) to apoptotis-inducing (such as Bax) proteins in a cell controls its apoptotic response (Korsmeyer *et al.*, 1993; Oltvai *et al.*, 1993). Thus, the differential expression of members of the bcl-2 gene family may regulate susceptibility to apoptosis during development.

Bcl-2 family proteins are found in the outer mitochondrial, outer nuclear, and endoplasmic reticular membranes (Yang and Korsmeyer, 1996), where they are thought to form pores that are open or closed under different conditions (Schendel *et al.*, 1997; Antonsson *et al.*, 1997). The pro-apoptotic protein Bax is soluble in the cytoplasm in living cells but becomes membrane-associated in cells undergoing apoptosis (Wolter *et al.*, 1997). It has been suggested that, under the influence of apoptosis-inducing stimuli, the flux of small molecules such as ions through the putative Bax channel might induce the changes in these organelles that are associated with cell death (Pettmann and Henderson, 1998). Since bcl-2 family members can form either homodimers or heterodimers, it is possible that the effects of the anti-apoptotic members of the family, such as Bcl-2 itself, arise because their heterodimerization with the pro-apoptotic members, such as Bax, generates pores that remain closed. As yet, this is still speculative.

In summary, neuronal death during development represents one pathway of differentiation that involves the expression of specific proteins. Our current knowledge indicates that neuronal death is regulated in part by neurotrophic molecules that act from outside the cell to repress its suicidal tendency. In this commonly accepted scheme, neurotrophic molecules promote survival by suppressing death, although there are likely to be other mechanisms involved in the regulation of neuronal death. For some neurons, death induced by neurotrophic factor withdrawal is regulated by the relative levels of expression of members of the bcl-2 family (Allsopp *et al.*, 1993; Bergeron and Yuan, 1998; Pettmann and Henderson, 1998). How the levels of expression of these modifiers of cell death are controlled in the developing nervous system is not yet clear.

3 NEUROTROPHIC FACTORS

Increased survival resulting from a substance located extracellularly that interacts with a cell is termed a trophic response, although many authors also use this term for growth-promoting effects. Neurotrophic factors are proteins that regulate the development, maintenance, and survival of neurons. Many have actions very early in neural development, on cell proliferation, and differentiation (Chapter 3). As will be discussed later, they are also implicated in synaptic plasticity. Many neurotrophic factors are small (with molecular weights between 13 and 24 kDa), soluble, and are active as homodimers. Table 6.2 lists many of the known neurotrophic factors and their receptors with selected references. These factors can be classified under the headings of growth factors and cytokines. This classification owes most to a knowledge of the receptors through which the factors operate, and a recognition that these receptors are similar to those of either growth factors (such as fibroblast growth factor, FGF, or platelet-derived growth factor, PDGF) or cytokines (such as leukaemia inhibitory factor, LIF, or interleukin-6, IL-6) that were originally identified in non-neural tissues (Ip and Yancopoulos, 1996). Both neural and non-neural growth factors bind to receptor tyrosine kinases, whereas neural and non-neural cytokines use distinct multicomponent receptor systems.

3.1 Growth factors. I. The neurotrophins

Nerve growth factor (NGF) was the first neurotrophic factor to be identified (Hamburger and Levi-Montalcini, 1949; Levi-Montalcini and Angeletti, 1968; Levi-Montalcini, 1987). It is now known that NGF is a member of a family of closely related peptide factors, called the neurotrophins, which includes

Table 6.2 Neurotrophic factors: a list of some of the currently recognized growth factors, cytokines, and their receptors that may play a part in cortical development.

Family	Member	Receptor	Selected References
Neurotrophins	Nerve growth factor (NGF)	TrkA, p75	Ip and Yancopoulos 1996; Lewin and Barde 1996; Lindsay *et al.* 1994; Chao and Hempstead 1995; Maness *et al.* 1994; Chao 1992; Meakin and Shooter 1992; Thoenen and Edgar 1985; Barde 1989
	Brain-derived neurotrophic factor (BDNF)	TrkB, p75	
	Neurotrophin-3 (NT-3)	TrkC, p75	
	Neurotrophin-4/5 (NT-4/5)	TrkB, p75	
	Neurotrophin-6 (NT-6)		
Fibroblast growth factors (FGFs)	Acidic FGF (aFGF or FGF-1)	FGF receptors 1–4 (FGFR-1–4)	Gonzalez *et al.*, 1996; Gomez-Pinilla and Cotman 1991; Tagashira *et al.* 1995; Eckenstein 1994; Vicario-Abejon *et al.* 1995
	Basic FGF (bFGF or FGF-2), FGF-3, FGF-4, FGF-5, FGF-6, FGF-7, FGF-8, FGF-9		
Insulin-like growth factors (IGFs)	IGF-I	IGF type I receptor (IGF1-R)	Ye *et al.* 1995; D'Costa *et al.* 1995; Stewart and Rotwein 1996; Collet-Solberg and Cohen 1996; D'Ercole 1996
	IGF-II	IGFR-I	
Epidermal growth factor (EGF)	Transforming growth factor alpha (TGFα)	Receptor tyrosine kinases $p185^{erbB2}$/HER2/ c-Neu and $p180^{erbB4}$/HER4	Mogi *et al.* 1994
	Glial growth factor (GFG)		Shah *et al.* 1994
Transforming growth factor beta (TGFβ)	TGFβ1, TGFβ2, TGFβ3	TGFβ type I, II, and III receptors	Massague 1996

Table 6.2

Family	Member	Receptor	Selected References
	Glial cell line-derived neurotrophic factor (GDNF)	Glycosylphosphati- dylinositol (GPI) linked protein and tyrosine kinase receptor (c-Ret protein)	Treanor *et al.* 1996
	Bone morphogenetic proteins (BMP)		See Table 3.2, Chapter 3
Neuropoietins	Interleukin-1 (IL-1), IL-2, IL-3, IL-6		Ide *et al.* 1996; Mogi *et al.* 1994; Pousset 1994
	Leukaemia inhibitory factor (LIF)	LIF receptor complex (gp130, LIFRβ subunits)	Yamakumi *et al.* 1996; Watanabe *et al.* 1996.
	Ciliary neurotrophic factor (CNTF)	CNTF receptor complex (CNTFRα, gp130, LIFRβ subunits)	Seniuk-Tatton *et al.* 1995; David and Yancopoulos 1993; Ip and Yancopoulos 1996; Stahl and Yancopoulos 1994
Other growth factors	Platelet-derived growth factor (PDGF)	PDGFα- and β-receptors	Oumesmar *et al.* 1997; Ellison *et al.* 1996
	Stem cell factor (mast cell growth factor)	c-kit proto-oncogene receptor	Wong and Licinio 1994
	Hepatocyte growth factor (HGF)	c-met proto-oncogene receptor	Honda *et al.* 1995; Jung *et al.* 1994
	Plasminogin activators Vascular endothelial growth factor (VEGF)		Dent *et al.* 1993

brain-derived neurotrophic factor (BDNF), neurotrophin-3 (NT-3), neurotrophin-4 (NT4), and neurotrophin-6 (NT-6) (Snider and Johnson, 1989; Eide *et al.*, 1993; Korsching, 1993; Snider, 1994; Gotz *et al.*, 1994). The neurotrophins act upon one of two types of receptors on the surface of their target neurons. Many of the effects of the neurotrophins on cell survival and neurite outgrowth are mediated by receptors known as the high affinity glycoprotein tyrosine receptor kinases ($K_d = 10^{-11} M$), Trk receptors. They consist of an extracellular domain containing the neurotrophin-binding site, a short transmembrane segment, and an intracellular domain encoding a tyrosine kinase. The neurotrophins selectively

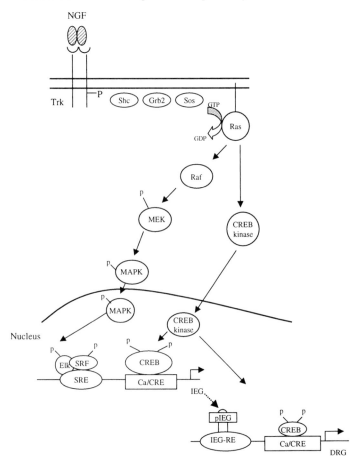

FIG. 6.2. Intracellular pathways activated by the neurotrophins. The binding of neurotrophin (nerve growth factor, NGF) causes receptor dimerization and activates the intrinsic tyrosine kinase activity of the Trk receptor. The Trk molecule itself is the initial substrate of Trk kinase; within the TrkA dimer, the individual molecules each catalyse the phosphorylation of the other. A protein, Shc, binds to its recognition site on the activated receptor and mediates a further association with additional proteins, Grb2 and Sos. These proteins are translocated from the cytoplasm to the plasma membrane where they activate the G protein Ras. One pathway following activation of Ras leads to the sequential activation of the kinases Raf and the mitogen activated protein kinase (MAPK). MAPK translocates to the nucleus where it phosphorylates transcription factors (such as Elk-1). Elk binds to the serum response factor (SRF) and the serum response element (SRE). A second pathway following activation of Ras leads to activation of cAMP regulatory element-binding protein (CREB) kinase, which is thought to translocate to the nucleus and phosphorylate CREB itself. CREB is a transcription factor which binds to the cAMP-Ca response element (Ca/CRE) and,

bind to the high affinity Trk receptors, which form homodimers and autophospho-rylate, triggering the intracellular cascade (Segal and Greenberg, 1996) (Fig. 6.2). There are three members of the Trk receptor family: TrkA, which is the receptor for NGF, TrkB, which is the receptor for BDNF and NT-4, and TrkC, which is the receptor for NT-3 (Bothwell, 1991, 1995; Segal and Greenberg, 1996). There are some truncated forms of the TrkB and TrkC receptors which lack the intracellu-lar tyrosine kinase domains; it is possible that these receptors are involved in the deactivation of neurotrophins (Bothwell, 1995; Lewin and Barde, 1996; Lindsay *et al.*, 1994; Meakin and Shooter, 1992).

All neurotrophins bind with relatively equal and low affinity ($K_d = 10^{-9}M$) to a membrane receptor known as $p75^{NGF}$ (low affinity NGF receptor) which is found on both neuronal and non-neuronal cells (Rodriguez-Tebar *et al.*, 1990, 1992). The p75 receptor lacks kinase activity, although it does appear to have signalling capabilities (Dobrowsky *et al.*, 1994; Itoh *et al.*, 1995). It has been implicated in apoptosis, as discussed above (Frade *et al.*, 1996; Casaccia-Bonnefil *et al.*, 1996), and may modulate cellular responses to the neurotrophins by enhancing the sensitivity of the Trk receptors (Davies *et al.*, 1993; Hantzopoulus *et al.*, 1994).

The neurotrophins have been implicated in a wide variety of developmental processes at numerous sites in the nervous system (Segal and Greenberg, 1996). They may play roles in very early development; for example, as described in Chapter 3, NT-3 has been shown to induce neuronal differentiation in neocor-tical precursors (Ghosh and Greenberg, 1995). They can enhance axonal growth, including that of cortical afferents and efferents, and affect the electrophysiological properties of neurons (Lotto and Price, 1995; Schnell *et al.*, 1994; Levine *et al.*, 1995). But their best-known roles are in the regulation of cell survival (Segal and Greenberg, 1996; Snider and Johnson, 1989; Korsching, 1993; Ghosh *et al.*, 1994; Meyer-Franke *et al.*, 1995; Bergeron and Yuan, 1998; Davies, 1997; Burek and Oppenheim, 1998; Oppenheim, 1991; Henderson, 1996; Pettmann and Henderson, 1998). Later in this chapter we shall describe what is known of their possible roles in the survival of specifically cortical neurons and their afferents and in the growth and refinement of connections to the cortex and within it.

---

in cooperation with the SRE complex, activates the transcription of immediate early genes (IEGs) such as the c-fos proto-oncogene. IEG products (pIEG) are transcription factors that bind to IEG-response elements (IEG-RE) and, in cooperation with phosphorylated CREB, activate transcription of delayed response genes (DRGs) (Segal and Greenberg, 1996). Some responses to neurotrophins occur independently of Ras and recent studies have elucidated novel intracellular pathways activated by these molecules (Toledo-Aral *et al.*, 1995; Peng *et al.*, 1995).

3.2   Growth factors. II. Other neurotrophic factors

Fibroblast growth factors (FGFs) play multiple roles in neural development, for example in early inductive interactions and the control of proliferation (see Chapter 3) as well as being neurotrophic factors (Walicke *et al.*, 1986; Walicke and Baird, 1988). They have actions similar to the neurotrophins in promoting the outgrowth and survival of neurons in the cortex and thalamus (Lotto and Price, 1995; Lotto *et al.*, 1997). There are at least nine different FGFs and their effects are mediated by a family of transmembrane tyrosine kinase receptors (FGFRs). These receptors are named FGFRs 1–4, but they have alternative names. FGFR-1 is also known as flg, bFGFR, or Cek1. FGFR-2 is also known as bek, K-sam, KGFR, or Cek3. FGFR-3 is also known as Cek2.

FGF signalling is mediated in a different way from that of the neurotrophins. It involves a low affinity binding site on heparan sulphate and a high affinity receptor that contains a tyrosine kinase (Fig. 6.3). The high affinity receptors contain three extracellular immunoglobulin domains and two intracellular tyrosine kinase domains. FGF binds with low affinity to a heparan sulphate proteoglycan FGF receptor which then facilitates binding of FGF monomers to the high affinity FGF receptor. This interaction leads to autophosphorylation and signal transduction.

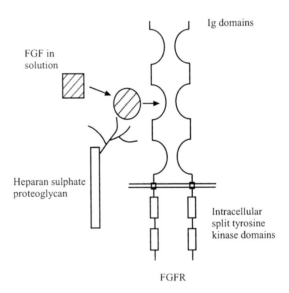

FGF in solution

Ig domains

Heparan sulphate proteoglycan

Intracellular split tyrosine kinase domains

FGFR

FIG. 6.3. Activation of the FGF receptor (FGFR). Binding of FGFs to heparan sulphate on heparan sulphate proteoglycan molecules (Chapter 3) may induce a conformational change in the FGF molecules. The altered form of FGF may have a conformation capable of promoting dimerization and tyrosine kinase activity of the high affinity receptor (Klagsbrun and Baird, 1991). Ig: immunoglobulin.

The signalling of other growth factors likely to be involved in cortical development is mediated by other types of molecule. GDNF uses a unique receptor system in which a novel glycosylphosphatidylinositol (GPI) linked protein is a ligand-binding component and tyrosine kinase receptor ret is a signalling component (Treanor *et al.*, 1996).

3.3 Cytokines

The receptor topology for the cytokines is very different from the neurotrophins and FGFs (Fig. 6.4). The transduction pathway for CNTF involves a tyrosine kinase but the receptor itself is not a tyrosine kinase. The receptor consists of three subunits, only one of which directly binds CNTF and the tyrosine kinase JAK/TYK, which associates with the CNTF receptor complex on the cytosolic side of the plasma

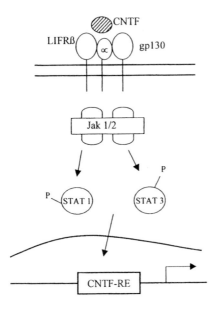

FIG. 6.4. Ciliary neurotrophic factor (CNTF) signalling involves the Jak-STAT pathway. A trimeric receptor, comprising the CNTF-specific α receptor, the leukaemia inhibitory factor receptor β (LIFRβ) subunit, and the related gp130 subunit (LIFRβ and gp130 make up the LIF receptor), is formed by CNTF. This activates the Janus tyrosine kinase (Jak1 or Jak2), which phosphorylates STAT-1 and/or STAT-3. These phosphorylated proteins translocate to the nucleus where they bind to CNTF-response elements (CNTF-RE) and initiate transcription of distinct subsets of immediate early genes and delayed response genes (Segal and Greenberg, 1996; Mulderry, 1994).

membrane. CNTF binds with low affinity to the specific CNTFα receptor moiety which has a transmembrane domain. This complex interacts with two membrane spanning signalling molecules gp130 and LIFRβ, thereby activating an associated tyrosine kinase (JAK/TYK) (David and Yancopoulos, 1993; Stahl and Yancopoulos, 1994). LIF contains a ligand binding and signal transducing subunit both of which belong to the gp130 family of cytokine receptors (Watanabe *et al.*, 1996).

4 REGULATION OF CELL DEATH IN THE DEVELOPING CORTEX AND ITS CONNECTIONS

4.1 The intracellular cell death machinery

Our understanding of the intracellular events that lead to programmed cell death has come from work on many types of cell. Some studies have been on neurons, but very few have focused specifically on the forebrain, let alone the cerebral cortex. Those experiments that have been carried out support the view that the processes that underlie cell death in other cell types are similar or the same as those that cause cell death in the forebrain. First, transgenic mice overexpressing the bcl-2 gene, which modulates the cell death process through its anti-apoptotic action (see above), show a reduction in neuronal loss in the brain (Martinou *et al.*, 1994). Secondly, bcl-2 is widely expressed in the embryonic murine brain (Merry *et al.*, 1994). Further studies of bcl-2 expression in the developing human cortex have suggested that bcl-2 levels are high in the early prenatal period but decline at a time which coincides with an elevation in levels of bax (a pro-apoptotic modulator) and with the onset of prominent apoptotic cell death (Wisniewski *et al.*, 1997).

4.2 Neurotrophic factors and their receptors

Although many neurotrophic molecules are expressed in the cortex, several types of experiment need to be carried out to demonstrate beyond reasonable doubt that a particular molecule has a role in promoting the survival of a group of cells. First, it is necessary to establish that the molecule in question is expressed in the cells. With regards to the cerebral cortex, this criterion is met by many of the molecules in Table 6.2. Secondly, it is useful to know whether the molecule in question is able to stimulate the survival of the cells in isolation in culture. Cortical and thalamic cells respond to a range of growth factors, some identified, others not, many of which enhance both their survival and process growth. A large number of neurotrophic factors have been discovered from work throughout the nervous system (Table 6.2), and some have been shown to affect survival in the cerebral cortex and its afferents in culture. Many of the molecules listed in Table 6.2 have not been tested on isolated cortical or thalamic cells. There are some notable exceptions. For example, brain-derived neurotrophic factor (BDNF) can stimulate the survival of isolated cortical cells in culture (Ghosh *et al.*, 1994). An interesting aspect of this study was the finding that BDNF production by cortical cells was enhanced by a depolarizing stimulus (elevation of potassium), and that blocking this enhancement of BDNF levels with antibodies prevented the survival-promoting effect of elevated potassium. These results suggest that neural activity has a role in the regulation of factors that influence the viability of cortical neurons.

Compared with our understanding of the factors regulating survival of cells in the peripheral nervous system, little is known about factors controlling cortical cell survival. Even less is known about the control of cortical afferent survival. The major afferent input to the cerebral cortex originates in the thalamus. Over the past few years, our work has shown that many neurotrophic factors, including the neurotrophins and fibroblast growth factors, are produced by embryonic thalamic cells and that these factors can enhance thalamic neuronal survival in culture (Lotto *et al.*, 1997). Moreover, our work has indicated that the survival of thalamic neurons in culture is enhanced by depolarizing stimuli, although what molecules mediate this effect is unclear (Magowan and Price, 1996).

These lines of evidence indicate that some of the known neurotrophic factors, and no doubt numerous as yet unidentified factors, some of which (such as GAGs) may act synergistically with neurotrophic factors, might regulate programmed cell death in the developing cerebral cortex and in structures that innervate it. Other essential tests of the involvement of these factors in regulating cell death in these regions have either yielded little or no supporting evidence, or have not been done. For example, blocking the actions of the neurotrophins or other growth factors, such as the FGFs, should block the ability of cortical or thalamic neurons to regulate their survival. Ghosh *et al.* (1994) have published evidence that blocking the activity of BDNF with antibodies added to cultured cortical cells prevents the depolarization-induced enhancement of viability that is found when the antibodies are not present. There are very few other reports of similar experiments, probably largely because proven effective blockers of the actions of these growth factors are not yet widely available. Another approach to blocking the actions of a particular growth factor is to create transgenic mice with a null-mutation of the corresponding gene. However, although a number of genes for growth factors and their receptors have been knocked out, none of the mutants has shown major abnormalities in the cerebral cortex nor the thalamus (Ernfors *et al.*, 1994a,b; Snider, 1994; Silos-Santiago *et al.*, 1997). It is likely that, unlike the peripheral nervous system, the central nervous system is able to compensate for the loss of just a single growth factor. This may arise because central neurons, which have larger numbers of targets than peripheral neurons, use multiple growth factors to regulate their survival. This may minimize the impact of the loss of just one factor.

Overall, very little is known about the regulation of cell survival in the cerebral cortex and thalamus. It is likely that at least some of the known growth factors are involved in controlling cell death in at least some stages of development, and that activity modulates this process.

4.3   The neurotrophic hypothesis for cell death; does it apply in the cerebral cortex?

One frequently proposed explanation for the substantial amount of neuronal death during development is that it is a way of matching the number of presynaptic cells to the number of postsynaptic cells by neurons competing for a supply of one or more neurotrophic factors produced by their target cells. It has been proposed that, during development, insufficient neurotrophic factor is produced to support the excessive numbers of neurons generated and those that are unsuccessful in the competition die. This has been termed the neurotrophic hypothesis (Oppenheim, 1991; Burek and Oppenheim, 1998). It arose from observations on cell death among developing motoneurons that innervate the limb bud. The work by Hamburger and colleagues showed that (i) there is substantial motoneuron death in normal development, (ii) removal of the limb bud in chick embryos causes increased death of the motoneurons whereas (iii) some of the motoneurons that would have died during normal development are rescued by grafting in an extra limb bud (Hamburger, 1958, 1975; Hamburger and Oppenheim, 1982; Oppenheim *et al.*, 1978; Oppenheim, 1991; Burek and Oppenheim, 1998). Similar findings have been reported in *Xenopus laevis* (Prestige, 1967, 1970; Lamb, 1979). The idea that there is a simple arithmetical matching of numbers of presynaptic cells to numbers of postsynaptic cells does not account for the results. When an additional limb is grafted onto an embryonic chick, the number of motoneurons that are rescued is less than would be predicted from this change in target size (Hollyday and Hamburger, 1976; Lamb, 1979). Lamb (1980) was able to increase the size of the population of presynaptic nerve cells. He amputated one hind limb bud of a *Xenopus* tadpole and then diverted the nerves that would have innervated it into the surviving limb, thereby providing this limb with double innervation, from both sides of the spinal cord. He found that the same proportion of motoneurons died as in normal development, so that in this experimental case the number of surviving motoneurons that innervate the single limb is twice as great as normal, even though the postsynaptic target had not changed in size. It is certainly true that motoneurons require a target for survival. Lamb (1981) axotomized newly growing *Xenopus* motoneurons by removing the limb bud. He found axons would regenerate when the limb bud was replaced immediately but the cells would die in the absence of the target.

The induction of abnormally high rates of death among motoneurons following target ablation can be prevented by addition of muscle extract and, to some extent, glial cell line-derived neurotrophic factor (GDNF) (Oppenheim, 1991; Caldero *et al.*, 1998). One interpretation of these observations is that the numbers of motoneurons that die during normal development is regulated by the amount of neurotrophic support available in the target tissue. There has been much other experimental work relevant to the neurotrophic hypothesis. Some is supportive, some has raised as yet unanswered questions. Recent support for the neurotrophic hypothesis has come from studies on the actions of various neurotrophins in regulating the survival of peripheral sensory neurons in the mouse. Inactivation of the genes encoding neurotrophic factors leads to neuronal loss in a gene-dose dependent manner (Ernfors *et al.*, 1994a,b; Snider, 1994), indicating that quantities of particular neurotrophic factors are limiting in some systems *in vivo*. The converse is also the case: increasing the levels of neurotrophic factors through their administration or overexpression can reduce cell death in these systems (Oakley *et al.*, 1997; Wright *et al.*, 1997).

A major unresolved question concerns the applicability of the neurotrophic hypothesis to the central nervous system. Some work is supportive. For example, decreasing the size of the cerebral cortex by making early lesions reduces the numbers of thalamic neurons; this result can be reversed by adding cortical-conditioned medium to the lesion site, implying that trophic factors in the cortex are necessary for thalamic cell survival (Cunningham *et al.*, 1987). There is also evidence that cortex-derived factors can promote the survival of thalamic neurons *in vitro* (Price *et al.*, 1995). The molecules that may mediate these effects have not yet been identified. A role for the neurotrophins has been postulated on the basis of their *in vitro* survival-promoting effects on cortical and thalamic neurons (Ghosh *et al.*, 1994; Lotto *et al.*, 1997), but studies of mice with the genes for one or more of these factors deleted have failed to show major neuronal loss in the forebrain (Ernfors *et al.*, 1994a,b; Snider, 1994; Silos-Santiago *et al.*, 1997). This could be because factors other than the neurotrophins are important for the promotion of cell survival in the developing cortex and among its afferents or because overlaps in the function of the various neurotrophins (Lotto *et al.*, 1997) lead to a high degree of redundancy in the actions of any one of them (Minichiello and Klein, 1996). Similar observations suggesting the involvement of multiple neurotrophic factors in neuronal survival and the possibility of redundancy have been made in other regions of the developing central nervous system. Neurons at many sites in the central nervous system have many more targets than peripheral neurons and motoneurons. Thus, the extent to which the neurotrophic hypothesis is applicable in the central nervous system and the exact roles of factors such as the neurotrophins in the survival of central neurons remain unclear.

5 THE MODIFICATION OF CORTICAL CONNECTIONS AND CIRCUITS BY ACTIVITY

The immature neural circuits generated early in embryogenesis undergo enormous transformations before adulthood, not only through the elimination of cells by death but also through more subtle changes, including alterations of synaptic strengths and numbers, rearrangements of axonal arbors, and elimination of synapses or entire projections. It has long been realized that much of this is achieved with the involvement of neural activity. As sensory cells mature and develop their connections, there are overall changes in levels of spontaneous or evoked activity as well as the emergence of increasingly elaborate patterns of activity. Much emphasis has been placed on the role of neural activity, particularly in the later stages of cortical development. It is important to recognize (i) that the ways in which activity acts to influence processes of refinement (for example, whether the activity instructs the changes or merely permits them to happen) are often not clear and (ii) that other factors (for example, genetic) may be the primary regulators of some refinements.

In the previous chapter we discussed the role of activity in map formation. We now discuss how activity can act at the level of the single synapse or single cell. We then discuss the possible involvement of specific molecules such as neurotrophic factors.

5.1   Long-term potentiation and long-term depression

Long-term potentiation

Activity in developing circuits, initially spontaneous and later evoked and patterned by external stimuli, plays a crucial role in changes of connectivity, as described in Chapter 5. But how does activity operate to change the morphology and physiology of connections? One strong possibility is that during development, activity induces synaptic changes similar to those that are thought to underlie learning and memory in the adult, namely long-term potentiation (LTP) (Bliss and Lomo, 1973; Bliss and Gardner-Medwin, 1973) and long-term depression (LTD) (Ito *et al.*, 1982), described initially in the adult hippocampus and cerebellum respectively.

In LTP, high frequency electrical stimulation of a neural pathway strengthens synapses, the effect lasting for long periods of time. This is thought to be caused by the coincidence of intense presynaptic stimulation with changes in the electrical properties of the postsynaptic cells that result from the stimulation. Long-term potentiation in vertebrates was discovered when experiments on rat hippocampus showed that, after activation of specific pathways by high frequency trains of impulses, the population spike (the summed excitatory postsynaptic potentials) recorded extracellularly from groups of pyramidal cells measured in response to a test pulse was greater than that recorded before the application of the high frequency activation. The effect of LTP induction can last for up to several weeks (Bliss and Collingridge, 1993).

Much of the work on LTP has been carried out on rat hippocampus using *in vitro* slice preparations. The most commonly investigated pathway is that involving CA3 pyramidal cells which innervate the CA1 pyramidal cells directly through the Schaffer collaterals for which the transmitter is the excitatory amino acid glutamate. CA1 cells contain both NMDA and non-NMDA (kainate and quisqualate) receptor subtypes. Non-NMDA receptors are activated during normal synaptic transmission while NMDA receptors are involved in the induction of LTP (Collingridge and Bliss, 1987). Application of the transmitter glutamate causes the non-NMDA receptors to open. In addition, glutamate binds to NMDA receptors which normally are blocked by magnesium. When the membrane is depolarized, the magnesium block is freed, allowing calcium ions to enter the postsynaptic membrane. This seems to induce LTP although the precise details of the mechanism at the molecular level are not absolutely clear. Two separate conditions must therefore be satisfied for LTP to be induced; activation of the NMDA receptor and sufficient depolarization of the postsynaptic membrane. Synaptic modification through the coincident action of presynaptic and postsynaptic signals had long been suspected. In 1949 the psychologist Hebb defined what has come to be called the Hebb synapse (Fig. 5.17a):

When an axon of cell A is near enough to excite cell B and repeatedly or persistently takes part in firing it, some growth process or metabolic change takes place in one or both cells such that A's efficiency, as one of the cells firing B, is increased.

(Hebb, 1949, p. 62.)

Long-term depression
Long-term depression of the parallel fibre synapses on the Purkinje cells of the cerebellar cortex was first described by Ito *et al.* (1982). The Purkinje cells of cerebellar cortex are innervated in an approximately one-to-one fashion by a strong climbing fibre input and in a many-to-many fashion by the parallel fibres of the granule cells (Eccles *et al.*, 1967). The conditions for induction of LTD is that the Purkinje cells receive input simultaneously from both parallel fibres and climbing fibres (Bear and Abraham, 1996).

The classical account of LTD induction is as follows. The release of the transmitter glutamate by the climbing fibre terminals activates the Purkinje cell AMPA receptors and causes a strong depolarization of the Purkinje cell membrane. One effect of this depolarization is influx of a large amount of calcium through voltage gated calcium channels on Purkinje cell dendrites. Active parallel fibres release glutamate that activates the AMPA receptors and also the metabotropic receptors of the Purkinje cells. Activation of metabotropic receptors has a number of effects, principally the formation of cytoplasmic diacyl glycerol. Together with an increase in calcium concentration, this results in activation of protein kinase C (PKC). Activated PKC phosphorylates the postsynaptic AMPA receptors, leading to a reduced sensitivity of the receptors to glutamate by decreasing their number. The consequence of this is a long-term depression of the excitatory postsynaptic potentials evoked by the parallel fibres, as a result of climbing fibre activity coupled with parallel fibre activity.

Since the discovery of LTP and LTD, both phenomena have been found widely in other systems. For example, low frequency stimulation of hippocampus can produce LTD (Bayer *et al.* 1994; see also Bliss and Collingridge 1993). LTP is also known in the adult neocortex (Markram *et al.*, 1997).

The question we examine here is whether activity-dependent effects at the synaptic level are known during development and whether in particular these effects correspond to those of LTP and LTD.

5.2 Neonatal cortical plasticity

Several investigators have looked at the role of neural activity in developing cortex at the cellular level (Fig. 6.5 a–c; Chapter 5, Section 5.2). Fregnac *et al.* (1988)

investigated, in kitten, the effects of artificially induced functional changes in neurons of area 17 which are responsive to two different types of stimuli, such as bar stimuli presented stimultaneously to the two eyes (for binocular cells) or stimuli of different orientations (for orientation selective cells). Iontophoretic current injection was used to increase artificially the response of the postsynaptic cell to one type of stimulus and decrease its response to a stimulus of the second type. On testing, the responsiveness of the cell to the stimulus paired with the reinforced response was found to be enhanced. These changes could be induced during the recording experiment. The largest changes were obtained during the critical period of the kitten although similar effects were obtained from adults. These experiments support the idea that a temporal correlation between pre- and postsynaptic activity is involved in the induction of long-term synaptic modifications during development. The experiments suggest a slightly different synaptic learning rule from that proposed by Hebb (1949) (see Section 5.3).

We have described how the induction of LTP in the hippocampus depends on activation of glutamate receptors of the N-methyl-D-aspartate (NMDA) type. Several authors have revealed a similar involvement of NMDA receptors during development. There is evidence that blockade of NMDA receptors in the developing visual cortex by infusion of amino phosphonovaleric acid (AP5) reduces the plasticity of ocular dominance columns (Bear *et al.*, 1990). This might be explained by disruption of LTP in the visual cortex. Both LTP and LTD are present in the developing visual cortex (Kirkwood *et al.*, 1993; Kirkwood and Bear, 1994b; Kato *et al.*, 1991b). Relationships between the critical period for cortical development and the period during which LTP can be elicited have been identified in rodents. When rats are reared in the dark, the critical period during which closing one eye shifts the ocular dominance of binocular cells in the visual cortex towards the non-deprived eye is lengthened, as is the period during which stimulation of the white matter elicits LTP in layer 4 (Kirkwood and Bear, 1994a; Kirkwood *et al.*, 1995). Similarly, in the developing barrel-field of the somatosensory cortex of rodents, LTP between thalamocortical afferents and cells in cortical layer 4 is found only early in life (Crair and Malenka, 1995). All of these observations suggest an important role for NMDA receptors and the phenomenon of LTP in the development and plasticity of the early cortex. It is not known, however, how activity causes persistent changes in synapses and connections in the developing cortex, nor whether NMDA receptors and LTP are always involved.

Continuous blockade of NMDA receptors by the antagonist AP5 disrupts map refinement in goldfish (Schmidt, 1990); and this also prevents segregation of afferents into ocular dominance stripes in the three-eyed tadpole (Cline *et al.*, 1987, 1990). Infusions of AP5 into cat visual cortex prevents the shift in ocular dominance following monocular deprivation (Kleinschmidt *et al.*, 1987; Bear *et al.*, 1990). These experiments are difficult to interpret because in some cases the blocking agent has more global effects such as on the overall level of activity and so general activity changes cannot be easily distinguished from specific changes to NMDA receptors.

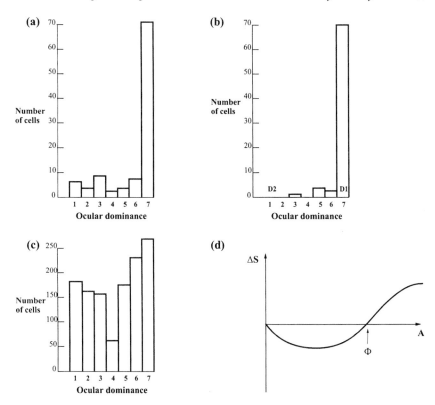

FIG. 6.5. (a–c) Showing the distribution of ocular dominance amongst cells of area 17 of monkey visual cortex. Results from three experimental configurations are shown. (Based on Wiesel, 1982. Reproduced with permission of *Nature*.) The degree of ocularity of individual cells is estimated on a scale of 1–7, where 1 is exclusively activated by the contralateral eye, 7 is exclusively activated by the ipsilateral eye and 4 is activated equally by both eyes. (a) Monocular deprivation: A two-week old monkey had the contralateral eye closed for 18 months (D=deprived). (b) Reverse suture: The ipsilateral eye was closed at 2 days for 3 weeks (D1) and then opened when the contralateral eye was closed for 8 months (D2). Nearly all neurons came to respond to the initially deprived eye. (c) Control data from normal monkeys. (d) The Bienenstock-Cooper-Munro (1982) model of synaptic modification. The magnitude of the synaptic change (ΔS) to be applied to activated synapses (i.e. those whose presynaptic neuron is active) depends on the postsynaptic activity, A. High activity leads to potentiation and low activity to depression. The threshold (Φ) between depression and potentiation is a variable and depends on the mean level of activity in the target cells. In addition, inactive synapses become gradually weakened. Configuration (a) results because the activated synapses from the undeprived eye increase in strength whereas the inactive synapses from the deprived eye weaken. Following reverse suture (b), the activity of the postsynaptic cell is low, lowering the threshold (Φ). This enables the initially low activity from the newly opened eye to bring about a strengthening of its synapses and allowing it to dominate.

Temporal relations in synaptic learning rules

There are now a number of reports from adult cortex showing that when synaptic modification in adult cortex is mediated by a coincident firing of depolarization of the presynaptic and the postsynaptic neurons, the form of the synaptic change will depend on the precise timing relation between presynaptic and postsynaptic stimuli: when the inputs arrived before the action potential, synaptic potentiation resulted; when they arrived afterwards there was depression (e.g. Markram *et al.*, 1997). Recent work on the development of the retinotectal projection in *Xenopus* has highlighted the importance of the temporal aspect of synaptic modification. Zhang *et al.* (1998) made *in vivo* whole cell recordings from neurons in the optic tectum in *Xenopus* tadpoles following repetitive electrical stimulation of retinal neurons in the contralateral eye (which projects to this tectum). They found effects analogous to those discovered previously in adult cortex. Synaptic potentiation resulted when presynaptic activation preceded the postsynaptic action potential by 20 ms; conversely depression resulted when the presynaptic signal succeeded the potential by the same amount of time. There is therefore a 40 ms window during which synaptic modification can take place. Outside this window there is neither potentiation nor depression.

5.3   Models for activity-dependent synaptic modification

A number of different types of models have been advanced to understand the computational power of different types of synaptic modification schemes. Most of them have been formulated in the context of associative memory theory to address the question of what combinations of potentiation and depresssion of synapses would allow the largest number of patterns of activity to be stored and retrieved from a network associative memory. They are known by the generic title of synaptic learning rules. The problem of how topographically ordered maps at least are developed might be thought of in associative memory terms: each input pattern (activity in a small circumscribed group of cells) must elicit a similar output; maximizing pattern storage corresponds to optimizing the precision of the map.

A family of learning rules has been considered in which the amount and sign of the synaptic modification depends on the states of the presynaptic and postsynaptic neurons. The rules differ according to which particular combination of presynaptic and postsynaptic states of the neurons give rise to which type of change in synaptic strength (Fig. 6.6). The earliest of these rules is the covariance rule due to Sejnowski (1977a,b) (Fig. 6.6c). He proposed that the change to be applied to a synaptic strength at any time is calculated from the difference between the presynaptic activity and mean firing rate multiplied by the difference in the postsynaptic activity compared to its mean rate. This means that when the activities in the two neurons are both abnormally high or abnormally low, synapses will be strengthened and when one activity is abnormally high and the other abnormally low the synapse will be weakened. This particular type of learning rule is a more general expression of the

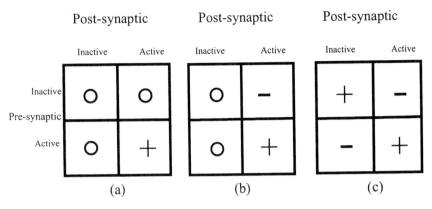

F I G .   6 . 6 .   Various types of synaptic learning rule, for the case when individual changes applied to a synapse are additive. The 2×2 tables show the changes to be applied depending on the states of the presynaptic and postsynaptic neurons, each regarded as existing in one of two states. (a) The Hebb (1949) rule. (b) The Stent (1973) Rule. (c) The optimum Covariance Rule (Sejnowski, 1977a,b; Dayan and Willshaw, 1991). $+$ indicates synaptic strengthening; $\circ$ indicates no change; $-$ indicates weakening.

simple correlation learning rule, called the Hopfield (1982) rule in artificial neural networks circles. According to the proposal due to Hebb (1949), synapses are potentiated only when both presynaptic and postsynaptic elements are concurrently active. According to the rule proposed by Stent (1973; see also Rauschecker and Singer, 1979) (Fig. 6.6b), synaptic modification occurs only when the postsynaptic neuron is active. There is potentiation if the presynaptic neuron is also active and depression if it is inactive.

For associative memories, it is possible to calculate what the best learning rule is for the simplest possible case when the presynaptic and the postsynaptic neurons can exist in just one of two states corresponding to, say, activity or inactivity in the neuron and there is a linear superposition of individual synaptic changes applied to the same synapse (Willshaw and Dayan, 1990; Dayan and Willshaw, 1991). They calculated by how much a synapse should be changed for each of these four possible configurations defining the states of the presynaptic and postsynaptic neurons. The learning rule which yields maximal performance provides for synaptic changes for all of these four states and is the covariance rule already mentioned (Sejnowski, 1977a,b). It has the property that the mean strength of synapses taken over the whole population of synapses is zero, which means that it must be possible for individual synapses to change from having positive to negative effects. The Hebb rule, which does not allow positive and negative changes, is not optimal (Fig. 6.6a).

One synaptic learning rule that has been advanced specifically to account for plasticity in cat visual cortex during the critical period (Wiesel and Hubel, 1963, 1965; Blakemore and Van Sluyters, 1974) is called the BCM rule, after its authors

(Bienenstock *et al.*, 1982). This rule was proposed to account for the findings that:

(a) Monocular deprivation during the critical period leads to a shift in ocular dominance of cortical neurons so that most respond to stimulation of the non-deprived eye (Fig. 6.5a).

(b) Binocular deprivation leaves cells responsive to stimulation through either eye.

(c) The effect of opening an eye that had been previously closed (at the same time closing the eye that had been open) was that the newly opened eye does not recover its ability to excite cortical cells before the newly closed eye has become functionally disconnected (Fig. 6.5b).

According to the BCM rule (Fig. 6.5d), synapses will be modified when the presynaptic neuron is active. Whether the change in synaptic efficacy is positive or negative depends on the level of activity in the postsynaptic neuron. High levels of activity lead to potentiation and low levels lead to depression. The transition between depression and potentiation is defined by a particular threshold level of activity which, according to this model, can change according to the time-averaged level of activity in the postsynaptic neuron. In addition, synapses which connect inactive cells are gradually weakened. These mechanisms make it possible for the basic results of monocular deprivation to be explained. However, empirical information is lacking about whether the modifiable threshold does in fact exist and it is a subject of current research. One possibility is that the threshold can be interpreted as a postsynaptic membrane potential related to the potential at which calcium influx induces LTP through NMDA receptors. In favour of this idea is that application of the NMDA antagonist AP5 disrupts the cellular consequences of monocular deprivation; against this is the suggestion that AP5 has other, more global effects, such as diminishing the level of activity.

5.4   Synaptic rearrangements that do not involve NMDA receptors

Elsewhere in the developing nervous system, the process of synaptic rearrangement can occur without NMDA receptors. A particularly striking example is the neuromuscular junction, which is a cholinergic synapse. In many vertebrate skeletal muscles each muscle fibre has a single endplate which in the adult is innervated by contact from a single motor neuron. It is well known that this pattern of innervation arises from an initial pattern of superinnervation in which there is innervation from a number of different axons at a single endplate (Fig. 6.7). During the first few weeks of neonatal life, contacts are withdrawn until adult configuration is reached (Redfern, 1970). A similar sequence of events has been found to occur at both central and peripheral sites (Crepel *et al.*, 1975; Lichtman, 1977). The same pattern of events takes place in the adult after transection of the motor nerve. In the initial stages of reinnervation, muscle fibres are superinnervated and this pattern is transformed into a pattern of single innervation after a few weeks (McArdle, 1975).

(a)   **Motor nerve axons**

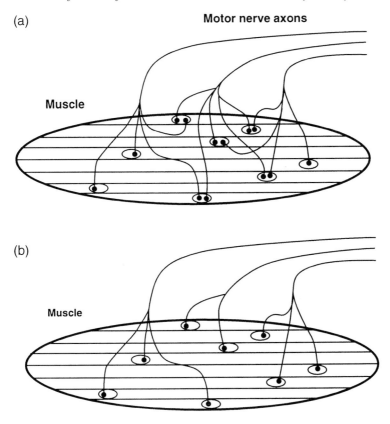

(b)

FIG.   6.7.   Schematic of the states of innervation of mammalian skeletal muscle showing (a) initial superinnervation (b) the adult state where each endplate has contact from a single axon. (After Rasmussen and Willshaw, 1993)

Activity-dependent effects
There is a long and established history of the role of activity during the development and regeneration of nerve connections in the neuromuscular system. For example, tenotomy delays the withdrawal of superinnervation by a moderate amount (Benoit and Changeux, 1975); muscle paralysis results in increased, long-lasting levels of polyneuronal innervation (Thompson *et al.*, 1979), as does application of TTX to the motor nerve (Taxt, 1983); chronic muscle stimulation accelerates the elimination of synapses during development (O'Brien *et al.*, 1978; Thompson, 1983). To investigate the selective effects of activity, experiments on the reinnervation of neuromuscular connections have been carried out on the fourth deep lumbrical muscle of the rat, which has two nerve supplies which can be manipulated independently. The rat lumbrical muscle has a major input, comprising about ten motor units, and a minor input comprising about one to four motor units (Betz *et al.*, 1979). A comprehensive series of experiments involving nerve cut or crush

combined with nerve block by continual perfusion of TTX through a cuff surrounding one or both of these nerves has enabled a systematic investigation of the effects of activity on elimination of superinnervation during regeneration of connections (e.g. Ribchester and Taxt, 1983, 1984; Ribchester, 1993). It turns out that active synapses (i.e. those whose activity has not been blocked by TTX) have an advantage over inactive synapses.

After cutting or crushing both nerves, the regenerating motor axons initially superinnervate the muscle fibres and over the following few weeks the pattern of single innervation is re-established. When just one nerve is cut or crushed, at the same time as these motor axons reinnervate the muscle, the motor unit sizes of the incumbent projection expand; i.e. the axons of this nerve come to innervate the endplates formerly occupied by the operated nerve. Over the next few weeks, motor units of the regenerated axons gradually increase in size, presumably pushing off the axons from the expanded projection. Broadly speaking, the effect of blocking one of the nerves by TTX during such manipulations is to assign a competitive advantage to the active synapses as against the inactive synapses (i.e. those made by the axons from the nerve blocked by TTX). For example, in the experiments in which a regenerating nerve can 'regain' its territory, its ability to regain territory is enhanced if the other nerve is blocked and is diminished if the regenerating nerve is blocked (Ribchester and Taxt, 1983, 1984). Activity is not the sole driving force behind the elimination of superinnervation as shown by the fact that a nerve blocked with TTX will still withdraw its innervation to make a pattern of singular innervation, albeit at a slower rate (Ribchester, 1993). Other experiments on rabbit soleus suggest a competitive advantage to inactivated motor axons (Callaway *et al.*, 1987, 1989).

Recent experiments by Ballice-Gordon and Lichtman (1994) have investigated how it is that terminals at the same endplate from the same axon behave differently from terminals from different axons. During the elimination of superinnervation, terminals from the same axon are either both eliminated or both remain; when two terminals are from different axons, just one of them is eliminated. They suggested that the basis for this effect is that terminals from the same axon are likely to be simultaneously active whereas terminals from different axons are not and it is the imbalance of activity that drives the withdrawal process. In support of their hypothesis, they showed that when part of the postsynaptic membrane at an endplate is blocked by focal application of the receptor blocker α-bungarotoxin, then the terminals above it (which have become inactive) are withdrawn, driven by a difference in activity between the unblocked and blocked terminals. In contrast, when the whole membrane is blocked or when none of it is blocked, creating no imbalance in activity, there is no effect.

5.5   Molecular link between activity and synaptic change

A crucial and unresolved issue concerns the nature of the molecules that translate activity into synaptic changes, for example following activation of NMDA receptors, or the nature of those that are the resource for which developing synapses compete. There is evidence that these molecules might be, or might include, the neurotrophins. Neurotrophins can very rapidly modulate the strengths of synapses in the hippocampus (Kang and Schumann, 1995; Figurov *et al.*, 1996) and at the neuromuscular junction (Lohof *et al.*, 1993). Therefore, they have been considered as strong candidates for retrograde signals, released by the postsynaptic cell in response to activation, that regulate the growth and strength of the presynaptic input. Moreover, there is evidence that neurotrophins can up-regulate the expression of their own receptors.

There is further evidence that the neurotrophins are involved in the longer-term synaptic rearrangement that occurs in the visual cortex during normal ocular dominance development or in response to visual deprivation. Neural activity regulates levels of the neurotrophin BDNF mRNA in rat visual cortex (Castren *et al.*, 1992). Several experiments have shown that infusion of neurotrophins into the developing visual cortex can prevent the formation of ocular dominance columns or shifts of ocular dominance towards the non-deprived eye following monocular deprivation (Cabelli *et al.*, 1995; Carmignoto *et al.*, 1993).

A theory proposed by Lamberto Maffei (Maffei *et al.*, 1992; Domenici *et al.*, 1994) is that during ocular dominance column segregation, the two eyes are in competition for neurotrophic factors. The production of these factors may be dependent on the number and pattern of spikes in the cortical afferents and the amount of trophic factor required by a neuron to maintain its viability or its axon may also depend on its level of activity. Thus, correlated activity may, via Hebbian processes, establish complex patterns of innervation, such as ocular dominance columns or clustered intrinsic connections between iso-orientation domains, and these mechanisms may operate within an environment in which competitive interactions are prominent. The fact that not only is correlated activity important but also competitive mechanisms are at work is suggested by challenges to the developing system that either assign a competitive advantage to one set of axons over another or alter the levels of factors for which the sets of axons may be competing. Monocular deprivation during the critical period of development produces the condition of amblyopia (blindness caused by disuse). Cortical territory is dominated by inputs from the non-deprived eye, whereas those afferents from the deprived eye have a correspondingly weak influence (Fig 6.5a). The receptive fields of cells in the deprived eye have reduced acuity, as assessed on the basis of their contrast-sensitivity function. However, if monocular deprivation during the critical period is accompanied by infusion of nerve growth factor into the cortex, the shift in ocular dominance and the loss of acuity is prevented. In addition, infusion of NGF prevents the reduction of cell soma diameter in the LGN that occurs after monocular deprivation. When endogenous NGF is blocked by placing hybridoma cells producing antibodies against NGF into the hemispheres, LGN cells shrink and acuity is impaired.

One possible explanation for these findings is that the competitive mechanisms that regulate the segregation of inputs from the two eyes during normal development, or the domination of cortical territory by inputs from a normal as opposed to a deprived eye, are abolished when the resource for which the inputs normally compete is present in excess. However, uncertainties remain. It is not clear whether the neurotrophins act directly on LGN axons in the infusion experiments. Different experiments have suggested roles for particular neurotrophins. Thus, Carmignoto *et al.* (1993) have evidence that NGF infusion blocks shifts in ocular dominance in response to monocular deprivation, yet the high affinity receptor for NGF, TrkA, is at best only weakly expressed in the LGN and cortex (Allendoerfer *et al.*, 1994; Lotto *et al.*, 1997). This raises the possibility that the NGF infused in these experiments is acting indirectly, via the NGF-sensitive basal forebrain cholinergic system, which is known to influence cortical plasticity (Kasamatsu and Pettigrew, 1976; Bear and Singer, 1986). Other infusion experiments have suggested that BDNF and NT4 may be more directly involved in ocular dominance development and plasticity (Cabelli *et al.*, 1995). The high affinity receptor for these ligands is present in the LGN and cortex (Allendoerfer *et al.*, 1994; Lotto *et al.*, 1997), but even so a direct action has not been proven. It is known that neurotrophins including BDNF and NT4 can influence the health and viability of developing thalamic and LGN neurons under normal or deprived conditions (Riddle *et al.*, 1995; Lotto *et al.*, 1997), and so there is a real possibility that the neurotrophins simply act in a permissive way, allowing other molecules to orchestrate appropriate responses to normal or abnormal patterns of activity.

If competition for a limited supply of a crucial target-derived resource is the basis for the synaptic changes that occur during the critical period of cortical development, one might predict that this period of rearrangement and plasticity would end if the endogenous supply of the resource by the cortex were to reach high enough levels. If thalamic explants are cultured with cortical explants, diffusible factors from the cortical explants can stimulate the growth of axons from the thalamus (Rennie *et al.*, 1994; Lotto and Price, 1994, 1995). The older the cortical explant, the greater the stimulatory effect, until a plateau of activity is reached at a time that coincides with the end of the period of plasticity of cortical afferent connections (i.e. the end of the critical period). These results are compatible with the idea that the cortex produces growth factors that are initially in limited supply but later increase in concentration to the point where competition is reduced and connections are stabilized. The factors mediating this *in vitro* effect are not known. There is evidence that the cortical production of several neurotrophic factors, including neurotrophins and FGFs, increases during the same period of time *in vivo*, suggesting these molecules as candidates (Price *et al.*, 1995). It is also possible that the ending of the critical period of rearrangement involves changes in the expression of molecules that somehow consolidate whatever changes have occurred by then or block further changes. There have been several studies that have identified transiently expressed molecules whose time of expression is compatible with such a role, but as yet there no strong evidence for their involvement (Sur *et al.*, 1988; Hendrickson *et al.*, 1991; Van Huizen *et al.*, 1988; Jia *et al.*, 1990; McIntosh *et al.*, 1990; Shoen *et al.*, 1990; Imamura *et al.*, 1992).

5.6   Models of competition

One problem with understanding how competitive effects can be mediated in the nervous system is that the term 'competition' has been used in many different and often conflicting ways. Constructing formal models of competition has the advantage that it will be clear what is meant by this term and what are the consequences of any competitive scheme.

In its dictionary sense, competition means 'act of seeking or striving for something in rivalry with others', each individual attempting to acquire as much of a fixed amount of some resource as possible and thus at the expense of the others. In the neurobiological context the individuals are the terminals of the axons that 'attempt to stabilize their contact on their target at the expense of others'.

In the first models of competition, the entity that was intended to be in fixed supply was some morphological property of the nervous system, such as numbers of synaptic contacts or extent of arborization. For example, in their model of competition for the development of nerve connections, Prestige and Willshaw (1975) assumed that presynaptic cells and postsynaptic cells each make only a limited number of contacts; i.e. the presynaptic cells compete to capture the contacts from the postsynaptic cells and *vice versa*. The number of contacts is therefore the resource that is conserved. Similarly in Swindale's (1980) model for the development of occularity stripes it is assumed that the axons originating from the two eyes compete for the limited number of termination sites available in the cortex. Smallheiser and Crain (1984) assumed that the number of contacts made by each motor neuron in innervating muscle fibres is limited. In their model for the development of nerve connections in cortex, Devor and Schneider (1975) assumed a conservation of arbor principle; that is, the spatial extent of each axonal arborization is limited. Many models of nerve connections define the mapping of one set of cells onto another in terms of the pattern of individual synaptic strengths. In many of these models the total amount of synaptic strength assigned to the contacts of each cell is often kept constant. This is a way of introducing competition into the system because as the strength of one synapse of an axon increases then the strength of another synapse made by that axon must decrease. This is referred to as synaptic normalization and ensures the stability of the system (von der Malsburg and Willshaw, 1981). A simple example of such a scheme is the model due to Willshaw (1981) for the elimination of superinnervation in the developing muscular system. Following experimental work due to O'Brien *et al.* (1978), he proposed that elimination of contacts proceeds under the action of two processes. First, each synapse emits a signal that degrades all terminals at its endplate, at a rate proportional to its own synaptic strength. Secondly, synaptic terminals become continually replenished so as to keep the sum of strengths of all the synapses available to each motor axon at a constant value. According to this very simple scheme, any pattern of superinnervation will be transformed to one of single innervation and other experimental facts, such as the decrease in variability of motor unit size over development (Brown *et al.*, 1976), are accounted for. However, like most schemes of this type, the process of synapse normalization is justified only at the general level of conservation of resources and not in terms of any underlying mechanism.

Such a mechanism can be quite complicated as it involves communication between all the spatially distributed terminals made by each axon.

In constructing models of competition, two basic questions need to be addressed. First, competition implies that there is some entity in limited supply which is the subject of the competition; if there is no such constraint there is no competition. For example, in the case modelled by Prestige and Willshaw (1975), if each cell can make a potentially infinite number of connections then no ordered map results. It must then be decided what this entity is. In the neurobiological case usually this is assumed to be something directly related to synaptic efficacy, such as the size of the terminal or the number of bound receptors.

Secondly, it must be decided how the process of competition acts. Schemes involving competition for a fixed amount of resource or competition for a resource which is generated at a fixed rate are both possible.

Fixed resource models

The model due to Willshaw (1981) cited above is of this type, the resource being the total strength of synapses made by each motor neuron. Another example is found in the model due to Gouzé *et al.* (1983), who assumed that each muscle has a fixed amount of factor which is taken up preferentially by the synapses innervating it. The rate of uptake by any particular synapse is an escalating function of its own strength. Under the operation of this mechanism, at each end plate one synapse acquires a very large amount of factor at the expense of the others. However, this model is extremely sensitive to the choice of parameter values, which have to be adjusted for different numbers of muscle fibres and motor neurons. Rasmussen and Willshaw (1993) developed the more sophisticated earlier model due to Bennett and Robinson (1989) for the elimination of hyperinnervation from developing muscle. In the Dual Constraint Model (Rasmussen and Willshaw, 1993) it is assumed that there are factors in both the motorneuron and the muscles for which the synapses compete. A synapse is thought to be formed by a reversible binding of a substance A, provided from the motor neuron, to a substance B, derived from the muscle. Both presynaptic and postsyaptic factors are assumed to be limited in supply. Plausible reaction equations were devised for the allocation of A to the terminals of each motorneuron and for the binding of A to B. Rasmussen and Willshaw showed how the phenomenon of 'intrinsic withdrawal' can be accounted for within this framework. Intrinsic withdrawal is an effect observed in muscles where removal of most of the motor units from the developing muscle gives rise to incomplete innervation of the adult muscle. It was found that motor unit size was independent of the number of surviving motor units (Fladby and Jansen, 1987). It was argued that if withdrawal of innervation is entirely a competitive process, the larger the number of competing motor neurons, the smaller the motor unit size should be and so this result suggests a process of withdrawal that is independent of the competition. This could mean that, when a single motor neuron innervates the muscle, there could be withdrawal of innervation at an endplate that already has contact from a single axon. The analysis of Rasmussen and Willshaw (1993) of the Dual Constraint Model (Fig. 6.8) showed that for a synapse to be stable it

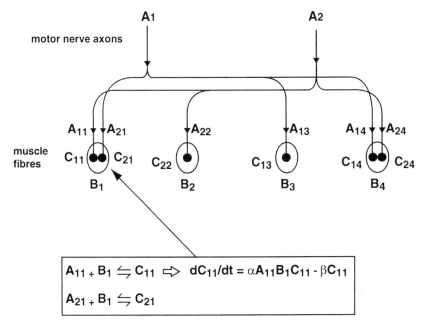

FIG. 6.8. The Dual Constraint Model for the elimination of superinnervation in developing muscle. Presynaptic factor, *A*, binds with postsynaptic factor, *B*, to make complex, *C*, that builds the synapse. The equation shown specifies how *A* and *B* are converted into *C* for the synapse made by axon terminal 1 at endplate 1. (After Rasmussen and Willshaw, 1993)

must be built of certain minimum amounts of presynaptic and postsynaptic factors. As the amounts of both presynaptic and postsynaptic factor available are limited, this means that a motor neuron can support only a certain maximum number of terminals. If this number is less than the number formed when the motor neuron initially innervates the muscle there is bound to be elimination of contacts. This provides an explanation for intrinsic withdrawal.

In this theoretical approach, one unanswered question concerns the identity of the presynaptic and postsynaptic factors which are assumed to interact to build the synapse. Joseph and Willshaw (1996) suggested that the protein Agrin (McMahan, 1990) could act as the presynaptic factor, binding to free acetylcholine receptors, the postsynaptic factor. The advantage of this scheme is that it explains naturally certain activity-dependent effects such as those involving partial or complete block of individual nerve terminals (Section 5.4) (Ballice-Gordon and Lichtman, 1994).

Competition for resources generated at fixed rate
Fixed resource models have the disadvantage that they will only work if there are no losses of any kind in the system. This seems biologically implausible. An alternative approach is that used in population biology and epidemiology where it is assumed that interactions between predators and preys are driven by the

(a)

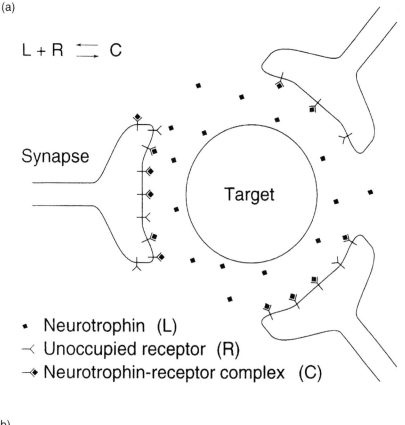

$$L + R \; \rightleftarrows \; C$$

Synapse

Target

• Neurotrophin (L)
⤙ Unoccupied receptor (R)
⤙• Neurotrophin-receptor complex (C)

(b)

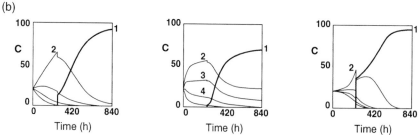

FIG. 6.9. The van Ooyen and Willshaw model (1999) for the development of nerve connections by up-regulation of receptors by neurotrophin. (a) A single target neuron innervated by a number of different axons. For nerve terminal i, presynaptic receptors R_i bind to neurotrophin L (ligand) to form complex C_i. For constant rate of neurotrophin production, σ, and variable receptor production, ϕ_i, the rates of production of C_i, R_i and L are $dC_i/dt = k_a L R_i - k_d C_i - \rho C_i$; $dR_i/dt = \phi_i - k_a L R_i + k_d C_i - \gamma R_i$; $dL/dt = \sigma - \delta L - k_a L R_i + k_d C_i$ where $k_a, k_d, \rho, \gamma, \delta$ are reaction and decay constants. The rate of production, ϕ_i, of receptor is $d\phi_i/dt + \phi_i = q(f(C_i))$ where q is a multiplying constant and $f()$ the up-regulation function, specifying how the steady state rate of production of receptors depends on the amount of bound neurotrophin, C. (b) Illustrating the effects of different up-regulation functions on the patterns of connections that develop.

competition for a resource or resources generated at fixed rate (Yodzis, 1989). In the neurobiological case, the competition can be thought in terms of a different number of predators (axonal terminals) taking up some resource that is generated at a fixed rate, converting it into synaptic structures, and being subject to absorption and other types of loss. Jeanprêtre *et al.* (1996) were the first to suggest such a scheme and they have examined its stability as applied to the development of neuromuscular connections. More recently, van Ooyen and Willshaw (1999) have proposed a model for the building of synapses by the reversible binding of target-derived neurotrophin (such as NGF or BDNF) to their presynaptic receptors (Fig. 6.9). They examined the case of a single target cell that initially is innervated by a number of different axons and they explored the hypothesis that the density of presynaptic receptors is up-regulated by the amount of bound neurotrophin (Bernd and Greene, 1984; Lindsay *et al.*, 1990; Holtzman *et al.*, 1992; Li *et al.*, 1995a; ElShamy *et al.*, 1996). Using conventional reaction dynamics with reaction constant values derived from the experimental literature for NGF, they devised equations showing how (i) the amount of available neurotrophin (L), (ii) the number of free receptors (R), (iii) the amount of bound receptor complex (C; taken to be the 'size' of the synapse) vary over time. In this scheme, the crucial component is the receptor up-regulation function; that is, how the rate of production of receptor varies with the amount of bound neurotrophin under steady state conditions. Van Ooyen and Willshaw (1999) showed that different types of up-regulation function lead to different patterns of innervation. For any particular up-regulation functions, they were able to show the effect of (1) a decrease in the supply of neurotrophin, (2) changes in the level of activity (there is evidence that this changes the amount of neurotrophin receptor (Birren *et al.*, 1992; Cohen-Cory *et al.*, 1993)), (3) whether the pattern of connections that is regenerated following severance of the nerve is the same or can be different from the pattern of innervation initially developed. For one of the up-regulation functions examined, under conditions when a pattern of single innervation is normally developed, after regeneration it is possible for dual innervation to occur. Persistent multiple innervation is found in partial denervation experiments after reinnervation and recovery from prolonged nerve

---

Changes of the amounts of binding complex, C, at different terminals over time in the case when initially there are 4 axons and a contact from a new axon, numbered 1, is introduced after 250 hours. *Left hand figure*: linear upregulation function. A pattern of single innervation is restored in which axon 1 has replaced axon 2. *Middle figure*: non-linear, up-regulation function of the Hill type. A pattern of multiple innervation is restored in which axon 1 has replaced axon 4. *Right hand figure*: non-linear up-regulation function of the Michaelis-Menten type. The pattern of multiple innervation has been replaced by one of single innervation. These figures illustrate that for some up-regulation functions the equilibrium pattern of innervation attained is independent of the initial conditions and for some functions it is dependent on the initial conditions (*right hand figure*). All reaction constants in the equations were assigned physiologically realistic values. See van Ooyen and Willshaw (1999) for more details.

conduction block (Barry and Ribchester, 1995). As interpreted on this model, the conduction block causes the systems to reach abnormal equilibrium states, thereby allowing multiple innervation. This analysis provides a framework which links the phenomenology of the innervation pattern formed and the underlying biochemistry. There is a need for quantitative evidence of the nature of the up-regulation function. For a particular developing system, if the form of the up-regulation function can be discovered then the pattern of innervation can be predicted.

6 THE REGULATION OF THE DENDRITIC GROWTH OF CORTICAL NEURONS

Each layer of the cerebral cortex contains neurons with characteristic connections, physiological properties, and dendritic arbors. The way in which a neuron's dendritic arbor develops will determine the number and pattern of synaptic connections that the neuron receives. The development of unique physiological properties (outlined in Chapter 7) is determined in at least large part by the elaboration of dendrites, since these are the sites of most synapses. Cortical neurons undergo extensive, highly regulated dendritic growth soon after they have completed migration. The final form of dendritic arbors is determined by intrinsic developmental programmes (Banker and Cowan, 1979; Bartlett and Banker, 1984) and local extracellular signals including levels and patterns of activity (Bailey and Kandel, 1993). However, the molecular signals that influence and instruct the development of dendritic patterns are largely unknown.

One group of molecules that has been examined for a possible role in this process are the neurotrophic factors. Members of this family of proteins and their receptors are expressed by neurons in the cerebral cortex and they have been shown to influence dendritic arborization patterns in the peripheral nervous system (Purves *et al.*, 1988; Ruit and Snider, 1991) and the arborization of axons in the optic nerve (Cohen-Cory and Fraser, 1995). Recent experiments suggest a role for the neurotrophins in influencing connectivity and dendritic arborizations within the cortex.

McAllister *et al.* (1995) used a technique called biolistics to label a proportion of the developing neurons in slices of cortex, by transfection with a gene for β galactosidase, and then showed that exogenous application of neurotrophins to the slices altered the growth and complexity of dendritic processes. Neurons within each layer of the cortex responded to a particular subset of neurotrophins, as follows.

Basal dendrites in each layer tended to be stimulated maximally by a specific factor. In layer 4, they were enhanced maximally by BDNF. Dendrites were longer, more numerous, more branched, and covered with more dendritic spines. In layer 5, they were enhanced maximally by NT4, and the effect was similar to that of BDNF on layer 4 neurons. In layer 6, they were enhanced maximally by NT4. This was the only layer in which there was any response to NT3 with an increase in length of dendritic spines. An unusual finding in layer 6 was that BDNF and NGF tended to decrease dendritic growth. Apical dendrites tended to respond to a wider range of neurotrophins than the basal dendrites.

Neurons in layer 4 responded to all four neurotrophins, although BDNF was still the most effective. The apical dendrites of neurons in layer 5 were most strongly affected by BDNF. In layer 6 results were similar to those for the basal dendrites although no negative effect of any of the neurotrophins was observed. These results indicate that the neurotrophins could be involved in establishing the final dendritic form of neurons in the cortex.

In more recent work, McAllister *et al.* (1997) looked at the effects of the neurotrophins endogenous to the cortex on dendritic growth. This was done by manipulating neurotrophin signalling in organotypic slices by addition of exogenous neurotrophins to increase levels or by addition of Trk-IgGs to neutralize endogenous neurotrophins. They found that blocking endogenous BDNF markedly reduced dendritic complexity in layer 4 with a greater effect on the basal dendrites. Blocking NGF receptors had little effect. Neutralizing the effects of endogenous NT3 had the surprising effect of increasing basal dendrite growth, suggesting that NT3 may play a role in limiting dendritic growth. It therefore appears that BDNF and NT3 have opposing effects on the dendritic growth of layer 4 neurons. In layer 6, BDNF and NT3 were found to have opposing effects but with reversed roles. These results suggest that both exogenous and endogenous neurotrophic factors modulate the dendritic arborisation patterns of pyramidal neurons in the visual cortex. It appears that the neurotrophins can function in both positive and negative directions to regulate dendritic growth.

7 MODELS OF DENDRITIC GROWTH

A variety of attempts have been made to construct complex models of the generation of the complex pattern of dendritic branches. The basic assumption is that the dendritic tree is developed from an initially unbranched structure by extra branches being generated at the tips of the dendrites to produce over time a more and more elaborate structure. Generally it is assumed that when branching occurs, just two branches are generated at each branch point, or node. This process has been modelled in two ways. In one approach, it is attempted to discover a set of simple principles by which the dendritic tree could have been generated, such as whether dendrites are grown by random branching. Sadler and Berry (1984) and Berry and Flinn (1984) examined the dendritic trees of Purkinje cells of the cerebellum at various developmental stages. There are three different possible types of branch point in each dendritic tree: (i) branch points which themselves lead to two further branch points; (ii) those that lead to one terminal node and one branch point; (iii) those that lead to two terminal nodes. They found that the numbers of nodes of these three types were inconsistent with those numbers that would be generated were dendritic branching at random. They concluded that Purkinje cells' dendritic trees

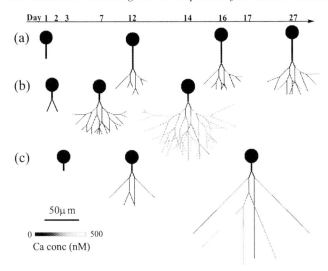

F I G .   6 . 1 0 . Shows various types of dendritic trees generated according to the model of Hely *et al.* (1999). The effect of varying the dephosphorylation reaction rates is to change the rate of branching over time. (a) Branching rate increases over time. (b) Branching rate is constant over time. (c) Branching rate decreases over time.

are sculpted by other factors, such as being crowded by growth of dendritic arbors of Purkinje cells nearby. This type of approach exemplifies the class of mathematical models of branching (van Pelt and Verwer, 1986; Kliemann, 1987; Burke *et al.*, 1992; Dityatev *et al.*, 1995; van Pelt *et al.*, 1997) where the emphasis is on attempting to account for the wide variety of branching patterns seen in different cells in terms of a set of probabilistic rules specified by as few parameters as possible.

The other approach attempts to develop a model for branching that is biologically justified. The drawback of this type of model is that it can account only for a small number of different types of arborization pattern (Li *et al.*, 1992; Albinet and Pelce, 1996; Hentschel and Fine, 1996). Hely *et al.* (1999) have developed a new compartmental model for dendritic branching involving the microtubule associated protein 2 (MAP2) (Fig. 6.10). MAP2 is found in dendrites and is a member of the MAP family of proteins (Maccioni and Cambiazo, 1995) which is involved in many aspects of microtubule dynamics. The model is based on the idea that phosphorylated MAP2 favours branching of dendrites whereas dephosphorylated MAP2 favours elongation. It is proposed that the rate of elongation and branching is determined by the relative concentrations of phosphorylated and dephosphorylated MAP2. This itself is dependent on the concentration of intracellular calcium through the action of calmoduline-dependent protein kinase 2 and calcineurin. The performance of the model compares favourably with other models of a more mathematical nature. As this model is based on the underlying biology there are predictions that can be made from it, particularly that dendritic branching patterns will be sensitive to changes in the concentrations of calcium and of phosphorylated MAP2.

7

Functional development of the cortex

1 OVERVIEW

In the preceding chapters, we discussed some of the mechanisms that control the early development of the cerebral cortex, including its emergence as a distinct region of the forebrain, the growth of its afferent and efferent axonal pathways, and its subdivision into cortical areas with different properties. We have seen how the biochemical processes that regulate events such as cell division, cell migration, axonal growth, and other features of differentiation (such as cell type, neurotransmitter phenotype, etc.) are controlled by factors within the cells, such as regulatory genes, and factors from their environment, such as intercellular signalling molecules. Essentially, most of our discussion has concerned the mechanisms that guide the development of the cellular structure of the cortex. What about the mechanisms that guide the development of cortical function? These two issues overlap considerably, since cellular structure underlies function. However much knowledge we have of the development of structure, we would need to have additional information to understand fully the generation of cortical function. We would also need to know about the functional properties of synapses, of the regions of the cell on which they are located, of the way in which impulses are transmitted through the postsynaptic cell, of how these impulses summate, and so on. In a sense, all of the work described in the previous chapters will contribute towards answering the question: what are the mechanisms that generate cortical function? But a full answer to that question will come only when we know about all the mechanisms that generate every single aspect of cortical structure, including all its cells, their connections, and their functional properties. Given that the human brain consists

(a)

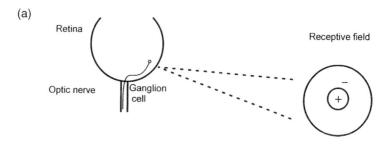

(b)

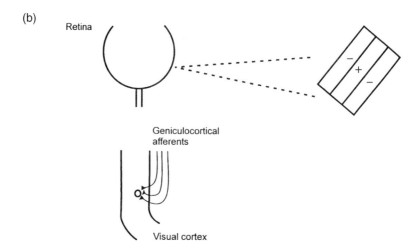

FIG. 7.1. Receptive fields in the adult visual system. (a) Diagram of the retina and optic nerve. Ganglion cells in the retina project to the lateral geniculate nucleus (Fig. 4.3, Chapter 4). In common with other sensory neurons, ganglion cells have a background rate of activity in the absence of stimulation. The activity of ganglion cells is regulated by the activity of the photoreceptors that are connected to it. If light is shone onto those photoreceptors, the ganglion cell responds either by increasing or decreasing its activity. The total area of the retina from which either a positive or negative response is the receptive field. The arrangement of the inhibitory and excitatory areas are shown for a typical ganglion cell (not all conform to this pattern). The receptive field is circular and light shone in the centre excites the cell whereas light shone in the surround inhibits it. The effects of light shone on centre and surround simultaneously cancel. (b) Receptive fields of cells in the visual cortex are the result of convergence of inputs from several geniculate cells (Fig. 5.2b, Chapter 5), whose receptive fields are similar to those in (a). Typical (not all) cortical cells have rectangular receptive fields; i.e. light shone on a rectangular shaped area of the retina (*top* of the diagram) will produce a response, either excitatory or inhibitory, in the cortical cell (*bottom* of the diagram). For some cortical cells, called simple cells, the receptive field has clearly segregated excitatory and inhibitory regions with a typical arrangement as shown here. The cell is excited optimally by a bar of light of the correct orientation and size to fit exactly over the excitatory region of the receptive field without straying into the inhibitory regions. Thus, the receptive field of the cell

of 10–15 billion cells connected by perhaps 100 000 billion synapses, the prospect of gaining all this information seems remote.

Nevertheless, the issue of functional development does have another side to it. It is possible to measure the functional properties of the cortex and its neurons as it develops. Essentially, this approach provides one way of observing development and the analysis can be done at the level of single cells or any higher level up to that of the entire structure. The functional methods that have been applied to the growing cortex have provided some insight into the mechanisms that may regulate cortical development, although their explanatory power is limited. Results are often interpreted in the light of findings in other types of study. In this chapter we first consider the development of the functional attributes of individual cortical cells in the sensory system (in particular the visual system). We then consider what conclusions about mechanisms of cortical development can be drawn from studies of the developing brain as a whole.

2   RECEPTIVE FIELD PROPERTIES IN SENSORY CORTEX

The receptive field of any sensory neuron, however many synapses removed it is from the sensory receptors, is defined as the area of the sensory surface that, when stimulated, evokes a response in that sensory neuron. Receptive fields have certain properties that may be relatively simple or highly complex; some examples of the simpler properties are given in Chapter 5. For example, in the visual system, cells in the retina or lateral geniculate nucleus typically have circular receptive fields divided into regions—light shone on circumscribed regions will activate the cell, light shone on other regions will inhibit it (Fig. 7.1a). Many cells in the visual cortex have rectangular receptive fields and these display a range of additional properties—for example, some have separate regions that activate or inhibit the cell, others do not (Fig. 7.1b). Neurons in the visual cortex are tuned to particular stimuli; in other words their response is strongest to a particular value of the stimulus and it declines monotonically as stimulus values depart from the optimum. For example, they may be tuned to the particular orientation of a line stimulus (as can often be predicted by the rectangular shape of their receptive fields; Fig. 7.1) (Hubel and Wiesel, 1962), to the direction of motion of the stimulus (Hubel and Wiesel, 1962; Dubner and Zeki, 1971) or to more elaborate stimuli

---

is said to be oriented, and the cortical cell has an orientation preference (i.e. it is tuned to a particular orientation). When the optimal stimulus is rotated, it will cease to stimulate some of the excitatory centre and start to activate the inhibitory flanking regions, giving a suboptimum response that will lessen further as the stimulus continues to rotate away from the optimum. Some cortical cells do not show segregated excitatory and inhibitory sub-regions and, although they may show orientation tuning, their responses are not necessarily predictable on the basis of their receptive field structure. Such cells are called complex cells.

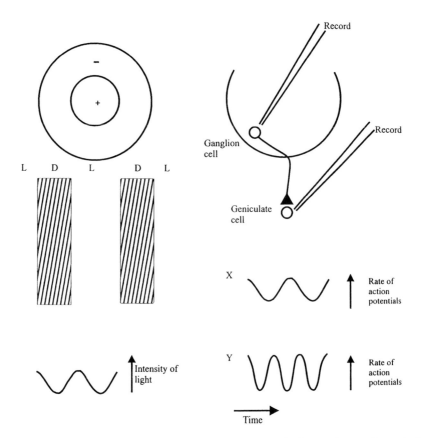

FIG. 7.2. Receptive fields of ganglion and lateral geniculate nucleus cells (typical example is shown *top left*) can be stimulated by repeating patterns, such as gratings of alternating light (L) and dark (D) stripes. The intensity of light may be made to vary in a stepwise fashion (square wave grating, *middle left*) or sinusoidally (*bottom left*). Such patterns can be moved across the receptive fields of ganglion cells or geniculate cells and their responses studied (*top right*). As the grating is moved, the activity of these cells varies. Some cells are maximally stimulated when the light bar falls over the excitatory region of the cell and the dark bars fall over the inhibitory region; they are maximally inhibited when the dark bar falls over the excitatory region and the light bars fall over the inhibitory region. The response of such cells to a moving sinusoidal grating fluctuates around the background activity level of the cell and the rate of action potential production is in phase with (and linearly related to the position of) the moving stimulus (*middle right*). Such cells are called X cells. The activity of other cells in response to a sinusoidal grating is not linearly related to the position of the stimulus (*bottom right*). Such cells may increase their mean firing rate and their activity may fluctuate with a higher frequency. The mechanisms that generate this response are not understood. Such cells are called Y cells. A third class of ganglion and geniculate cells has been discovered; these respond sluggishly to light and are called W cells (not illustrated).

such as faces (Perrett *et al.*, 1982; Sergent *et al.*, 1992). In the same way, neurons are tuned to specific stimuli in other sensory areas of the cortex; for example, many somatosensory neurons are tuned to the frequency of vibration (Talbot *et al.*, 1968; Mountcastle *et al.*, 1969) and many auditory neurons are tuned to the frequency of a sound (Kiang *et al.*, 1965) (Fig. 5.1c, Chapter 5).

The visual detection of spatially repeating patterns, such as a sinusoidally varying pattern of intensity (illustrated in Fig. 7.2), both by human observers (in psychophysical tests) and by single neurons has been studied intensively. In the retina and lateral geniculate nucleus, the use of such stimuli led to the identification of two classes of cell, termed X and Y in cat, as described in the next section. Grating patterns have also proved extremely useful for comparing the functional properties of single visual cortical cells with those of the entire system (Parker and Hawken, 1985; Hawken and Parker, 1990). The conclusion from such studies is that at least some cortical neurons can perform as well as the entire organism in discriminating sensory stimuli (Parker and Newsome, 1998).

The receptive field properties of cortical sensory neurons are the product of the convergent input that they receive. An obvious example of this is the presence of cells that can be activated through either eye (i.e. binocular cells) in the visual cortex. These binocular receptive fields are created through the convergence of largely monocular afferents from the lateral geniculate nucleus onto individual cortical cells. Models have been proposed to explain how convergence of afferents representing several receptive field positions on the retina creates oriented cortical receptive fields (Fig. 5.2b, see also Chapter 5). In principle, information on how the receptive field properties of cortical cells develop, as described in the next section, is interpretable in terms of changes in the convergence and nature of the inputs to those cells. Understanding these synaptic changes ought to give considerable insight into the mechanisms that generate the perceptual abilities of the system as a whole. We are still a long way from such an understanding.

3 DEVELOPMENT OF RECEPTIVE FIELD PROPERTIES IN THE VISUAL CORTEX

We now discuss the development of receptive field properties of cells that are more complex than those discussed in Chapter 5. The maturation of receptive field properties has been studied extensively using electrophysiological methods in both the striate and extrastriate cortex of the cat and monkey (for example Blakemore and Van Sluyters, 1975; Blakemore *et al.*, 1978; Albus and Wolf, 1984; Blakemore and Price, 1987a; Price *et al.*, 1988; Blakemore, 1988; Zumbroich *et al.*, 1988a). The receptive field properties of visual cortical neurons mature rapidly as the afferent pathways develop. Visual responses have been recorded from the cortex of kittens as young as six days postnatal. In both striate and extrastriate cortex, visually responsive neurons are found primarily in deep cortical layers in kittens aged 14 days or less; during this period, almost all cells in the superficial part of the cortex remain unresponsive to visual stimuli. The eyelids of kittens normally separate at around postnatal day 10, but even in visually inexperienced kittens aged six or seven days (with eyelids opened under anaesthesia immediately before recording), many of the responsive cells that lie deep in the cortex display an innate orientation preference.

The receptive fields of cells in the visual cortex have been divided into two classes, simple and complex (Hubel and Wiesel, 1962, 1963). Simple cells have mutually antagonistic, spatially segregated subregions within their receptive fields, and their preferred stimulus can be predicted from a knowledge of the arrangement of these subregions following their delineation with a small spot of light. Within the subregions, be they excitatory or inhibitory, there is spatial summation so that the larger the stimulus, the greater the response. It is not possible to predict the preferred stimulus of complex cells in the same fashion, and they often respond at all points in their receptive fields when a spot of light is turned both on and off. The studies of Blakemore and Van Sluyters (1975) and Blakemore and Price (1987a) suggest that most of the selective cortical responses in very young kittens are from cells that are clearly dissimilar to complex cells and have some, but not all, of the characteristics of adult simple cells. These cells have been called immature simple cells (Blakemore and Price, 1987a).

As the kitten matures, the proportion of visually responsive cells in the deep cortical layers increases and receptive field properties become progressively more refined. Complex cells appear and orientation tuning becomes narrower (Blakemore and Price, 1987a). The development of the superficial cortical layers initially lags behind that of the deep layers, but later catches up after the second postnatal week. Between weeks two and four, substantial numbers of cells in the superficial layers rapidly become visually responsive, and orientation-selective receptive field properties mature (Blakemore and Price, 1987a).

The difference in the responsiveness and specificity of neurons in superficial and deep parts of the cortex of kittens aged two weeks or less is probably related to the fact that geniculocortical afferents are distributed mainly in deep layers shortly after birth. During this time the superficial layers are still forming. Most corticocortical afferents do not reach the superficial layers until the second postnatal week (Price and Zumbroich, 1989). It seems likely that the receptive field properties of cells in the superficial cortical layers are generated by intrinsic connections within each cortical area and by corticocortical projections, and that the development of the superficial laminae is delayed because the formation of intracerebral connections occurs later than the maturation of the thalamocortical afferents.

The neurons in the cat LGN that project to the visual cortex are classified as X, Y, and W cells, according to their response characteristics, receptive field sizes, cell body and axon diameters, and conduction velocities (Fig. 7.2) (reviewed by Stone, 1983; Enroth-Cugell and Robson, 1966). The response to a drifting grating moving across the receptive field of an X cell is linearly related to the stimulus and fluctuates at the same frequency; in other words, there is linear spatial summation across the receptive field. Y cells do not display linear spatial summation. They also have larger receptive fields, cell bodies, and axon diameters, and conduct action potentials more rapidly. W cells share some of the properties of Y cells, but respond only very sluggishly to visual stimuli. A number of anatomical and physiological studies in the cat have shown that each visual cortical area receives inputs from characteristic proportions of X, Y, and W cells, and in the projections to some areas geniculocortical projections arise predominantly from one particular type of cell. While area 17 receives afferents from X, Y, and W cells, area 18 and the PMLS are innervated exclusively by Y and W cells (Stone, 1983; Berson, 1985). It has been suggested that the development of the geniculate X cells differs from that of the Y cells. Daniels *et al.* (1978) found that the receptive field properties of Y cells in the LGN mature more slowly than those of X cells. Furthermore, Sherman *et al.* (1972) reported a decrease in the ratio of the number of Y cells to the number of X cells in samples of neurons studied along microelectrode penetrations through the LGN of monocularly, and to a lesser extent, binocularly, deprived cats. Whether this decreased ratio is due to Y cell loss or shrinkage is not clear (Stone, 1983), but whatever the cause it seems likely that visual deprivation has different effects on X and Y cells in the LGN.

Blakemore and Van Sluyters (1975) suggested that the earliest, innate orientation selective cells that develop in area 17 of the newborn kitten are usually simple in type, and may be produced by the convergence of afferents from X cells; in their hypothesis, Y cells initially contribute only a very weak excitatory input to the cortex. The early X cell inputs may condition the subsequent development of the receptive fields of cortical cells dominated by Y cell afferents. This is an attractive suggestion, but against it is the more recent finding that areas of the visual cortex that receive no direct X cell input, such as area 18 and PMLS (Fig. 5.14a, Chapter 5), develop in a very similar fashion to area 17 (Blakemore and Price, 1987a; Price *et al.*, 1988). Innately orientation selective cells can be found in these extrastriate regions even from the earliest postnatal ages, demonstrating that the presence of a direct X cell input is not necessary for the establishment of the earliest specific receptive field properties. Whatever the processes that produce the microcircuitry required to generate the receptive field properties of visual cortical neurons, they may be similar for different visual areas and for different types of afferents. Although it seems likely that an initial framework of early afferent connections guides the development of other inputs, any such framework is probably not composed exclusively of X, Y, or W cells.

Even in kittens as young as seven days, electrophysiological studies have revealed that those cells that are visually responsive (some of which demonstrate orientation selectivity) are grouped into rudimentary ocular dominance and orientation columns (Blakemore and Van Sluyters, 1975; Albus and Wolf, 1984; Blakemore and Price, 1987a). It is interesting to note that the techniques involving the transneuronal transport of intraocularly injected tracers fail to demonstrate the segregation of geniculocortical afferents until a later date. It seems that there is a variation in function throughout the early extensive terminal arborizations of the geniculocortical afferents, allowing one eye to dominate particular regions of the immature cortex despite the anatomical presence of inputs from the other eye.

Full radial columnar organization matures rapidly during the third postnatal week in the cat, and it seems likely that the early rudimentary organization, present almost exclusively in the deep layers, forms a framework for the future columnar development (Blakemore and Van Sluyters, 1975; Blakemore and Price, 1987a).

4   CONTROL OF RECEPTIVE FIELD DEVELOPMENT

In earlier chapters we described how neural activity plays an important role in corticogenesis. Initially, the neural activity is spontaneous (Galli and Maffei, 1988), but later it becomes evoked by external stimuli. Sensory receptor stimulation from the environment conveys increasingly complex patterns of activity to the cortex. As described earlier, a role for neural activity in the refinement of cortical connections, for example in the formation of ocular dominance columns in the visual cortex or the formation of barrels in the somatosensory cortex, is well-established. Our earlier discussions in Chapter 5 focused on the innervation of specific populations of cortical neurons by populations of axons. Here we consider the development of the elaborate receptive field properties of individual neurons through the convergence of multiple afferents, and the role that neural activity plays in this process.

In general, it seems that visual deprivation, which influences patterns and/or overall levels of neural activity in the visual cortex, has its most devastating effects on the development of the detailed circuitry required for the normal functional properties of visual cortical neurons. For example, in visual areas of the cat and ferret, the normal appearance of a large proportion of orientation selective cells is prevented by dark-rearing or by binocular eyelid suture (e.g. Blakemore and Van Sluyters, 1975; Cynader *et al.*, 1976; Blakemore and Price, 1987b; Chapman and Stryker, 1993). Studies in both cats and primates have shown that, before the neonate has received any visual experience, geniculocortical fibres find their main target, layer 4, and converge to generate immature orientation selective cells clustered into rudimentary orientation columns (Blakemore and Van Sluyters, 1975; Albus and Wolf, 1984; Blakemore and Price, 1987a). Visual deprivation early in life, during the critical period, does not abolish these features of early organization, but prevents their elaboration and the consequent emergence of the full richness of functional architecture and receptive field properties normally found in the adult visual cortex.

Although it has long been recognized that neural activity plays a role in regulating the development of the higher-order receptive field properties of cortical neurons, it is not so clear whether activity permits this development or whether it instructs it. Thus, neural activity may be essential to allow innate developmental programs to control the emergence of specific patterns of innervation (the permissive role). Alternatively, innate mechanisms may require instructions in the form of patterned activity to complete the development of neural circuits (the instructive role). Most visual deprivation experiments reduce overall electrical activity as well as abolishing or altering patterns of activity, and so it is not possible to identify unambiguously the cause of the resulting receptive field changes. In a recent series of experiments, Weliky and Katz (1997) artificially stimulated the developing visual pathway of ferret with electrodes around the optic nerve, to disrupt patterns of activity without suppressing overall levels of activity. They found that artificial, synchronous activation reduced the proportions of orientation and direction selective cells in the visual cortex, although the patterns of orientation and direction domains and retinotopic maps were unaltered (feature maps are discussed extensively in Chapter 5). These results indicate that the generation of an adequate level of neural activity is insufficient to permit the emergence of higher-order receptive fields. The afferent activity must be patterned, for example by correlations in spontaneous retinal activity, for mature receptive field properties to develop. Although demonstrating the importance of patterned activity, these recent results do not exclude the possibility that patterned activity permits innately controlled processes of development. Thus, the exact role of patterned activity in the regulation of receptive field development is far from clear.

One of the major problems with work on this subject to date is that current techniques cannot follow the development of the receptive field properties of individual cortical neurons over time. If this were possible, we could directly test the hypothesis that individual neurons have properties, such as orientation selectivity, determined by patterns of afferent activity, and that changes in these 'instructions' during the critical period alter receptive field properties. Although work by Blakemore and Cooper (1970) and Hirsch and Spinelli (1971) has indicated that exposure of neonates to an environment comprising bars of a specific orientation can generate a visual cortex that responds primarily to bars of that orientation, it is not clear whether this is because failure to stimulate with orthogonal bars does not permit cells with those receptive fields to develop or whether cells that would normally develop a different preference are instructed to develop differently.

5   INVESTIGATION OF THE FUNCTIONAL DEVELOPMENT OF THE CORTEX AS A WHOLE

Despite major progress in recent years on the mechanisms that regulate cortical development, there is enormous ignorance about the ways in which neural networks develop to generate the functional properties of individual cortical cells and multicellular cortical circuits. These functional properties underlie our perceptual, cognitive, and motor abilities. Attempts to understand how they generate our mental life are central to much current research, particularly in the field of cognitive neuroscience. An understanding of the mechanisms controlling the development of cortical neural networks has been sought both experimentally and theoretically.

5.1   Experimental methodologies

A profound understanding of the mechanisms that generate the functional properties of cortical cells and circuits, from relatively simple two-cell circuits to that linking all the cells in the cortex, is hampered in several ways. In large part, the problem is one of size and complexity. In the adult brain, a typical cortical neuron is contacted by many thousands of other neurons, and the way in which it responds to activity in those neurons depends on many factors such as the positions of their synapses on its cell body or dendrites, the electrical properties of its cell body or dendrites, the type of neurotransmitter released from each synapse, the degree of temporal coincidence in the activity of the synapses, and so on. At present, it is simply not possible to describe how the functional properties of cortical neurons develop at such a detailed level, let alone explain the mechanisms that guide such fine developmental processes. Despite this fundamental difficulty, there have been many studies of the functional development of the brain and cerebral cortex, in which researchers have measured those functional properties that our current technology can measure. Such studies can be grouped into two sets.

(i) Those in which the activity of cells or groups of cells are monitored, by recording their electrical impulses. This might be by using:

Electrodes implanted into the cortex of animals to study the activity of individual cells or small groups of cells.

Electroencephalography in humans to study the activity of the population of cells.

Other markers of multicellular activity within discrete brain regions (e.g. fluctuations in the blood flow to cortical areas).

(ii) Those in which the behaviour of the whole brain is monitored.

These types of studies fall within the fields of neurophysiology and psychology. In recent years, the overlap between these fields has increased greatly. One reason is that, for those studying human psychology, there are now new techniques, in addition to electroencephalography, for scanning the activity of brain regions in humans, such as functional magnetic resonance imaging and positron emission tomography. Their availability has prompted a search for the regions of the brain that are active during complex perceptual, cognitive, or motor behaviours and for abnormalities that underlie psychiatric disorders, both in adults and in children. On the positive side, this work indicates an ever increasing willingness to find the neural substrates that generate normal and abnormal behaviour. They should help to take the fields of psychology and psychiatry further away from traditional beliefs that some normal cognitive processes and some psychiatric disorders defy explanation in terms of brain anatomy and physiology. However, technologically advanced though they are, methods for scanning the activity of the entire brain or its regions offers only very crude information on the cellular processes that underlie behaviour or the changes that occur during development. Some of what has been learnt from the use of brain scanning techniques was predictable on the basis of our knowledge from studies of brain lesions, brain anatomy, and electrophysiology in humans and other mammals.

Clearly, one of the main functions of the cerebral cortex is in the generation of a perception of the outside world. It is possible to study the functional development of the cerebral cortex by taking a holistic approach and observing the changing properties of the entire system as it grows, using behavioural or psychological methods. A review of the enormous amount of work that has been done on the development of behaviour in both non-human species and in humans is outside the scope of this book. In attempting to understand the mechanisms that generate the cerebral cortex, the behavioural approach has limitations. First, it is difficult to be sure whether a particular behaviour is controlled primarily by the cortex and whether changes in that behaviour during development are caused by changes at a cortical level. The use of new methods for functional brain scanning described above may help with this problem in the future. Secondly, behavioural approaches can seek to distinguish the origins of the different influences that drive brain development, for example whether they are innate or environmental, and can be combined with a genetic approach to try and distinguish genetic from epigenetic factors. However, by their very nature, they do not address the molecular and cellular nature of the machinery that causes the behaviours.

Another way to study the functional development of the cerebral cortex is first to ask to what extent the functional properties of the system when it operates as a whole are distinguishable in the functional properties of its individual components. Work on the development of the receptive fields of individual cells is described above. Several studies have sought to explain brain function on the basis of the activities of individual neurons, focusing largely on perception, particularly by the visual system. Comparisons have been made between the receptive field properties of individual neurons and the perceptual ability of the system as a whole. While some high-level functions traditionally attributed to the cerebral cortex, such as consciousness, speech, and so on, are likely to be the product of networks of neurons and are not likely to be found as the properties of individual cells (Ryle, 1967), there is considerable evidence that even very complex perceptual tasks can be carried out by individual neurons (Parker and Newsome, 1998). This holds out the prospect that we could understand a lot about the mechanisms underlying functional development of the cerebral cortex by studying the way in which the properties of individual cells are created.

5.2   Theoretical approaches—constructivism

There has been much recent interest in relating the development of cognitive processes with that of neural processes under the name neural constructivism. This is derived from constructivism, a term that reflects Piaget's view that there is an active interaction between the developing system and the environment in which it develops (Quartz and Sejnowski, 1997).

The driving force behind neural constructivism derives most immediately from work in neural network research, which is concerned with devising networks of simple computing units modelled loosely on the architecture of the brain that are to learn specific input/output relationships (Hertz *et al.*, 1991). Most neural network applications are to problems in pattern recognition, classification, and prediction

(Bishop, 1995). Programming such devices, which usually exist as simulation programs, involves presenting many examples of the input/output pairings to be learnt and gradually altering the strengths of the connections ('synapses') between individual computing units. Whether a given task can be learnt (or in fact whether it will be learnt at all) depends on the structure of the network. In recent work, methods have been developed for building the network whilst the task is being learnt, which in many cases yields better performance than training a network with a fixed architecture (Gallant, 1986; Frean, 1990; Hertz *et al.*, 1991). By analogy, neural constructivism describes the idea that the development of structures such as the neocortex involves a dynamic interaction between the mechanisms of growth and environmentally driven neural activity. How information is represented in the cortex depends on the particular computational task being learnt.

Neural constructivism lies between the extreme versions of the theories of chemoaffinity (Sperry, 1943, 1944, 1963) (the entire blueprint of the nervous system is specified in the genome; see Chapter 5, Section 3.2) and a tabula rasa theory (nothing is prespecified). It has been contrasted with the doctrine of selectionism, which Quartz and Sejnowski (1997) take to be the idea that neural development proceeds by initial overproduction of neural structure followed by the selective pruning away of the inappropriate parts. Neural constructivism is concerned specifically with how neural activity guides the development of connections, the patterns of activity being generated from the external environment rather than through, for example, spontaneous activity. It is suggested that, as neocortex evolved in mammals, there was a progression toward more flexible representational structures, rather than there being an increase in the number and complexity of innate, specialized circuits.

Different types of evidence is cited in favour of neural constructivism:

(i) Changes in synaptic number
During development in primates the number of synapses rises and eventually falls but there is no decrease until post-puberty. This modifies the view first developed by Rakic *et al.* (1986) that there is significant loss of synapses during development. (Huttenlocher, 1979, 1990; Huttenlocher and de Courten, 1987; Bourgeois *et al.* 1989, 1994)

(ii) Axonal growth
In the visual system during the period of activity-dependent development there is evidence for axonal growth (Antonini and Stryker, 1993), contrary to the doctrine of selectionism.

(iii) Dendritic growth
Dendrites grow at a much slower rate than axons, over a longer time scale, stretching over the period of time when according to selectionism they should not be growing. Dendritic morphology can be moulded by the patterned neural activity incident upon it.

(iv) The extent of cortical development
Human cortical postnatal development is also more extensive and protracted than generally supposed, suggesting that cortex has evolved so as to maximize the

capacity of environmental structure to shape its structure and function through constructive learning.

5. The power of constructive neural networks

As already mentioned above, the computational power of neural networks that develop their structure whilst they are being trained may be much greater than that of fixed architecture neural networks.

Recently neural constructivism has become a fashionable subject amongst theoretical neurobiologists and psychologists particularly. It emphasizes the dynamic interaction between the developing system and the developmental 'task' to be accomplished. However, like the doctrine of selectionism, it focuses on the activity-dependent stages of neural development and therefore does not address any phenomenon that can best be explained in molecular terms. It is questionable whether a polarized debate between the merits of neural constructivism versus selectionism is useful. It is fairly straightforward to find phenomena to fit each of these two doctrines. In the neuromuscular system, there is very strong evidence for initial hyperinnervation of developing muscle followed by withdrawal of connections (an example of selectionism, as defined here); conversely, the development of retinotectal connections in lower vertebrates involves, at the same time, both the formation of connections and their withdrawal, an example of neural constructivism.

6 ACQUISITION OF THE HIGHEST LEVELS OF CORTICAL FUNCTION: DEVELOPMENT OF LANGUAGE

Finally, what of the mechanisms that regulate the development of the very highest levels of cortical function? A discussion of much of the psychological literature relevant to this issue, or of philosophical issues such as the development of consciousness, is outside the scope of this book. A few comments on the acquisition of language will serve to illustrate the importance of the postnatal environment to the development of even the most phylogenetically advanced regions of the human cerebral cortex. Conclusions regarding the role of neural activity in the development of the functional properties of individual cortical cells are often mirrored by observations on entire high-level systems.

The human cortex has discrete areas that are essential for language, including Broca's area in the frontal lobe and Wernicke's area in the temporal lobe (Geschwind, 1970). Key regions for language are usually found in the left hemisphere. As described in the following section on brain lesions, the position of these language areas is not determined at birth. The development of cortical centres for language involves a lengthy postnatal period during which environmental factors can act. In studies of the importance of the postnatal environment, work on animal models has severe limitations due to the rudimentary nature of auditory communication in non-human species. However, there is evidence from cases of deprived children that this growth and remodelling occurs during a limited window of opportunity (the critical period) for language learning. There have been instances of children who have spent their early years without human contact and sound. Even after years of therapy and language training, such individuals were unable to develop normal language skills, indicating that the acquisition of the complex features of language requires exposure to speech before a certain age (Lea, 1984).

As discussed by Pinker (1994), children are born with the innate ability to distinguish phonemes (the units of sound that are strung together to form syllables and words). Psychological experiments by Einas *et al.* (1971) have shown that these distinctions are made through an awareness of phonetic differences important in speech perception and not merely on the basis of acoustic differences, which were ignored by babies. In fact, infants during the first few months of life can discriminate all the phonetic contrasts, irrespective of whether they are used in their native language. Infants start with an ability that equips them with the potential to respond to all the languages in the world. This ability is lost during the first year of life (Kuhl *et al.*, 1992). For example, Japanese does not distinguish between 'r' and 'l', but whereas Japanese adults cannot hear the difference between these sounds, Japanese infants do. Infants under six months who are learning English can distinguish phenomes used in a variety of other languages such as Czech or Hindi, whereas English-speaking adults cannot even after extensive training.

Although current research to identify the possible neural substrates for these behavioural findings is some way from reaching a conclusion (e.g. Dehaene-Lambertz and Dehaene, 1994), it is clear that even the most complex of human behaviours develops through the controlling influence of the environment on an initially multipotent neural system. The environment sculpts the brain by restricting the scope of its circuitry, presumably allowing some neural networks to grow and elaborate at the expense of others. The way in which language is acquired provides one of the clearest and most fascinating examples of how innate mechanisms of embryonic development described in the early chapters of this book generate a newborn brain that has enormous adaptability to its particular environment.

7 EFFECTS OF LESIONS ON DEVELOPMENT OF CORTICAL FUNCTION IN HUMANS

In Chapters 5 and 6 we discussed the mechanisms that may underlie the plasticity of the cerebral cortex. This plasticity is apparent in recent studies using brain scanning to examine the development of the cortex in humans following lesions to the brain in early childhood. A major conclusion from such studies is that the newborn human cortex retains sufficient plasticity to allow cortical regions not normally associated with particular high-level processes to take on those functions in response to early cortical damage. This ability to compensate for lesions lessens with age. Examples of this have been found in the pathways for the perception of faces and for language.

7.1   Face-perception

The human visual system is in a highly immature state at birth. For example, the number of cells in the fovea of the eye has still to develop to that required for the perception of fine details (Goldstein, 1989). Nevertheless, many of the basic elements of perception are present in the first few days. Although the ability to recognize complex patterns seems to come only with experience, there is evidence that infants may be innately tuned to perceive at least one important complex pattern in the human face (Johnson *et al.*, 1991).

    The processing of faces by the brain has been well studied, as a good example of the existence of a complex system specialized in the processing of a specific category of objects (Perrett *et al.*, 1982; Sergent *et al.*, 1992; Tovee, 1995, 1998). Studies with brain imaging have shown that in most face tasks particular cortical regions in adults are activated. This raises the question of how cortical regions become specified for this task. There is evidence that neonates pay particular attention to faces over other similar objects and that they have a preference for the mother's face from as young as three days (Goren *et al.*, 1975; Johnson *et al.*, 1991; Pascalis and De Schonen, 1994). There is a right hemisphere dominance in the processing of faces in infants from four months (de Schonen and Mathivet, 1989, Johnson, 1997). Neuroimaging of developing human infants and studies of the effects of early brain lesions have indicated that there is a gradual emergence of face processing within the cortex rather than an innate circuitry (de Schonen and Mancini, 1995; Mancini *et al.*, 1994). It is possible, following early lesions to regions normally associated with face recognition, for the brain to develop the ability to process faces through other routes (Johnson, 1997).

7.2   Language

There is much debate over the degree to which the newborn human brain is innately specified to learn language. Chomsky (1957) suggested that humans are born with a 'language acquisition device' that is used to understand and construct their native language. Others have argued that such a device does not exist (Bates *et al.*, 1992). Since the neural basis of language is poorly understood, controversy is likely to continue for some time. At the heart of this issue is whether the neonatal cortex contains regions that are irreversibly committed, perhaps by genetic mechanisms, to develop into language centres. Evidence from lesions of young children has indicated that this is not the case.

    Research on the effects of cortical injuries in childhood has suggested that either the right or the left hemisphere can support normal language abilities if damage is early in life. Early lesions to key regions of the left hemisphere can cause delays in the development of language, but reorganization of the brain eventually compensates. Unlike adults, who show chronic and severe aphasic symptoms after focal left cortical damage, children rarely demonstrate persistent disruption of speech and language function following such lesions (Vargha Khadem, 1998; Vargha Khadem *et al.*, 1997; Muter *et al.*, 1997; Isaacs *et al.*, 1996). It is certainly possible that, in normal development, there is some preference for particular regions of the left hemisphere to become associated with language. This may be a consequence of regional variations in information processing that is related to language. However, the observations on the effects of early lesions illustrate a theme that has emerged throughout studies of cortical development, namely that different regions of the cortex may be specified to particular fates from a very early age, but they are not determined (i.e. irreversibly committed) in the neonate. Their commitment increases as the brain ages under the influence of its environment, although plasticity may never be completely lost even in adults (Buonomano and Merzenich, 1998). The newborn cortex is a highly adaptable structure that can undergo extensive modifications in response to its environment and to early damage, at all levels of processing.

Bibliography

Acampora, D., Mazan, S., Lallemand, Y., Avantaggiato, V., *et al.* (1995). Forebrain and midbrain regions are deleted in Otx2-/- mutants due to a defective anterior neurectoderm specification during gastrulation. *Development*, **121**, 3279–3290.

Adelmann, H.B. (1936a). The problem of cyclopia. *Q. Rev. Biol.*, **11**, 116–182.

Adelmann, H.B. (1936b). The problem of cyclopia. *Q. Rev. Biol.*, **11**, 284–304.

Agmon, A., Young, L.T., Jones, E.G., and O'Dowd, D.K. (1995). Topological precision in the thalamic projection to neonatal mouse barrel cortex. *J. Neurosci.*, **15**, 549–561.

Akam, M. (1987). The molecular basis for metameric pattern in the Drosophila embryo. *Development*, **101**, 1–22.

Akbarian, S., Kim, J.J., Potkin, S.G., Hetrick, W.P., Bunney, W.E., and Jones, E.G. (1996a). Maldistribution of interstitial neurons in prefrontal white matter of the brains of schizophrenic subjects. *Arch. Gen. Psychiatry*, **53**, 425–436.

Akbarian, S., Sucher, N.J., Bradley, D., Tafazzoli, A., *et al.* (1996b). Selective alterations in gene expression for NMDA receptor subunits in prefrontal cortex of schizophrenics. *J. Neurosci.*, **16**, 19–30.

Alberts, B., Bray, D., Lewis, J., Raff, M., Roberts, K., and Watson, J.D. (1994). *Molecular biology of the cell.* Garland Publishing Inc., New York, USA.

Albinet, G. and Pelce, P. (1996). Computer simulation of neurite outgrowth. *Europhys. Lett.*, **33**, 569–574.

Albus, K. and Wolf, W. (1984). Early post-natal development of neuronal function in the kitten's visual cortex: a laminar analysis. *J. Physiol.*, **348**, 153–185.

Allendoerfer, K.L. and Shatz, C.J. (1994). The subplate, a transient neocortical structure: its role in the development of connections between the thalamus and the cortex. *Annu. Rev. Neurosci.*, **17**, 185–218.

Allendoerfer, K.L., Cabelli, R.J., Escandon, E., Kaplan, D.R., Nikolics, K., and Shatz, C.J. (1994). Regulation of neurotrophin receptors during the maturation of the mammalian visual system. *J. Neurosci.*, **14**, 1795–1811.

Allendorfer, K.L. and Shatz, C.J. (1994). The subplate, a transient neocortical structure: its role in the development of connections between thalamus and cortex. *Annu. Rev. Neurosci.*, **17**, 185–218.

Allsopp, T.E., Wyatt, S., Paterson, H.F., and Davies, A.M. (1993). The proto-oncogene bcl-2 can selectively rescue neurotrophic factor dependent neurons from apoptosis. *Cell*, **73**, 295–307.

Altman, J. and Bayer, S.A. (1989a). Development of the rat thalamus. IV. the intermediate lobule of the thalamic neuroepithelium, and the time and site of origin and settling pattern of neurons of the ventral nuclear complex. *J. Comp. Neurol.*, **284**, 534–566.

Altman, J. and Bayer, S.A. (1989b). Development of the rat thalamus. VI. the posterior lobule of the thalamic neuroepithelium, and the time and site of origin and settling pattern of neurons of the lateral geniculate and lateral posterior nuclei. *J. Comp. Neurol.*, **284**, 581–601.

Amari, S. (1980). Topographic organization of nerve fields. *Bull. Math. Biol.*, **42**, 339–364.

Amari, S. (1983). Field theory of self-organizing nets. *IEEE Trans. Syst., Man, Cybernetics*, **13**, 741–748.

Anders, J.J. and Hibbard, E. (1974). The optic system of the teleost *Cichlasoma meeki*. *J. Comp. Neurol.*, **158**, 145–154.

Anderson, S.A., Eisenstat, D.D., Shi, L., and Rubenstein, J.L.R. (1997). Interneuron migration from basal forebrain to neocortex: dependence on Dlx genes. *Science*, **278**, 474–476.

Ang, S.-L., Jin, O., Rhinn, M., Daigle, N., Stevenson, L., and Rossant, J. (1996). A targeted mouse Otx2 mutation leads to severe defects in gastrulation and formation of axial mesoderm and to deletion of rostral brain. *Development*, **122**, 243–252.

Angevine, J.B. and Sidman, R.L. (1961). Autoradiographic study of cell migration during histogenesis of cerebral cortex in the mouse. *Nature*, **192**, 766–768.

Anton, E.S., Marchionni, M.A., Lee, K.F., and Rakic, P. (1997). Role of GGF/Neuregulin signaling in interactions between migrating neurons and radial glia in the developing cerebral cortex. *Development*, **124**, 3501–3510.

Antonini, A. and Stryker, M.P. (1993). Rapid remodeling of axonal arbors in the visual cortex. *Science*, **260**, 1819–1821.

Antonopoulos, J., Pappas, I.S., and Parnavelas, J.G. (1997). Activation of the GABAA receptor inhibits the proliferative effects of bFGF in cortical progenitor cells. *Eur. J. Neurosci.*, **9**, 291–298.

Antonsson, B., Conti, F., Ciavatta, A., Montessuit, S., *et al.* (1997). Inhibition of bax channel-forming activity by Bcl-2. *Science*, **277**, 370–372.

Apter, J.T. (1945). Projection of the retina on superior colliculus of cats. *J. Neurophysiol.*, **8**, 123–134.

Arimatsu, Y., Ishida, M., Takiguchi-Hayashi, K., and Uratani, Y. (1999). Cerebral cortical specification by early potential restriction of progenitor cells and later phenotype control of postmitotic neurons. *Development*, **126**, 629–638.

Arnett, D.W. (1978). Statistical dependence between neighbouring retinal ganglion cells in goldfish. *Exp. Brain Res.*, **32**, 49–53.

Attardi, D.G. and Sperry, R.W. (1963). Preferential selection of central pathways by regenerating optic fibers. *Exp. Neurol.*, **7**, 46–64.

Austin, C.O. and Cepko, C.L. (1990). Cellular migration patterns in the developing mouse cerebral cortex. *Development*, **110**, 713–732.

Ba-Charvet, K.T.N., von Boxberg, Y., Guazzi, S., Boncinelli, E., and Godement, P. (1998). A potential role for the Otx2 homeoprotein in creating early 'highways' for axon extension in the rostral brain. *Development*, **125**, 4273–4282.

Bagnard, D., Lohrum, M., Uziel, D., Puschel, A.W., and Bolz, J. (1998). Semaphorins act as attractive and repulsive guidance signals during the development of cortical projections. *Development*, **125**, 5043–5053.

Baier, H., Klostermann, S., Trowe, T., Karlstrom, R.O., Nusslein-Volhard, C. and Bonhoeffer, F. (1996). Genetic dissection of the retinotectal projection. *Development*, **123**, 415–425.

Bailey, C.H. and Kandel, E.R. (1993). Structural changes accompanying memory storage. *Ann. Rev. Physiol.*, **55**, 397–426.

Balice-Gordon, R.J. and Lichtman, J.W. (1994). Long-term synapse loss induced by focal blockade of postsynaptic receptors. *Nature*, **372**, 519–524.

Banker, G.A. and Cowan, W.M. (1979). Further observations on hippocampal neurons in dispersed cell culture. *J. Comp. Neurol.*, **187**, 69–93.

Bar I., Lambert de Rouvroit, C., Royaux, I., Kritzman, D.B., Dernoncourt, C., Ruelle, D., Beckers, M.C. and Goffinet, A.M. (1995). A YAC contig containing the *reeler* locus with preliminary characterization of candidate gene fragments. *Genomics*, **26**, 543–549.

Barbe, M.F. and Levitt, P. (1992). Attraction of specific thalamic input by cerebral grafts depends on the molecular identity of the implant. *Proc. Natl. Acad. Sci. USA*, **89**, 3706–3710.

Barde, Y.-A. (1989). Trophic factors and neuronal survival. *Neuron*, **2**, 1525–1534.

Barone, P., Dehay, C., Berland, M., Bullier, J., and Kennedy, H. (1995). Developmental remodeling of primate visual cortical pathways. *Cereb. Cortex*, **5**, 22–38.

Barone, P., Dehay, C., Berland, M., and Kennedy, H. (1996). Role of directed growth and target selection in the formation of cortical pathways: prenatal development of the projection of area V2 to area V4 in the monkey. *J. Comp. Neurol.*, **374**, 1–20.

Barry, J.A. and Ribchester, R.R. (1995). Persistent polyneuronal innervation in partially denervated rat muscle after reinnervation and recovery from prolonged nerve-conduction block. *J. Neurosci.*, **15**, 6327–6339.

Bartlett, W.P. and Banker, G.A. (1984). An electron microscopic study of the development of axons and dendrites by hippocampal neurons in culture. I. Cells which develop without intercellular contacts. *J. Neurosci.*, **4**, 1944–1953.

Batardiere, A., Barone, P., Dehay, C., and Kennedy, H. (1998). Area-specific laminar distribution of cortical feedback neurons projecting to cat area 17: Quantitative analysis in the adult and during ontogeny. *J. Comp. Neurol.*, **396**, 493–510.

Bates, C.A. and Killackey, H.P. (1984). The emergence of a discretely distributed pattern of corticospinal projection neurons. *Dev. Brain Res.*, **13**, 265–273.

Bates, E., Thal, D. and Jankowsky, J.S. (1992). Early language development and its neural correlates. In *Handbook of Neuropsychology* (eds. I. Rapin and S. Segalowitz), vol. 7, pp. 69–110. Elsevier, Amsterdam.

Bayer, M.C. and Valenco, R.C. (1994). Synaptic plasticity, LTP and LTD. *Current Opinions in Biology*, **4**, 38–399.

234   *Bibliography*

Bayer, S.A. and Altman, J. (1990). Development of layer I and the subplate in the rat neocortex. *Exp. Neurol.*, **107**, 48–62.

Bayer, S.A. and Altman, J. (1991). *Neocortical development*. Raven Press, New York.

Bear, M.F. and Abraham, W.C. (1996). Long-term depression in hippocampus. *Annu. Rev. Neurosci.*, **19**, 437–462.

Bear, M.F. and Singer, W. (1986). Modulation of visual cortical plasticity by acetylcholine and noradrenaline. *Nature*, **320**, 172–176.

Bear, M.F., Kleinschmidt, A., Gu, Q.A., and Singer, W. (1990). Disruption of experience-dependent synaptic modifications in striate cortex by infusion of an NMDA receptor antagonist. *J. Neurosci.*, **10**, 909–925.

Beazley, L.D. (1975). Factors determining decussation at the optic chiasma by developing retinotectal fibres in *Xenopus*. *Exp. Brain Res.*, **23**, 491–504.

Beazley, L.D. (1977). Abnormalities in the visual system of *Xenopus* after larval optic nerve section. *Exp. Brain Res.*, **30**, 369–385.

Bedlack, R.S., Wei, M.-D., and Loew, L.M. (1992). Localized membrane depolarizations and localized calcium influx during electric field-guided neurite growth. *Neuron*, **9**, 393–403.

Benes, F.M., Vincent, S.L., Marie, A., and Khan, Y. (1996). Up-regulation of GABA-A receptor binding on neurons of the prefrontal cortex in schizophrenic subjects. *Neuroscience*, **75**, 1021–1031.

Benjelloum Toumi, S., Jacque, C.M., Derer, P., *et al.* (1985). Evidence that mouse astrocytes may be derived from radial glia: An immunohistochemical study of the cerebellum in the normal and reeler mouse. *J. Neuroimmunol.*, **9**, 87–97.

Bennett, M.R. and Robinson, J. (1989). Growth and elimination of nerve terminals at synaptic sites during polyneuronal innervation of muscle cells: a trophic hypothesis. *Proc. R. Soc. London B*, **235**, 299–320.

Benoit, P. and Changeux, J.-P. (1975). Consequences of tenotomy on the evolution of multiinnervation of developing rat soleus muscle. *Brain Res.*, **99**, 354–358.

Bentley, D. and Caudy, M. (1983). Pioneer axons lose directed growth after selective killing of guidepost cells. *Nature*, **304**, 62–65.

Bergeron, L. and Yuan, J. (1998). Sealing one's fate: control of cell death in neurons. *Curr. Opin. Neurobiol.*, **8**, 55–63.

Berlucchi, G. (1972). Anatomical and physiological aspects of visual functions of corpus callosum. *Brain Res.*, **37**, 371–392.

Bernd, P. and Greene, L.A. (1984). Association of 125I-nerve growth factor with PC12 pheochromocytoma cells. Evidence for internalisation via high affinity receptors only and for long term regulation by nerve growth factor of both high- and low-affinity receptors. *J. Biol. Chem.*, **259**, 15509–15516.

Berry, M and Flinn, R. (1984). Vertex analysis of Purkinje cell dendrites in the cerebellum of the rat. *Proc. R. Soc. London B*, **221**, 321–348.

Berson, D.M. (1985). Cat lateral suprasylvian cortex: Y-cell inputs and corticotectal projection. *J. Neurophysiol.*, **53**, 544–556.

Betz, W.J., Caldwell, J.H., and Ribchester, R.R. (1979). The size of motor units during post-natal development of rat lumbrical muscle. *J. Physiol.*, **297**, 463–478.

Bicknese, A.R., Sheppard, A.M., O'Leary, D.D.M., and Pearlman, A.L. (1994). Thalamocortical axons extend along a chondroitin sulfate proteoglycan-enriched pathway coincident with the neocortical subplate and distinct from the efferent path. *J. Neurosci.*, **14**, 3500–3510.

Bienenstock, E.L., Cooper, L.N., and Munro, P.W. (1982). Theory for the development of neuron selectivity: orientation specificity and binocular interaction in visual cortex. *J. Neurosci.*, **2**, 32–48.

Birren, S.J., Verdi, J.M. and Anderson, D.J. (1992). Membrane depolarization induces p140[trk] and NGF responsiveness, but not p75[LNGFR], in MAH cell. *Science*, **257**, 395–397.

Bishop, C.M. (1995). *Neural networks for pattern recognition.* Clarendon Press, Oxford.

Blakemore, C. (1988). The sensitive periods of the monkey's visual cortex. In *Strabismus and amblyopia* (eds. G. Lennerstrand, G.K. von Noorden, and E.C. Campos). Macmillan Press, London.

Blakemore, C. and Cooper, G.F. (1970). Development of the brain depends on the visual environment. *Nature*, **228**, 477–478.

Blakemore, C. and Molnar, Z. (1990). Factors involved in the establishment of specific interconnections between thalamus and cerebral cortex. *Cold Spring Harbour Symp on Quant Biol*, **55**, 491–504.

Blakemore, C. and Price, D.J. (1987a). The organisation and postnatal development of area 18 of the cat's visual cortex. *J. Physiol.*, **384**, 263–292.

Blakemore, C. and Price, D.J. (1987b). Effects of dark-rearing on the development of area 18 of the cat's visual cortex. *J. Physiol.*, **384**, 293–309.

Blakemore, C. and Van Sluyters, R.C. (1974). Reversal of the physiological effects of monocular deprivation in kittens. Further evidence for a sensitive period. *J. Physiol. (Lond.)*, **237**, 195–216.

Blakemore, C. and Van Sluyters, R.C. (1975). Innate and environmental factors in the development of the kitten's visual cortex. *J. Physiol.*, **248**, 663–716.

Blakemore, C., Garey, L.J., and Vital-Durand, F. (1978). The physiological effect of monocular deprivation and their reversal in the monkey's visual cortex. *J. Physiol.*, **283**, 223–262.

Blaschke, A.J., Staley, K., and Chun, J. (1996). Widespread programmed cell death in proliferative and postmitotic regions of the fetal cerebral cortex. *Development*, **122**, 1165–1174.

Blaschke, A.J., Weiner, J.A., and Chun, J. (1998). Programmed cell death is a universal feature of embryonic and postnatal neuroproliferative regions throughout the central nervous system. *J. Comp. Neurol.*, **396**, 39–50.

Blasdel, G.G. and Salama, G. (1986). Voltage sensitive dyes reveal a modular organization in the monkey striate cortex. *Nature*, **321**, 579–585.

Bliss, T.V.P. and Collingridge, G.L. (1993). A synaptic model of memory: long-term potentiation in the hippocampus. *Nature*, **361**, 31–39.

Bliss, T.V.P. and Gardner-Medwin, A.R. (1973). Long-lasting potentiation of synaptic transmission in the dentate area of the unanaesthetized rabbit following stimulation of the perforant path. *J. Physiol. (Lond.)*, **232**, 357–374.

Bliss, T.V.P. and Lomo, T. (1973). Long-term potentiation of synaptic transmission in the dentate area of the anaesthetised rabbit following stimulation of the perforant path. *J. Physiol. (Lond.)*, **232**, 331–356.

Bohner, A.P., Akers, R.M., and McConnell, S.K. (1997). Induction of deep layer cortical neurons *in vitro*. *Development*, **124**, 915–923.

Bolz, J., Novak, N., Gotz, M., and Bonhoeffer, T. (1990). Formation of target-specific neuronal projections in organotypic slice cultures from rat visual cortex. *Nature*, **346**, 359–362.

Bolz, J., Gotz, M., Hubener, M., and Novak, N. (1993). Reconstructing cortical connections in a dish. *Trends Neurosci.*, **16**, 310–316.

Bolz, J., Kossel, A., and Bagnard, D. (1995). The specificity of interactions between the cortex and the thalamus. In *Development of the cerebral cortex* (eds. G. Bock and G. Cardew), pp. 173–191. Wiley, New York, USA.

Boncinelli, E., Gulisano, M., and Broccoli, V. (1993). Emx and Otx homeobox genes in the developing mouse brain. *J. Neurobiol.*, **24**, 1356–1366.

Boncinelli, E., Gulisano, M., Spada, F., and Broccoli, V. (1995). Emx and Otx gene expression in the developing mouse brain. In *Development of the cerebral cortex* (eds. G. Bock and G. Cardew). Wiley (Ciba Foundation Symposium 193).

Bonhoeffer, T. and Grinvald, A. (1991). Orientation columns in cats are organized in a pin-wheel like pattern. *Nature*, **353**, 429–431.

Bopp, D., Burri, M., Baumgartner, S., Frigerio, G., and Noll, M. (1986). Conservation of a large protein domain in the segmentation gene paired and in functionally related genes of Drosophila. *Cell*, **47**, 1033–1040.

Bothwell, M. (1991). Keeping track of neurotrophin receptors. *Cell*, **65**, 915–918.

Bothwell, M. (1995). Functional interactions of neurotrophins and neurotrophin receptors. *Annu. Rev. Neurosci.*, **18**, 223–253.

Bottjer, S.W. and Arnold, A.P. (1997). Developmental plasticity in neural circuits for a learned behaviour. *Annu. Rev. Neurosci.*, **20**, 459–481.

Bourgeois, J.P., Goldman-Rakic, P.S. and Rakic, P. (1994). Synaptogenesis in the prefrontal cortex of rhesus monkeys. *Cerebr. Cortex*, **4**, 78–96.

Bourgeois, J.P., Jastreboff, P.J. and Rakic, P. (1989). Synaptogenesis in visual cortex of normal and preterm monkeys: evidence for intrinsic regulation of synaptic overproduction. *Proc. Natl. Acad. Sci. USA*, **86**, 4297–4301.

Bouwmeester, T., Kim, S.-H., Sasai, Y., Lu, B., and DeRobertis, E.M. (1996). Cerberus is a head-inducing secreted factor expressed in the anterior endoderm of Spemann's organizer. *Nature*, **382**, 595–601.

Bredesen, D.E. (1995). Neural apoptosis. *Ann. Neurol.*, **38**, 839–851.

Breedlove, S.M. and Arnold, A.P. (1983). Hormonal control of a develop-ing neuromuscular system. II. Sensitive periods for the androgen-induced masculinization of the rat spinal nucleus of the bulbocavernosus. *J. Neurosci.*, **3**, 424–432.

Briata, P., Di Blas, E., Gulisano, M., Mallamaci, A., *et al.* (1996). EMX1 homeoprotein is expressed in cell nuclei of the developing cerebral cortex and in the axons of the olfactory sensory neurons. *Mech. Dev.*, **57**, 169–180.

Broadie, K., Sink, H., VanVactor, D., and Fambrough, D. (1993). From growth cone to synapse: the life history of the RP3 motor neuron. *Development 1993 Supplement*, pp. 227–238.

Brodal, P. (1992). *The central nervous system.* Oxford University Press, New York, Oxford.

Brodmann, K. (1909). *Vergleichende Lokalisationslehre der Groshirnrinde in ihren Prinzipien dargestellt auf Grund des Zellenbaues.* J.A. Barth, Leipzig.

Brown, M.C., Jansen, J.K.S., and Van Essen, D.C. (1976). Polyneuronal innervation of skeletal muscle in new-born rats and its elimination during maturation. *J. Physiol.*, **261**, 387–422.

Brummendorf, T., Kenwrick, S., and Rathjen, F.G. (1998). Neural cell recognition molecule L1: from cell biology to human hereditary brain malformations. *Curr. Opin. Neurobiol.*, **8**, 87–97.

Brustle, O., Maskos, U., and McKay, R.D.G. (1995). Host-guided migration allows targeted introduction of neurons into the embryonic brain. *Neuron*, **6**, 1275–1285.

Bulfone, A., Kim, H.-J., Puelles, L., Porteus, M.H., Grippo, J.F., and Rubenstein, J.L.R. (1993). The mouse Dlx-2 (Tes-1) gene is expressed in spatially restricted domains of the forebrain, face and limbs in midgestation mouse embryos. *Mech. Dev.*, **40**, 129–140.

Bulfone, A., Smiga, S.M., Shimamura, K., Peterson, A., Puelles, L., and Rubenstein, J.L.R. (1995). T-brain-1: A homolog of brachyury whose expression defines molecularly distinct domains within the cerebral cortex. *Neuron*, **15**, 63–78.

Bullier, J., Kennedy, H., and Salinger, W. (1984). Branching and laminar origin of projections between visual cortical areas in the cat. *J. Comp. Neurol.*, **228**, 329–341.

Bunt, S.M. (1982). Retinotopic and temporal organisation of the optic nerve and tracts in the adult goldfish. *J. Comp. Neurol.*, **206**, 209–226.

Buonomano, D.V. and Merzenich, M.M. (1998). Cortical plasticity: from synapses to maps. *Annu. Rev. Neurosci.*, **21**, 149–186.

Burek, M.J. and Oppenheim, R.W. (1998). Cellular interaction that regulate programmed cell death in the developing vertebrate nervous system. In *Cell death and diseases of the nervous system* (eds. V. Koliatsos and R. Ratan). Humana Press, Totowa, NJ.

Burke, R.E., Marks, W.B., and Ulfhake, B. (1992). A parsimonious description of motoneuron dendritic morphology using computer simulation. *J. Neurosci.*, **12**, 2403–2416.

Burrows, R.C., Wancio, D., Levitt, P., and Lillien, L. (1997). Response diversity and the timing of progenitor cell maturation are regulated by developmental changes in EGF-R expression in the cortex. *Neuron*, **19**, 251–267.

Cabelli, R.J., Hohn, A., and Shatz, C.J. (1995). Inhibition of ocular dominance column formation by infusion of NT-4/5 or BDNF. *Science*, **267**, 1662–1666.

Cajal, R. (1893). La retine des vertebres. *La Cellule*, **9**, 119–258.

Cajal, S.R. (1911). *Histologie du système nerveux de l'homme et des vertébrés.* vol II. Instituto Ramon y Cajal, Madrid.

Caldero, J., Prevette, D., Mei, X., Oakley, R.A., Li, L., *et al.* (1998). Peripheral target regulation of the development and survival of spinal sensory and motor neurons in the chick embryo. *J. Neurosci.*, **18**, 356–370.

Callaway, E.M. and Katz, L.C. (1990). Emergence and refinement of clustered horizontal connections in rat striate cortex. *J. Neurosci.*, **10**, 1134–1153.

Callaway, E.M. and Katz, L.C. (1991). Effects of binocular definition on the development of clusteral horizontal connections in rat striate cortex. *Proc. Natl. Acad. Sci. USA*, **88**, 745–749.

Callaway, E.M. and Katz, L.C. (1992). Development of axonal arbors of spiny neurons in cat striate cortex. *J. Neurosci.*, **12**, 570–582.

Callaway, E., Soha, J.M., and Van Essen, D.C. (1987). Competition favouring inactive over active motor neurons during synapse elimination. *Nature*, **328**, 422–426.

Callaway, E.M., Soha, J.M., and Van Essen, D.C. (1989). Differential loss of neuromuscular connections according to activity level and spinal position of neuronatal rabbit soleus motor neurons. *J. Neurosci.*, **9**, 1806–1824.

Cameron, R.S. and Rakic, P. (1991). Glial cell lineage in the cerebral cortex: A review and synthesis. *Glia*, **4**, 124–137.

Campbell, K., Olsson, M., and Bjorklund, A. (1995). Regional incorporation and site-specific differentiation of striatal precursors transplanted to the embryonic forebrain ventricle. *Neuron*, **15**, 1259–1273.

Caric, D. and Price, D.J. (1996). The organization of visual corticocortical connections in early postnatal kittens. *Neuroscience*, **73**, 817–829.

Caric, D. and Price, D.J. (1999). Evidence that the lateral geniculate nucleus regulates the normal development of visual corticortical projections in the cat. *Exp. Neurol.*, **156**, 353–362.

Caric, D., Gooday, D., Hill, R.E., McConnell, S.K., and Price, D.J. (1997). Determination of the migratory capacity of embryonic cortical cells lacking the transcription factor Pax-6. *Development*, **124**, 5087–5096.

Carmignoto, G., Canella, R., Candeo, P., Comelli, M.C., and Maffei, L. (1993). Effects of nerve growth factor on neuronal plasticity of the kitten visual cortex. *J. Physiol.*, **464**, 343–360.

Casaccia-Bonnefil, P., Carter, B.D., Dobrowsky, R.T., and Chao, M.V. (1996). Death of oligodendrocytes mediated by the interaction of nerve growth factor with its receptor p.75. *Nature*, **383**, 716–719.

Cases, O., Vitalis, T., Seif, I., De Maeyer, R., Sotelo, C., and Gaspar, P. (1996). Lack of barrels in the somatosensory cortex of monoamine oxidase A deficient mice: Role of serotonin excess during the critical period. *Neuron*, **16**, 297–307.

Castren, E., Zafra, F., Thoenen, H., and Lindholm, D. (1992). Light regulates expression of brain-derived neurotrophic factor mRNA in rat visual cortex. *Proc. Natl. Acad. Sci. USA*, **89**, 9444–9448.

Catalano, S.M., Robertson, R.T., and Killacky, H.P. (1991). Early ingrowth of thalamocortical afferents to the neocortex of the prenatal rat. *Proc. Natl. Acad. Sci. USA*, **88**, 2999–3003.

Catsicas, M., Pequignot, Y., and Clarke, P.G.H. (1992). Rapid onset of neuronal death induced by blockade of either axoplasmic transport or action potentials in afferent fibers during brain development. *J. Neurosci.*, **12**, 4642–4650.

Cavanagh, J.F.R., Mione, M.C., Pappas, I.S., and Parnavelas, J.G. (1997). Basic fibroblast growth factor prolongs the proliferation of rat cortical progenitor cells *in vitro* without altering their cell cycle parameters. *Cerebral Cortex*, **7**, 293–302.

Caviness, V.S. and Rakic, P. (1978). Mechanisms of cortical development: a view from mutations in mice. *Annu. Rev. Neurosci.*, **1**, 297–326.

Caviness, V.S., Takahashi, T., and Nowakowski, R.S. (1997). Cell proliferation in cortical development. In *Normal and abnormal development of cortex* (eds. A. Galaburda and Y. Christen), pp. 1–24. Springer-Verlag, Berlin.

Caviness, V.S. Jr. (1988). Architecture and development of the thalamocortical projection in the mouse. In *Cellular Thalamic Mechanisms* (eds. Bentivoglio and R. Spreafico), pp. 489–499. Excerpta Medica, Amsterdam–New York.

Caviness, V.S., Jr. and Frost, D.O. (1980). Tangential organization of thalamic projections of the neocortex in the mouse. *J. Comp. Neurol.*, **194**, 355–367.

Caviness, V.S., Jr., Takahashi, T., and Nowakowski, R.S. (1995). Numbers, time and neocortical neurogenesis: a general developmental and evolutionary model. *Trends Neurosci.*, **18**, 379–383.

Chalepakis, G., Wijnholds, J., Giese, P., Schachner, M., and Gruss, P. (1994). Characterization of Pax6 and Hoxa-1 binding to the promoter region of the neural cell adhesion molecule L1. DNA. *Cell Biol.*, **13**, 891–900.

Chalupa, L.M., Killacky, H.P., Snider, C.J., and Lia, B. (1989). Callosal projection neurons in area 17 of the fetal rhesus monkey. *Dev. Brain Res.*, **46**, 303–308.

Chao, M.V. (1992). Neurotrophin receptors: a window into neuronal differentiation. *Neuron*, **9**, 583–593.

Chao, M.V. and Hempstead, B.L. (1995). p75 and Trk: a two-receptor system. *Trends Neurosci.*, **18**, 321–326.

Chapman, B. and Stryker, M.P. (1993). Development of orientation selectivity in ferret visual cortex and effects of deprivation. *J. Neurosci.*, **13**, 5251–5262.

Chapman, B., Stryker, M.P., and Bonhoeffer, T. (1996). Development of orientation preference maps in ferret primary visual cortex. *J. Neurosci.*, **16**, 6443–6453.

Chedotal, A., Del Rio, J.A., Ruiz, M., He, Z., Borrell, V., de Castro, F., Ezan, F., Goodman, C.S., Tessier-Lavigne, M., Sotelo, C., and Soriano, E. (1998).

Semaphorins III and IV repel hippocampal axons via two distinct receptors. *Development*, **125**, 4313–4323.

Cheng, H.J., Nakamoto, M., Bergemann, A.D., and Flanagan, J.G. (1995). Complementary gradients in expression and binding of Elf-1 and Mek4 in development of the topographic retinotectal projection map. *Cell*, **82**, 371–381.

Cheng, H.-J. and Flanagan, J.G. (1994). Identification and cloning of ELF-1, a development expressed ligand for the Mek4 and Sek receptor tyrosine kinases. *Cell*, **79**, 157–168.

Chenn, A. and McConnell, S.K. (1995). Cleavage orientation and the asymmetric inheritance of Notch 1 immunoreactivity in mammalian neurogenesis. *Cell*, **82**, 631–641.

Chiang, C., Litingtung, Y., Lee, E., Young, K.E., Corden, J.L., Westphal, H., and Beachy, P.A. (1996). Cyclopia and defective axial patterning in mice lacking Sonic hedgehog gene function. *Nature*, **383**, 407–413.

Chomsky, N. (1957). *Syntactic structures*. The Hague: Morton.

Chun, J.J.M. and Shatz, C.J. (1988). A fibronectin-like molecule is present within the developing cat cerebral cortex and is correlated with subplate neurons. *J. Cell. Biol.*, **106**, 857–872.

Chun, J.J., Nakamura, M.J., and Shatz, C.J. (1987). Transient cells of the developing mammalian telencephalon are peptide-immunoreactive neurons. *Nature*, **325**, 617–620.

Chung, S.-H. (1974). In search of the rules for nerve connections. *Cell*, **3**, 201–205.

Chung, S.-H. and Cooke, J. (1975). Polarity of structure and of ordered nerve connections in the developing amphibian brain. *Nature*, **258**, 126–132.

Chung, S.-H. and Cooke, J. (1978). Observations on the formation of the brain and nerve connections following embryonic manipulation of the amphibian neural tube. *Proc. R. Soc. London B.*, **201**, 335–373.

Chung, W.W., Lagenaur, C.F., Yan, Y.M., and Lund, J.S. (1991). Developmental expression of neuronal cell adhesion molecules in the mouse neocortex and olfactory bulb. *J. Comp. Neurol.*, **314**, 290–305.

Clarke, P.G.H. (1998). Apoptosis versus necrosis. In *Cell death and diseases of the nervous system* (eds. V. Koliatsos and R. Ratan). Humana Press, Totowa, NJ.

Clarke, S. and Innocenti, G.M. (1986). Organization of immature intrahemispheric connections. *J. Comp. Neurol.*, **251**, 1–22.

Clasca, F., Angelucci, A., and Sur, M. (1994). Layer 5 neurons establish the first cortical projection to the dorsal thalamus in ferrets. *Soc. Neurosci. Abstr.*, **20**, 98.

Clasca, F., Angelucci, A., and Sur, M. (1995). Layer-specific programs of development in neocortical projection neurons. *Proc. Natl. Acad. Sci. USA*, **92**, 11145–11149.

Cline, H.T. and Constantine-Paton, M. (1989). NMDA receptor antagonists disrupt the retinotectal topographic map. *Neuron*, **3**, 413–426.

Cline, H.T. and Constantine-Paton, M. (1990). The different influence of protein kinase inhibitors on retinal arbor morphology and eye specific stripes. *Neuron*, **4**, 899–908.

Cline, H.T., Debski, E.A., and Constantine-Paton, M. (1987). N-methyl-D-aspartate receptor antagonist desegregates eye specific stripes. *Proc. Natl. Acad. Sci. USA*, **84**, 4342–4345.

Cline, H.T., Debski, E.A., and Constantine-Paton, M. (1990). NMDA receptor agonists and antagonists alter retinal ganglion cell arbor structure in the developing frog retinotectal projection. *J. Neurosci.*, **10**, 1197–1215.

Cohen, S. (1960). Purification of a nerve-growth promoting protein from the mouse salivary gland and its antiserum. *Proc. Natl. Acad. Sci. USA*, **46**, 302–311.

Cohen-Cory, S. and Fraser, S.E. (1995). Effects of brain-derived neurotrophic factor on optic axon branching and remodelling *in vivo*. *Nature*, **378**, 192–196.

Cohen-Cory, S., Elliott, R.C., Dreyfus, C.F., and Black, I.B. (1993). Depolarizing influences increased low-affinity NGF receptor gene expression in cultured Purkinje neurons. *Exp. Neurol.*, **119**, 165–173.

Cohen-Tannoudji, M., Babinet, C., and Wassef, M. (1994). Early determination of a mouse somatosensory cortex marker. *Nature*, **368**, 460–463.

Colamarino, S.A. and Tessier-Lavigne, M. (1995). The axonal chemoattractant netrin-1 is also a chemorepellent for trochlear motor axons. *Cell*, **81**, 621–629.

Collet-Solberg, P.F. and Cohen, P. (1996). The role of the insulin-like growth factor binding proteins and the IGFBP proteases in modulating IGF action. *Growth and Growth Disorders*, **25**, 591–611.

Collingridge, G.L. and Bliss, T.V.P. (1987). NMDA receptors—their role in long-term potentiation. *Trends Neurosci.*, **10**, 288–293.

Constantine-Paton, M. and Law, M.I. (1978). Eye-specific termination bands in tecta of three-eyed frogs. *Science*, **202**, 639–641.

Coogan, T.A. and Burkhalter, A. (1988). Segmental development of connections between striate and extrastriate visual cortical areas in the rat. *J. Comp. Neurol.*, **278**, 242–252.

Cook, J.E. (1987). A sharp retinal image increases the topographic precision of the goldfish retinotectal projection during optic nerve regeneration in stroboscopic light. *Exp. Brain Res.*, **68**, 319–328.

Cook, J.E. (1988). Topographic refinement of the goldfish retinotectal projection: sensitivity to stroboscopic light at different periods during optic nerve regeneration. *Exp. Brain Res.*, **70**, 109–116.

Cook, J.E. and Becker D.L. (1988). Retinotopical refinement of the regenerating goldfish optic tract is not linked to activity-dependent refinement of the retinotectal map. *Development*, **104**, 321–329.

Cook, J.E. and Horder, T.J. (1974). Interactions between optic fibres in their regeneration to specific sites in the goldfish tectum. *J. Physiol.*, **242**, 89–90.

Cook, J.E. and Rankin, E.E.C. (1984). Use of a lethin-peroxidase conjugate (WGA-HRP) to assess the retinotopic precision of goldfish optic terminals. *Neurosci. Lett.*, **48**, 61–66.

Cook, J.E. and Rankin, E.C.C. (1986). Impaired refinement of the regenerated retinotectal projection of the goldfish in stroboscopic light: a quantitative WGA-HRP study. *Exp. Brain Res.*, **63**, 421–430.

Cooke, B., Hegstrom, C.D., Villeneuve, L.S., and Breedlove, S.M. (1998). Sexual differentiation of the vertebrate brain: principles and mechanisms. *Front. Neuroendocrinol.*, **19**, 232–263.

Cooke, J. and Zeeman E.C. (1976). A clock and wave-front model for control of the number of repeated structures during animal morphogenesis. *J. Theor. Biol.*, **58**, 455–476.

Cowan, J.D. and Friedman, A.E. (1990). Development and regeneration of eye-brain maps: a computational model. In *Advances in neural information processing systems* (ed. Touretzky), vol. 2, pp. 3–10. Morgan Kaufman Publishers, San Mateo, California 94403.

Cowan, W.M., Fawcett, J.W., O'Leary, D.D.M., and Stanfield, B. (1984). Regressive events in neurogenesis. *Science*, **225**, 1258–1265.

Cowey, A. (1979). Cortical maps and visual perception. *Qua. Jou. Exper. Psychol.*, **31**, 1–17.

Cox, E.C. Muller, B. and Bonhoeffer, F. (1990). Axonal guidance in the chick visual system: posterior tectal membranes induce collapse of growth cones from temporal retina. *Neuron*, **2**, 31–37.

Crair, M.C. and Malenka, R.C. (1995). A critical period for long-term potentiation at thalamocortical synapses. *Nature*, **375**, 277–278.

Crandall, J.E. and Caviness, V.S. (1984a). Axon strata in the cerebral wall in embryonic mice. *Dev. Brain Res.*, **14**, 185–195.

Crandall, J.E. and Caviness, V.S. (1984b). Thalamocortical connections in newborn mice. *J. Comp. Neurol.*, **228**, 542–556.

Crandall, J.E. and Herrup, K. (1990). Patterns of cell lineage in the cerebral cortex reveal evidence for developmental boundaries. *Exp. Neurol.*, **109**, 131–139.

Crepel, F., Mariani, J., and Delhaye-Bouchaud, N. (1975). Evidence for a multiple innervation of Purkinje cells by climbing fibers in the immature rat cerebellum. *J. Neurobiol.*, **7**, 567–578.

Creutzfeldt, O.D. (1977). Generality of the functional structure of the neocortex. *Naturwissenschaften*, **64**, 507–517.

Crick, F. (1970). Diffusion in embryogenesis. *Nature*, **225**, 420–422.

Crossley, P.H., Martinez, S., and Martin, G.R. (1996). Midbrain development induced by FGF8 in the chick embryo. *Nature*, **380**, 66–68.

Culican, S., Baumrind, N., Yammamoto, M., and Pearlman, A. (1990). Cortical radial glia: Identification in tissue culture and evidence for their transformation to astrocytes. *J. Neurosci.*, **10**, 684–692.

Cunningham, T.J., Haun, F., and Chantler, P.D. (1987). Diffusible proteins prolong survival of dorsal lateral geniculate neurons following occipital cortex lesions in newborn rats. *Dev. Brain Res.*, **37**, 133–141.

Cynader, M., Berman, N., and Hein, A. (1976). Recovery of function in cat visual cortex following prolonged deprivation. *Exp. Brain Res.*, **25**, 139–156.

Da Silva Filho, A.R.C. (1992). Investigation of a generalised version of Amari's continuous model for neural networks. Ph.D. thesis, University of Sussex, UK.

Dale, J.K., Vesque, C., Lints, T.J., Sampath, T.K., Furley, A., Dodds, J., and Placzek, M. (1997). Cooperation of BMP7 and SHH in the induction of forebrain ventral midline cells by prechordal mesoderm. *Cell*, **90**, 257–269.

Daniels, J.D., Pettigrew, J.D., and Norman, J.L. (1978). Development of single-neuron responses in the kitten's lateral geniculate nucleus. *J. Neurophysiol.*, **41**, 1373–1393.

D'Arcangelo, G., Miao, G.G., Chen, S.-C., Soares, H.D., Morgan, J.I., and Curran, T. (1995). A protein related to extracellular matrix proteins deleted in the mouse mutant reeler. *Nature*, **374**, 719–723.

D'Arcangelo, G., Nakajima, K., Miyata, T., Ogawa, M., *et al.* (1997). Reelin is a secreted glycoprotein recognized by the CR-50 monoclonal antibody. *J. Neurosci.*, **17**, 23–31.

Davis, S. and Yancopoulos, G.D. (1993). The molecular biology of the CNTF receptor. *Curr. Opin. Cell Biol.*, **5**, 281–285.

Davidson, D. (1995). The function and evolution of Msx genes: pointers and paradoxes. *Trends Genet.*, **11**, 405–411.

Davies, A.M. (1997). Neurotrophin switching: where does it stand? *Curr. Opin. Neurobiol.*, **7**, 110–118.

Davies, A.M., Lee, K.F., and Jaenisch, R. (1993). p75-deficient trigeminal sensory neurons have an altered response to NGF but not to other neurotrophins. *Neuron*, **11**, 565–574.

Davies, J.A., Cook, G.M.W., Stern, C.D., and Keynes, R.J. (1990). Isolation from chick somites of a glycoprotein fraction that causes collapse of dorsal root growth cones. *Neuron*, **4**, 11–20.

Davis, A. and Temple, S. (1994). A self-renewing multipotential stem cell in embryonic rat cerebral cortex. *Nature*, **372**, 263–266.

Dawson, D.R. and Killackey, H.P. (1985). Distinguishing topography and somatotopy in the thalamocortical projections of the developing rat. *Dev. Brain Res.*, **17**, 309–313.

Dayan, P.S. and Willshaw, D.J. (1991). Optimising synaptic learning rules in linear associative memories. *Biol. Cybern.*, **65**, 253–265.

D'Costa, A.P., Xu, X., Ingram, R.L., and Sonntag, W.E. (1995). Insulin-like growth factor-1 stimulation of protein synthesis is attenuated in cerebral cortex of ageing rats. *Neuroscience*, **65**, 805–813.

De Carlos, J.A. and O'Leary, D.D.M. (1992). Growth and targeting of sub-plate axons and establishment of major cortical pathways. *J. Neurosci.*, **12**, 1194–1211.

De Carlos, J.A., Lopez-Mascaraque, L., and Valverde, F. (1996). Dynamics of cell migration from the lateral ganglionic eminence in the rat. *J. Neurosci.*, **16**, 6146–6156.

De la Pompa, J.L., Wakeham, A., Correia, K.M., Samper, E., *et al.* (1997). Conservation of the Notch signalling pathway in mammalian neurogenesis. *Development*, **124**, 1139–1148.

de Schonen, S. and Mancini, J. (1995). About functional brain specialization: the development of face recognition. *Develop. Cogn. Neurosci. Technical Report no. 95.1.*

de Schonen, S. and Mathivet, H. (1989). First come, first served: a scenario about the development of hemispheric specialization in face recognition during infancy. *Eur. Bull. Cogn. Psychol.*, **9**, 3–44.

DeAngelis, G.C. Ohazawa, I. Freeman, R.D. (1995). Receptive-field dynamics in the central visual pathways. *Trends Neurosci.*, **18**, 451–458.

Dechant, G. and Barde, Y.A. (1997). Signalling through the neurotrophin receptor p75NTR. *Curr. Opin. Neurobiol.*, **7**, 413–418.

Dehaene-Lambertz, G. and Dehaene, S. (1994). Speech and cerebral correlates of syllable discrimination in infants. *Nature*, **370**, 292–295.

Dehay, C., Bullier, J., and Kennedy, H. (1984). Transient projections from the fronto-parietal and temporal cortex to areas 17, 18 and 19 in the kitten. *Exp. Brain Res.*, **57**, 208–212.

Dehay, C., Kennedy, H., and Bullier, J. (1986). Callosal connectivity of areas V1 and V2 in the newborn monkey. *J. Comp. Neurol.*, **254**, 20–33.

Dehay, C., Kennedy, H., and Bullier, J. (1988a). Characterization of transient cortical projections from auditory, somatosensory and motor cortices to visual areas 17, 18 and 19 in the kitten. *J. Comp. Neurol.*, **272**, 68–89.

Dehay, C., Kennedy, H., Bullier, J., and Berland, M (1988b). Absence of interhemispheric connections of area 17 during development in the monkey. *Nature*, **331**, 348–350.

Dehay, C., Giroud, P., Berland, M., Smart, I., and Kennedy, H. (1993). Modulation of the cell cycle contributes to the parcellation of the primate visual cortex. *Nature*, **366**, 464–466.

Del Rio, J.A., Heimrich, B., Borrell, V., Forster, E., Drakew, A., *et al.* (1997). A role for Cajal-Retzius cells and reelin in the development of hippocampal connections. *Nature*, **385**, 70–74.

Dent, M.A., Sumi, Y., Morris, R.J., and Seeley, P.J. (1993). Urokinase-type plasminogen activator expression by neurons and oligodendrocytes during process outgrowth in developing rat brain. *Eur. J. Neurosci.*, **5**, 633–647.

D'Ercole, A.J. (1996). Insulin-like growth factors and their receptors in growth. *Growth and Growth Disorders*, **25**, 573–590.

Derer, P. and Nakanishi, S. (1983). Extracellular matrix distribution during neocortical wall ontogenesis in normal and reeler mice. *J. Hirnforsch.*, **24**, 209–224.

Devor, M. and Schneider, G.E. (1975). Neuroanatomical plasticity: the principle of conservation of total axonal arborization. *Les Colloques de l'INSERM*, **43**, 191–200.

Dityatev, A., Chmykhova, N., Studer, L., Karamian, O., Kozhanov, V., and Clamann, H.P. (1995). Comparison of the topology and growth rules of motoneuronal dendrites. *J. Comp. Neurol.*, **363**, 505–516.

Dobrowsky, R., Werner, M., Castellino, A., Chao, M., and Hannun, Y. (1994). Activation of the sphingomyelin cycle through the low affinity neurotrophin receptor. *Science*, **265**, 1596–1599.

Domenici, L., Cellerino, A., Berardi, N., Cattanco, A., and Maffei, L. (1994). Antibodies to nerve growth factor (NGF) prolong the sensitive period for monocular deprivation in the rat. *Neuroreport*, **5**, 2041–2044.

Doniach, T. (1995). Basic FGF as an inducer of anteroposterior neural pattern. *Cell*, **83**, 1067–1070.

Dono, R., Texido, G., Dussel, R., Ehmke, H., and Zeller, R. (1998). Impaired cerebral cortex development and blood pressure regulation in FGF-2-deficient mice. *EMBO J.*, **17**, 4213–4225.

Dreher, B. and Cottee, L.J. (1975). Visual receptive-field properties of cells in area 18 of cat's cerebral cortex before and after acute lesions in area 17. *J. Neurophysiol.*, **38**, 735–750.

Drescher, U., Kremoser, C., Handwerker, C., Loschinger, J., Noda, M., and Bonhoeffer, F. (1995). *In vitro* guidance of retinal ganglion-cell axons by RAGS, a 25 KDa tectal protein related to ligands for Eph receptor tyrosine kinases. *Cell*, **82**, 359–370.

Dubner, R. and Zeki, S. (1971). Response properties and receptive fields of cells in an anatomically defined region of the superior temporal sulcus. *Brain Res.*, **35**, 528–532.

Dunn-Meynell, A.A. and Sharma, S.C. (1986). The visual system of channel catfish (*Icatalurus-punctatus*) 1. Retinal ganglion cell morphology. *J. Comp. Neurol.*, **247**, 32–55.

Durbin, R. and Mitchison, G. (1990). A dimension reduction framework for understanding cortical maps. *Nature*, **343**, 644–647.

Durbin, R. and Willshaw, D.J. (1987). An analogue approach to the travelling salesman problem using an elastic net method. *Nature*, **126**, 689–691.

Eagleson, G.W. and Harris, W.A. (1990). Mapping of the presumptive brain regions in the neural plate of *Xenopus Laevis*. *J. Neurobiol.*, **21**, 427–440.

Eagleson, K.L., Ferri, R.T., and Levitt, P. (1996). Complementary distribution of collagen type IV and the epidermal growth factor receptor in the rat embryonic telencephalon. *Cereb. Cortex*, **6**, 540–549.

Eccles, J.C., Ito, M., and Szentagothai, J. (1967). *The cerebellum as a neuronal machine*. Springer-Verlag, Berlin.

Echelard, Y., Epstein, D.J., St-Jaques, B., Shen, L., Mohler, J., McMahon, J.A., and McMahon, A.P. (1993). Sonic hedgehog, a member of a family of putative signalling molecules, is implicated in the regulation of CNS polarity. *Cell*, **75**, 1417–1430.

Eckenstein, F.P. (1994). Fibroblast growth factors in the nervous system. *J. Neurobiol.*, **25**, 1467–1480.

Eckhorn, R., Bauer, R., Jordan, W., Brosch, M., Kruse, W., Munk, M., and Reitboeck, M.J. (1988). Coherent oscillations: a mechanism of feature linking in the visual cortex? *Biol. Cybern.*, **60**, 121–130.

Edds, M.V. (1979). Plasticity of retinotectal connections in fishes and amphibians. *Neurosci. Res. Prog. Bull.*, **17**, 251–272.

Edelman, G.M. and Crossin, K.L. (1991). Cell adhesion molecules: implications for a molecular histology. *Annu. Rev. Biochem.*, **60**, 155–190.

Edelman, G.M. and Jones, F.S. (1995). Developmental control of NCAM expression by Hox and Pax gene products. *Phil. Trans. R. Soc. Lond. B. Biol. Sci.*, **17**, 305–312.

Egar, M. and Singer, M. (1972). The role of the ependyma in spinal cord regeneration in the urodele *triturus*. *Exp. Neurol.*, **37**, 422–430.

Eide, F.F., Lowenstein, D.H., and Reichardt, L.F. (1993). Neurotrophins and their receptors—current concepts and implication for neurologic disease. *Exp. Neurol.*, **121**, 200–214.

Einas, P.D., Siqueland, E.R., Jusczyck, P., and Vigorito, J. (1971). Speech perception in infants. *Science*, **171**, 303–306.

Ellison, J.A., Scully, S.A., and de Vellis, J. (1996). Evidence for neuronal regulation of oligodendrocyte development: cellular localisation of platelet-derived growth factor alpha receptor and A-chain RNA during cerebral cortical development in the rat. *J. Neurosci. Res.*, **45**, 28–39.

Ellmeier, W., Aguzzi, A., Kleiner, E., Kurzbauer, R., and Weith, A. (1992). Mutally exclusive expression of a helix-loop-helix gene and N-myc in human neuroblastomas and in normal development. *EMBO J.*, **11**, 2563–2571.

ElShamy, W.M., Linnarsson, S., Lee, K.-F., Janeisch, R., and Ernfors, P. (1996). Prenatal and postnatal requirements of NT-3 for sympathetic neuroblast survival and innervation of specific targets. *Development*, **122**, 491–500.

Engel, A.K., König, P., Kreiter, A.K., and Singer, W. (1991). Interhemispheric synchronization of oscillatory neuronal responses in cat visual cortex. *Science*, **252**, 1177–1179.

Enroth-Cugell, C. and Robson, J.G. (1966). The contrast sensitivity of retinal ganglion cells of the cat. *J. Physiol.*, **187**, 517–552.

Ericson, J., Muhr, J., Placzek, M., Lints, T., *et al.* (1995). Sonic hedgehog induces the differentiation of ventral forebrain neurons: a common signal for ventral patterning within the neural tube. *Cell*, **81**, 747–758.

Ericson, J., Rashbass, P., Schedl, A., Brenner-Morton, S., *et al.* (1997). Pax6 controls progenitor cell identity and neuronal fate in response to graded Shh signaling. *Cell*, **90**, 169–180.

Ernfors, P., Lee, K.F., and Jaenisch, R. (1994a). Mice lacking brain-derived neurotrophic factor develop with sensory deficits. *Nature*, **368**, 147–150.

Ernfors, P., Lee, K.F., Kucera, J., and Jaenisch, R. (1994b). Lack of neurotrophin-3 leads to deficiencies in the peripheral nervous system and loss of limb proprioceptive afferents. *Cell*, **77**, 503–512.

Erwin, E., Obermayer, K., and Schulten, K. (1995). Models of orientation and ocular dominance columns in the visual cortex: a critical comparison. *Neural Computation*, **7**, 425–468.

Erzurumlu, R.S. and Jhaveri, S. (1990). Thalamic axons confer a blueprint of the sensory periphery onto the developing rat somatosensory cortex. *Dev. Brain Res.*, **56**, 229–234.

Erzurumlu, R.S. and Jhaveri, S. (1992). Emergence of connectivity in the embryonic rat parietal cortex. *Cerebral Cortex*, **2**, 336–352.

Evrard, P., Marret, S., and Gressens, P. (1997). Genetic and environmental determinants of neocortical development: clinical applications. In *Normal and abnormal development of the cortex* (eds. A. Galaburda and Y. Christen), pp. 165–178. Springer-Verlag.

Fawcett, J.W. and Willshaw, D.J. (1982). Compound eyes project stripes onto the optic tectum. *Nature*, **296**, 350–352.

Feldman, J.D. and Gaze, R.M. (1975). The development of half-eyes in *Xenopus* tadpoles. *J. Comp. Neurol.*, **162**, 13–22.

Ferrer, J.M.R., Price, D.J., and Blakemore, C. (1988). The organization of cortico-cortical projections from area 17 to area 18 of the cat's visual cortex. *Proc. R. Soc. London Ser. B*, **233**, 77–98.

Ferrer, J.M.R., Kato, N., and Price, D.J. (1992). The organisation of association projections from area 17 to areas 18 and 19 and to suprasylvian areas in the cat's visual cortex. *J. Comp. Neurol.*, **316**, 261–278.

Figurov, A., Pozzo-Miller, L.D., Olafson, P., Wang, T, and Lu, B. (1996). Regulation of synaptic responses to high-frequency stimulation and LTP by neurotrophins in the hippocampus. *Nature*, **381**, 706–709.

Filosa, S., Rivera-Perez, J.A., Gomez, A.P., Gansmuller, A., *et al.* (1997). Goosecoid and HNF-3b genetically interact to regulate neural tube patterning during mouse embryogenesis. *Development*, **124**, 2843–2854.

Finlay, B.L. and Pallas, S.L. (1989). Control of cell number in the developing mammalian visual system. *Prog. Neurobiol.*, **32**, 207–234.

Finlay, B.L. and Slattery, M. (1983). Local differences in amount of early cell death in neocortex predict adult local specializations. *Science*, **219**, 1349–1351.

Fishell, G. (1995). Striatal precursors adopt cortical identities in response to local cues. *Development*, **121**, 803–812.

Fishell, G. (1997). Regionalization in the mammalian telencephalon. *Curr. Opin. Neurobiol.*, **7**, 62–69.

Fishell, G. and Hatten, M.E. (1991). Astrotactin provides a receptor system for CNS neuronal migration. *Development*, **113**, 755–765.

Fishell, G., Rossant, J., and van der Kooy, D. (1990). Neuronal lineages in chimaeric mouse forebrain are segregated between compartments and in the rostrocandal and radial planes. *Dev. Biol.*, **141**, 70–83.

Fishell, G., Mason, C.A., and Hatton, M.E. (1993). Dispersion of neural progenitors within the germinal zones of the forebrain. *Nature*, **362**, 636–638.

Fitzgerald, M., Kwiat, G.C., Middleton, J., and Pini, A. (1993). Ventral spinal cord inhibition of neurite outgrowth from embryonic rat dorsal root ganglion. *Development*, **117**, 1377–1384.

Fladby, T. and Jansen, J.K.S. (1987). Postnatal loss of synaptic terminals in the partially denervated mouse soleus muscle. *Acta Physiol. Scand.*, **129**, 239–246.

Flanagan, J.G. and Vanderhaeghen, P. (1998). The ephrins and Eph receptors in neural development. *Annu. Rev. Neurosci.*, **21**, 309–345.

Ford, M., Bartlett, P.F., and Nurcombe, V. (1994). Co-localization of FGF-2 and a novel mouse heparan sulfate proteoglycan in embryonic mouse brain. *Neuroreport*, **5**, 565–568.

Forscher, P. (1988). Calcium and polyphosphoinositide control of cytoskeletal dynamics. *Trends Neurosci.*, **12**(11), 468–479.

Forscher, P. and Smith, S.J. (1988). Actions of cytochalasins on the organization of actin filaments and microtubules in a neuronal growth cone. *J. Cell Biol.*, **107**, 1505–1516.

Frade, J.M., Rodriguez-Tebar, A., and Barde, Y.A. (1996). Induction of cell death by endogenous nerve growth factor through its p75 receptor. *Nature*, **383**, 166–168.

Frantz, G.D. and McConnell, S.K. (1996). Restriction of late cerebral cortical progenitors to an upper-layer fate. *Neuron*, **17**, 55–61.

Frantz, G.D., Bohner, A.P., Akers, R.M., and McConnell, S.K. (1994a). Regulation of the POU domain gene SCIP during cerebral cortical development. *J. Neurosci.*, **14**, 472–485.

Frantz, G.D., Weimann, J.M., Levin, M.E., and McConnell, S.K. (1994b). Otx1 and Otx2 define layers and regions in developing cerebral cortex and cerebellum. *J. Neurosci.*, **14**, 5725–5740.

Franz, T. (1994). Extra-toes (xt) homozygous mutant mice demonstrate a role for the gli-3 gene in the development of the forebrain. *Acta Anat.*, **150**, 38–44.

Fraser, A., Keynes, R., and Lumsden, A. (1990). Segmentation in the chick embryo hindbrain is defined by cell lineage restrictions. *Nature*, **344**, 431–435.

Fraser, S.E. (1981). A different adhesion approach to the patterning of neural connections. *Dev. Bio.*, **79**, 453–464.

Fraser, S.E. and Hunt, R.K. (1980). Retinotectal specificity: models and experiments in search of a mapping function. *Annu. Rev. Neurosci.*, **3**, 319–352.

Frean, M. (1990). The upstart algorithm: a method for constructing and training feedforward neural networks. *Neural Comp.*, **2**, 198–200.

Frégnac, Y., Shulz, D., Thorpe, S., and Bienenstock, E. (1988). A cellular analogue of visual cortical plasticity. *Nature*, **333**, 367–370.

Friauf, E., McConnell, S.K., and Shatz, C.J. (1990). Functional synaptic circuits in the subplate during fetal and early postnatal development of cat visual cortex. *J. Neurosci.*, **10**, 2601–2613.

Friedlander, M.J. and Martin, K.A.C. (1989). Development of Y-axon innnervation of cortical area 18 in the cat. *J. Physiol.*, **416**, 183–214.

Friedman, G.C. and O'Leary, D.D.M. (1996). Retroviral misexpression of engrailed genes in the chick optic tectum perturbs the topographic targeting of retinal axons. *J. Neurosci.*, **16**, 5498–5509.

Frigerio, G., Burri, M., Bopp, D., Baumgartner, S., and Noll, M. (1986). Structure of the segmentation gene paired and the Drosophila PRD gene set as part of a gene network. *Cell*, **47**, 735–746.

Frost, D.O. and Metin, C. (1985). Introduction of functional retinal projections to the somatosensory system. *Nature*, **317**, 162–164.

Frotscher, M. and Soriano, E. (1998). Different functions of Cajal-Retzius cells and reelin in cortical development. *Eur. J. Neurosci.*, **S10**, 102.

Fujita, S. (1964). Analysis of neuron differentiation in the central nervous system by tritiated thymidine autoradiography. *J. Comp. Neurol.*, **122**, 311–328.

Fukuda, T., Kawano, H., Ohyama, K., Li, H.P., Takda, Y., Oohira, A., and Kawamura, K. (1997). Immunohistochemical localization of neurocan and L1 in the formation of thalamocortical pathway of developing rats. *J. Comp. Neurol.*, **382**, 141–152.

Furuta, Y., Piston, D.W., and Hogan, B.L.M. (1997). Bone morphogenetic proteins (BMPs) as regulators of dorsal forebrain development. *Development*, **124**, 2203–2212.

Gabriel, S.M., Haroutunian, V., Powchik, P., Honer, W.G., *et al.* (1997). Increased concentrations of presynaptic proteins in the cingulate cortex of subjects with schizophrenia. *Arch. Gen. Psychiatry*, **54**, 559–566.

Gadisseux, J.F., Evrard, P., Misson, J.P., and Cariness, V.S. (1989). Dynamic structure of the radial glial fibre system of the developing murine cerebral wall. an immunocytochemical analysis. *Dev. Brain Res.*, **50**, 55–67.

Gadisseux, J.-F., Goffinet, A.M., Lyon, G., and Evrard, P. (1992). The human transient subpial granular layer: an optical, immunohistochemical, and ultrastructural analysis. *J. Comp. Neurol.*, **324**, 94–114.

Galaburda, A.M. (1997). Toxicity of plasticity. Lessons from a model of developmental learning disorder. In *Normal and abnormal development of the cortex* (ed. A. Galaburda and Y. Christen), pp. 135–144. Springer-Verlag.

Gallant, S.I. (1986). Three constructive algorithms for network learning. Proc. Eight Annual Conference of the Cognitive Science Society, Amherst, MA, Aug. 15–17, 1986, 652–660.

Galli, L. and Maffei, L. (1988). Spontaneous impulse activity of rat retinal ganglion cells in prenatal life. *Science*, **242**, 90–91.

Garcia Bellido, A., Lawrence, P.A., and Morata, G. (1979). Compartments in animal development. *Sci. Am.*, **241**, 102–111.

Garrity, P.A., Rao, Y., Salecker, I., McGlade, J., Pawson, T. and Zipursky, S.L. (1996). Drosophila photoreceptor axon guidance and targeting requires the dreadlocks SH2/SH3 adaptor protein. *Cell*, **85**, 639–650.

Gaze, R.M. (1958). The representation of the retina on the optic lobe of the frog. *Qu. J. Exp. Physiol.*, **43**, 209–224.

Gaze, R.M. (1960). Regeneration of the optic nerve in Amphibia. *Int. Rev. Neurobiol.*, **2**, 1–40.

Gaze, R.M. (1970). The formation of nerve connections. London: Academic Press.

Gaze, R.M. and Hope, R.A. (1983). The visuotectal projection following translocation of grafts within an optic tectum in the goldfish. *J. Physiol.*, **344**, 257.

Gaze, R.M. and Keating, M.J. (1972). The visual system and 'neuronal specificity'. *Nature*, **237**, 375–378.

Gaze, R.M. and Sharma, S.C. (1970). Axial differences in the reinnervation of the goldfish optic tectum by regenerating optic nerve fibres. *Exp. Brain Res.*, **10**, 171–181.

Gaze, R.M., Jacobson, M., and Szekely (1963). The retinotectal projection in *Xenopus* with compound eyes. *J. Physiol. Lond.*, **165**, 384–499.

Gaze, R.M., Keating, M.J., and Chung, S.H. (1974). The evolution of the retinotectal map during development in *Xenopus*. *Proc. R. Soc. London B*, **185**, 301–330.

Gaze, R.M., Feldman, J.D., Cooke, J., and Chung, S.-H. (1979a). The orientation of the visuo-tectal map in *Xenopus*: development aspects. *J. Embryol. Exp. Morph.*, **53**, 39–66.

Gaze, R.M., Keating, M.J., Ostberg, A., and Chung (1979b). The relationship between retinal and tectal growth in larval *Xenopus*: implications for the development of the retino-tectal projection. *J. Embryol. Exp. Morph.*, **53**, 103–143.

Gaze, R.M. and Straznicky, C. (1980). Regeneration of optic nerve fibres from a compound eye to both tecta in *Xenopus*: evidence relating to the state of specification of the eye and the tectum. *J. Embryol. Exp. Morph.*, **60**, 125–140.

Gearhart, J. (1998). New potential for human embryonic stem cells. *Science*, **282**, 1061–1062.

Gehring, W. (1986). On the homeobox and its significance. *Bioessays*, **5**, 3–4.

Geschwind, N. (1970). The organisation of language and the brain. *Science*, **170**, 940–944.

Ghosh, A. and Greenberg, M.E. (1995). Distinct roles for bFGF and NT-3 in the regulation of cortical neurogenesis. *Neuron*, **15**, 89–103.

Ghosh, A. and Shatz, C. (1992a). Pathfinding and target selection by developing geniculocortical axons. *J. Neurosci.*, **12**, 39–55.

Ghosh, A. and Shatz, C. (1992b). Involvement of subplate neurons in the formation of ocular dominance columns. *Science*, **255**, 1441–1443.

Ghosh, A., Antonini, A., McConnell, S.K., and Shatz, C.J. (1990). Requirement for subplate neurons in the formation of thalamocortical connections. *Nature*, **347**, 179–181.

Ghosh, A., Carnahan, J., and Greenberg, M.E. (1994). Requirement for BDNF in activity-dependent survival of cortical neurons. *Science*, **263**, 1618–1623.

Gierer, A. (1983). Model for the retinotectal projection. *Proc. R. Soc. London B*, **218**, 77–93.

Gierer, A. and Meinhardt, H. (1972). A theory of biological pattern formation. *Kybernetik*, **12**, 30–39.

Giger, R.J., Wolfer, D.P., DeWit, G.M.J., and Verhaagen, J. (1996). Anatomy of rat semaphorin III collapsin-1 mRNA expression and relationship to developing nerve tracts during neuroembryogenesis. *J. Comp. Neurol.*, **375**, 378–392.

Gilbert, C.D. and Wiesel, T.N. (1981). Laminar specialisation and intracortical connections in cat primary visual cortex. In *The organisation of the cerebral cortex* (eds. F.O. Schmitt, F.G. Worden, G. Edelman, and S.G. Dennis). MIT Press, Cambridge, MA.

Gilbert, C.D. and Wiesel, T.N. (1983). Clustered intrinsic connections in cat visual cortex. *J. Neurosci.*, **3**, 1116–1133.

Gilbert, C.D. and Wiesel, T.N. (1989). Columnar specificity of intrinsic horizontal connections in cat visual cortex. *J. Neurosci.*, **9**, 2432–2442.

Gillies, K. and Price, D.J. (1993a). The fates of cells in the developing cerebral cortex of normal and methylazoxymethanol acetate-lesioned mice. *Eur. J. Neurosci.*, **5**, 73–84.

Gillies, K. and Price, D.J. (1993b). Cell migration and subplate loss in explant cultures of murine cerebral cortex. *Neuroreport*, **4**, 911–914.

Glantz, L.A. and Lewis, D.A. (1997). Reduction of synaptophysin immunore-activity in the prefrontal cortex of subjects with schizophrenia – regional and diagnostic specificity. *Arch. Gen. Psychiatry*, **54**, 660–669.

Gleeson, J.G. and Walsh, C.A. (1997). New genetic insights into cerebral cortical development. In *Normal and abnormal development of the cortex* (ed. A. Galaburda and Y. Christen), pp. 145–164. Springer-Verlag.

Godement, P., Vanselow, J., Thanos, S., and Bonhoeffer, F. (1987). A study in developing visual systems with a new method of staining neurones and their processes in fixed tissue. *Development*, **101**, 697–713.

Godfraind, C., Schachner, M., and Goffinet, A.M. (1988). Immunohistochemical localization of cell adhesion molecules L1, J1, N-CAM and their common carbohydrate L2 in the embryonic cortex of normal and reeler mice. *Dev. Brain Res.*, **42**, 99–111.

Goffinet, A.M. (1984). Events governing organization of postmigratory neurons: studies on brain development in normal and reeler mice. *Brain Res. Rev.*, **7**, 261–296.

Golden, J.A. and Cepko, C.L. (1996). Clones in the chick diencephalon contain mutliple cell types and siblings are widely dispersed. *Development*, **122**, 65–78.

Goldman, J.E. and Vaysse, P.J.-J. (1991). Tracing glial cell lineages in the mammalian forebrain. *Glia*, **4**, 149–156.

Goldstein, B. (1989). *Sensation and perception*. Belmont, CA: Wadsworth, third edition.

Gomez-Pinilla, F. and Cotman, C.W. (1993). Distribution of fibroblast growth factor-5 mRNA in the rat brain: an *in situ* hybridisation study. *Brain Res.*, **606**, 79–86.

Gonzales, A.M., Hill, D.J., Logan, A., Maher, P.A., and Baird, A. (1996). Distribution of fibroblast growth factor (FGF)-2 and FGF receptor-1 messenger RNA expression and protein presence in the mid-trimester human foetus. *Paediatric Research*, **39**, 375–385.

Goodhill, G.J. (1993). Topography and ocular dominance: a model exploring positive correlations. *Biol. Cybern.*, **69**, 109–118.

Goodhill, G.J. (1997). Diffusion in axon guidance. *Eur. J. Neurosci.*, **9**, 1414–1421.

Goodhill, G.J. and Willshaw, D.J. (1990). Application of the elastic net algorithm to the formation of ocular dominance stripes. *Network*, **1**, 41–59.

Goodhill, G.J. and Baier, H. (1998). Axon guidance: stretching gradients to the limit. *Neural Computation*, **10**, 521–527.

Goodhill, G.J. and Loewel, S. (1995). Theory meets experiment: correlated neural activity helps determine ocular dominance column periodicity. *Trends Neurosci.*, **18**, 437–439.

Goodhill, G.J. and Richards, L.J. (1999). Retinotectal maps: molecules, models and misplaced data. *Trends Neurosci.*, **22**, 529–534.

Goodman, C.S. and Shatz, C.J. (1992). Developmental mechanisms that generate precise patterns of neuronal connectivity. *Cell (Supplement)*, **72**, 77–98.

Goren, C.C., Sarty, M. and Wu, P.Y.K. (1975). Visual following and pattern discrimination of face-like stimuli by newborn infants. *Pediatrics*, **56**, 544–549.

Gottlieb, D., Rock, K., and Glaser, L. (1976). A gradient of adhesive specificity in developing avian retina. *Proc. Natl. Acad. Sci. USA*, **73**, 410–414.

Götz, M., Novak, N., Bastmayer, M., and Bolz, J. (1992). Membrane-bound molecules in rat cerebral cortex regulate thalamic innervation. *Development*, **116**, 507–519.

Götz, M., Wizenmann, A., Reinhardt, S., Lumsden, A., and Price, J. (1996). Selective adhesion of cells from different telencephalic regions. *Neuron*, **16**, 551–564.

Götz, M., Stoykova, A., and Gruss, P. (1998). Pax6 controls radial glia differentiation in the cerebral cortex. *Neuron*, **21**, 1031–1044.

Götz, R., Koster, R., Winkler, C., Raulf, F., Lattspeich, F., *et al.* (1994). Neurotrophin-6 is a new member of the nerve growth factor family. *Nature*, **372**, 266–269.

Gouzé, J. L., Lasry, J.M., and Changeux, J.P. (1983). Selective stabilization of muscle innervation during development: A mathematical model. *Biol. Cybern.*, **46**, 207–215.

Gradwohl, G., Fode, C., and Guillemot, F. (1996). Restricted expression of a novel murine atonal-related bHLH protein in undifferentiated neural precursors. *Dev. Biol.*, **180**, 227–241.

Graff, J.M., Bansal, A., and Melton, D.A. (1996). *Xenopus* mad proteins transduce distinct subsets of signals for the TGF-beta superfamily. *Cell*, **85**, 479–487.

Graham, A., Papalopulu, N., and Krumlauf, R. (1989). The murine and *Drosophila* homeobox gene complexes have common features of organization and expression. *Cell*, **57**, 367–378.

Graybiel, A.M. and Berson, D.M. (1981). Families of related cortical areas in the extrastriate visual system. In Cortical sensory organisation, vol 2, Multiple visual areas (ed. C. Woolsey). Humana Press, Clifton, NJ.

Gressens, P., Richelme, C., Kadhim, H., Gadisseux, J.F., and Evrard, P. (1992). The germinative zone produces most cortical astrocytes after neuronal migration in developing mammalian brain. *Biol. Neonate*, **61**, 4–24.

Gross, R.E., Mehler, M.F., Mabie, P.C., Zang, Z., Santschi, L., and Kessler, J. (1996). Bone morphogenetic proteins promote astroglial lineage commitment by mammalian subventricular zone progenitor cells. *Neuron*, **17**, 595–606.

Grove, E.A., Williams, B.P., Li, D.-Q., Hajihosseini, M., Friedrich, A., and Price, J. (1993). Multiple restricted lineages in the embryonic rat cerebral cortex. *Development*, **117**, 553–561.

Grove, E.A., Tole, S., Limon, J., Yip, L-W, and Ragsdale, C.W. (1998). The hem of the embryonic cerebral cortex is defined by the expression of multiple Wnt genes and is compromised in Gli3-deficient mice. *Development*, **125**, 2315–2325.

Guillery, R.W. (1974). Visual pathways in albinos. *Sci. Am.*, **230**, 44–54.

Gulisano, M., Broccoli, V., Pardini, C., and Boncinelli, E. (1996). Emx1 and Emx2 show different patterns of expression during proliferation and differentiation of the developing cerebral cortex in the mouse. *Eur. J. Neurosci.*, **8**, 1037–1050.

Gundersen, R.W. and Barrett, J.N. (1979). Neuronal chemotaxis: chick dorsal root axons turn toward high concentrations of nerve growth factor. *Science*, **206**, 1079–1080.

Guthrie, S. (1992). Lineage in the cerebral cortex: when is a clone not a clone? *Trends Neurosci.*, **15**, 273–276.

Hale, A.J., Smith, C.A., Sutherland, L.C., Stoneman, V.E.A., Longthorne, V.L., Culhane, A.C., and Williams, G.T. (1996). Apoptosis: molecular regulation of cell death. *Eur. J. Biochem.*, **236**, 1–26.

Halfter, W., Claviez, M., and Schwarz, U. (1981). Preferential adhesion of tectal membranes to anterior embryonic chick retina neurites. *Nature*, **292**, 67–70.

Hamburger, V. (1958). Regression versus peripheral control of differentiation in motor hypoplasia. *Am. J. Anat.*, **102**, 365–410.

Hamburger, V. (1975). Cell death in the development of the lateral motor column of the chick embryo. *J. Comp. Neuro.*, **160**, 535–546.

Hamburger, V. and Levi-Montalcini, R. (1949). Proliferation, differentiation and degeneration in the spinal ganglia of the chick embryo under normal and experimental conditions. *J. Exp. Zool.*, **111**, 457–501.

Hamburger, V. and Oppenheim, R.W. (1982). Naturally occurring neuronal death in vertebrates. *Neurosci. Comment*, **1**, 39–55.

Hamelin, M., Zhou, Y., Su, M.-W., Scott, I.M. and Culotti, J.G. (1993). Expression of the unc-5 guidance receptor in the touch neurons of *C. elegans* steers their axons dorsally. *Nature*, **364**, 327–330.

Hantzopoulus, P., Suri, C., Glass, D., Goldfarb, M., and Yancopoulos, G. (1994). The low affinity NGF receptor, p75, can collaborate with each of the Trks to potentiate functional response to the neurotrophins. *Neuron*, **13**, 187–201.

Harris, W.A. (1980). The effect of eliminating impulse activity on the development of the retino-tectal projection in salamanders. *J. Comp. Neurol.*, **194**, 303–317.

Harrison, R.G. (1910). The outgrowth of the nerve fiber as a mode of protoplasmic movement. *J. Exp. Zool.*, **9**, 787–845.

Harrison, R.G. (1914). The reaction of embryonic cells to solid structures. *J. Exp. Zool.*, **17**, 521–544.

Harrison, R.G. (1918). Experiments on the development of the forelimb of *ambystoma*, a self-differentiating equipotential system. *J. Exp. Zool.*, **25**, 413–461.

Hartwell, L.H. and Weinert, T.A. (1989). Checkpoints: controls that ensure the order of cell cycle events. *Science*, **246**, 614–621.

Hatanaka, Y., Uratani, Y., Takaguchi-Hayashi, K, *et al.* (1994). Intracortical regionality represented by specific transcription for a novel protein, latexin. *Eur. J. Neurosci.*, **6**, 973–982.

Hatini, V., Tao, W., and Lai, E. (1994). Expression of winged helix genes, BF-1 and BF-2, define adjacent domains within the developing forebrain and retina. *J. Neurobiol.*, **25**, 1293–1309.

Hatten, M.E. (1993). The role of migration in central nervous system neuronal development. *Curr. Opin. Neurobiol.*, **3**, 38–44.

Haukin, M.H. and Silver, J. (1988). Development of intersecting CNS fiber tracts: the corpus callosum and its perforating fiber pathway. *J. Comp. Neurol.*, **272**, 177–190.

Haun, F. and Cunningham, T. (1993). Recovery of frontal cortex-mediated visual behaviors following neurotrophic rescue of axotomised neurons in medial frontal cortex. *J. Neurosci.*, **13**, 614–622.

Hawken, M. and Parker, A.J. (1990). Detection and discrimination mechanisms in the striate cortex of the old-world monkey. In *Vision: coding and efficiency* (ed. C. Blakemore). Cambridge University Press, Cambridge.

He, X., Treacy, M.N., Simmons, D.M., Ingraham, H.A., Swanson, L.W., and Rosenfeld, M.G. (1989). Expression of a large family of POU-domain regulatory genes in mammalian brain development. *Nature*, **340**, 35–41.

Hebb, D.O. (1949). The organisation of behavior. Wiley, New York.

Heffner, C.D., Lumsden, A.G.S., and O'Leary, D.D.M. (1990). Target control of collateral extension and directional axon growth in the mammalian brain. *Science*, **247**, 217–220.

Hely, T.A. (1999). Computational models of developing neural systems. PhD thesis, University of Edinburgh.

Hely, T.A., Graham, B.C., and van Ooyen, A. (1999). A computational model of dendrite elongation and branching based on MAP2 phosphorylation. *paper submitted*.

Hemmati-Brivanlou, A. and Melton, D. (1997). Vertebrate neural induction. *Annu. Rev. Neurosci.*, **20**, 43–60.

Henderson, C.E. (1996). Programmed cell death in the developing nervous system. *Neuron*, **17**, 579–585.

Henderson, Z. and Blakemore, C. (1986). Organization of the visual pathways in the newborn kitten. *Neurosci. Res.*, **3**, 628–659.

Hendrickson, A.E., Van Brederode, J.F.M., Mulligan, K.A., and Celio, M.R. (1991). Development of the calcium-binding proteins parvalbumin and calbindin in monkey striate cortex. *J. Comp. Neurol.*, **307**, 626–646.

Henke-Fahle, S., Mann, F., Gotz, M., Wild, K., and Bolz, J. (1996). Dual action of a carbohydrate epitope on afferent and efferent axons in cortical development. *J. Neurosci.*, **16**, 4195–4206.

Hentschel, H.G.E. and Fine, A. (1996). Diffusion-regulated control of cellular dendritic morphogenesis. *Proc. Natl. Acad. Sci. USA*, **263**, 1–8.

Hermann, K., Antonini, A., and Shatz, C.J. (1994). Ultrastructural evidence for synpatic interactions between thalamocortical axons and subplate neurons. *Eur. J. Neurosci.*, **6**, 1729–1742.

Herrick, C.J. (1948). *The brain of the tiger salamander*. University of Chicago Press, Chicago.

Herrmann, B.G., Labeit, S., Poustka, A., King, T.R., and Lehrach, H. (1990). Cloning of the T-gene required in mesoderm formation in the mouse. *Nature*, **343**, 617–622.

Hertz, J.A., Krogh and Palmer, R.G. (1991). *Introduction to the theory of neural computation*. Addison Wesley, Redwood City.

Hickey, T.L. and Hitchcock, P.F. (1984). Genesis of neurons in the dorsal lateral geniculate nucleus of the cat. *J. Comp. Neurol.*, **228**, 186–199.

Hill, R.E., Favor, J., Hogan, B.L.M., Ton, C.C.T., Saunders, G.F., Hanson, I.M., Prosser, J., Jordan, T., Hastie, N.D., and van Heyningen, V. (1991). Small eye results from mutations in a paired-like homeobox-containing gene. *Nature*, **354**, 522–525.

Hirotsune, S., Takahara, T., Sasaki, N., Hirose, K., Yoshiki, A., Ohashi, T., Kusukabe, M., Murakami, Y., Muramatsu, M., Watanabe, S., Nakao, K., Katsuki, M. and Hayashizaki, Y. (1995). The reeler gene encodes a protein with an EGF-like motif expressed by pioneer neurons. *Nat. Genet.*, **10**, 77–83.

Hirsch, H.V.B. and Spinelli, D.N. (1971). Modification of the distribution of receptive filed orientation in cats by selective visual exposure during development. *Exp. Brain Res.*, **13**, 509–527.

Hitchcock, P.F. and Hickey, T.L. (1980). Ocular dominance columns: evidence for their presence in humans. *Brain Res.*, **182**, 176–179.

Hogan, B.L.M. (1996). Bone morphogenesis proteins: multifunctional regulators of vertebrate development. *Genes Dev.*, **10**, 1580–1594.

Hohn, A., Allendoerfer, K.L., Toroian-Raymond, A., and Shatz, C.J. (1993). Survival of subplate neurons in cultures of developing neocortex. *Soc. Neurosci. Abstr.*, **19**, 620.7.

Hollyday, M. (1981). Rules of motor innervation in chick-embryos with supernumerary limbs. *J. Comp. Neurol.*, **202**, 439–465.

Hollyday, M. and Hamburger, V. (1976). Reduction of the naturally occurring motor neuron loss by enlargement of the periphery. *J. Comp. Neurol.*, **170**, 311–320.

Holst, B.D., Wang, Y., Jones, F.S., and Edelman, G.M. (1997). A binding site for Pax proteins regulates expression of the gene for the neural cell adhesion molecule in the embryonic spinal cord. *Proc. Natl. Acad. Sci. USA*, **94**(4), 1465–1470.

Holt, C.E. (1984). Does timing of axon outgrowth influence retinotectal topography in *Xenopus*? *J. Neurosci.*, **4**, 1130–1152.

Holt, C.E., Bertsch, T.W., Ellis, H., and Harris, W.A. (1988). Cellular determination in the *Xenopus* retina is independent of lineage and birth date. *Neuron*, **1**, 15–26.

Holtzman, D.M., Li, Y., Parada, L.F., Kinsman, S., Chen, C.-K., Valletta, J.S., Zhou, J., Long, J.B., and Mobley, W.C. (1992). p140trk mRNA marks NGF-responsive forebrain neurones: evidence that trk gene expression is induced by NGF. *Neuron*, **9**, 465–478.

Honda, S., Kagoshima, M., Wanaka, A., Tohyama, M., Matsumoto, K., and Nakamura, T. (1995). Localisation and funtional coupling of HGF and C-Met/HGF receptor in rat brain: implication as a neurotrophic factor. *Mol. Brain Res.*, **32**, 197–210.

Honig, M.G. and Hume, R.I. (1986). Fluorescent carbocyanine dyes allow living cells of identified origin to be studied in long-term cultures. *J. Cell. Biol.*, **103**, 171–187.

Hoodless, P.A., Haerry, T., Abdollah, S., Stapleton, M., *et al.* (1996). MADR1, a MAD-related protein that functions in BMP2 signaling pathways. *Cell*, **85**, 489–500.

Hope, R.A., Hammond, B.J., and Gaze, R.M. (1976). The arrow model: retino-tectal specificity and map formation in the goldfish visual system. *Proc. R. Soc. London B*, **194**, 447–466.

Hopfield, J.J. (1982). Neural networks and physical systems with emergent collective computational abilities. *P.N.A.S.*, **79**, 2554–2558.

Horder, T.J. (1971). Retention, by fish optic nerve fibres regenerating to new terminal sites in the tectum, of 'chemospecific' affinity for their original sites. *J. Physiol. Lond.*, **216**, 53–55.

Horder, T.J. and Martin, K.C. (1979). Morphogenetics as an alternative to chemospecificity in the formation of nerve connections. *Symp. Soc. Exp. Biol.*, **32**, 275–539.

Hotary, K.B. and Robinson, K.R. (1990). Endogenous electric currents and the resultant voltage gradients in the chick embryo. *Dev. Biol.*, **140**, 149–160.

Hotary, K.B. and Robinson, K.R. (1994). Endogenous electric currents and voltage gradients in *Xenopus* neurons and the consequences of their disruption. *Dev. Biol.*, **166**, 1789–1800.

Houart, C., Westerfield, M., and Wilson, S.W. (1998). A small population of anterior cells patterns the forebrain during zebrafish gastrulation. *Nature*, **391**, 788–792.

Howell, B.W., Hawkes, R., Soriano, P., and Cooper, J.A. (1997). Neuronal position in the developing brain is regulated by mouse disabled-1. *Nature*, **389**, 733–737.

Hsieh-Li, H.M., Witte, D.P., Szucsik, J.C., Weinstein, M., Li, H., and Potter, S.S. (1995). Gsh-2, a murine homeobox gene expressed in the developing brain. *Mech. Dev.*, **50**, 177–186.

Hubel, D.H. and Wiesel, T.N. (1962). Receptive fields, binocular interaction and functional architecture in the cat's visual cortex. *J. Physiol.*, **160**, 106–154.

Hubel, D.H. and Wiesel, T.N. (1963). Receptive fields of cells in striate cortex of very young, visually inexperienced kittens. *J. Neurophysiol.*, **26**, 994–1002.

Hubel, D.H. and Wiesel, T.N. (1965). Binocular interaction in striate cortex of kittens reared with artificial squint. *J. Neurophysiol.*, **28**, 1041–1059.

Hubel, D.H. and Wiesel, T.N. (1971). Aberrant visual projections in the siamese cat. *J. Physiol.*, **218**, 33–62.

Hubel, D.H. and Wiesel, T.N. (1974). Sequence regularity and geometry of orientation columns in the monkey striate cortex. *J. Comp. Neurol.*, **158**, 267–293.

Hubel, D.H. and Wiesel, T.N. (1977). Ferrier lecture. Functional architecture of macaque monkey visual cortex. *Proc. R. Soc. London B*, **198**, 1–59.

Hubel, D.H., Wiesel, T.N., and LeVay, S. (1977). Plasticity of ocular dominance columns in monkey striate cortex. *Phil. Trans. R. Soc. London Ser. B*, **278**, 377–409.

Hübener, M., Shoham, D., Grinvald, A. and Bonhoeffer, T. (1997). Spatial relationships among three columnar systems in cat area 17. *J. Neurosci.*, **17**, 9270–9284.

Humphrey, A.L., Sur, M., Uhlrich, D.J., and Sherman, S.M. (1985). Projection patterns of individual X- and Y-cell axons from the lateral geniculate nucleus to cortical area 17 in the cat. *J. Comp. Neurol.*, **233**, 159–189.

Hunt, R.K. and Frank, E.D. (1975). Neuronal locus specificity: trans-repolarisation of *Xenopus* embryonic retina after the time of axial specification. *Science*, **189**, 563–565.

Huttenlocher, P.R. (1979). Synaptic density in human frontal cortex-development changes and effects of aging. *Brain Res.*, **163**, 195–205.

Huttenlocher. P.R. (1990). Morphometric study of human cerebral cortex development. *Neuropsych.*, **28**, 517–527.

Huttenlocher, P.R. and de Courten, C. (1987). The development of synapses in striate cortex in man. *Human Neurobiol.*, **6**, 1–9.

Ide, C.F., Fraser, S.E., and Meyer, R.L. (1983). Eye dominance columns formed by an isogenic double-nasal frog eye. *Science*, **221**, 293–295.

Ide, C.F., Scripter, J.L., Coltman, B.W., Dotson, R.S, Snyder, D.C., and Jelaso, A. (1996). Cellular and molecular correlates to plasticity during recovery from injury in the developing mammalian brain. *Prog. Brain Res.*, **108**, 365–377.

Imamura, K., Shirao, T., Mori, K., and Obata, K. (1992). Changes in drebrin expression in the visual cortex of the cat during development. *Neurosci. Res.*, **13**, 33–41.

Innocenti, G.M. (1981). Growth and reshaping of axons in the establishment of visual callosal connections. *Science*, **212**, 824–827.

Innocenti, G.M. and Clarke, S. (1984a). Bilateral transitory projection to visual areas from auditory cortex in kittens. *Dev. Brain Res.*, **14**, 143–148.

Innocenti, G.M. and Clarke, S. (1984b). The organization of immature callosal connections. *J. Comp. Neurol.*, **230**, 287–309.

Innocenti, G.M. and Tettoni, L. (1997). Exuberant growth, specificity, and selection in the differentiation of cortical axons. In *Normal and Abnormal Development of the Cortex* (eds. A. Galaburda and Y. Christen). Springer-Verlag, Heidelberg.

Innocenti, G.M., Fiore, L., and Caminiti, R. (1977). Exuberant connections into the corpus callosum from the visual cortex of newborn cats. *Neurosci. Lett.*, **4**, 237–242.

Innocenti, G.M., Clarke, S., and Kraftsik, R. (1986). Interchange of callosal and association projections in the developing visual cortex. *J. Neurosci.*, **6**, 1384–1409.

Innocenti, G.M., Berbel, P., and Clarke, S. (1988). Development of projections from auditory to visual areas in the cat. *J. Comp. Neurol.*, **272**, 242–259.

Ip, N.Y. and Yancopoulos, G.D. (1996). The neurotrophins and CNTF: two families of collaborative neurotrophic factors. *Annu. Rev. Neurosci.*, **19**, 491–515.

Isaacs, E., Christie, D., Vargha-Khadem, F., and Mishkin, M. (1996). Effects of hemispheric side of injury, age at injury, and presence of seizure disorder on functional ear and hand asymmetries in hemiplegic children. *Neuropsychologia*, **34**, 127–137.

Ishii, N., Wadsworth, W.G., Stern, B.D., Culotti, J.G. and Hedgecock, E.M. (1992). UNC-6, a laminin-related protein, guides cell and pioneer axon migrations in *C. elegans. Neuron*, **9**, 873–881.

Itasaki, N. and Nakamura, H. (1992). Rostro-caudal polarity of the optic tectum in birds—correlation of en gradient and topographic order in retinotectal projection. *Neuron*, **8**, 787–798.

Itasaki, N. and Nakamura, H. (1996). A role for gradient en expression in positional specification on the optic tectum. *Neuron*, **16**, 55–62.

Ito, M., Sakurai, M., and Tongroach, P. (1982). Climbing fibre induced depression of both mossy fibre responsiveness and glutamate sensitivity of cerebellar purkinje cells. *J. Physiol.*, **324**, 133–134.

Itoh, K., Brackenbury, R., and Akeson, R. (1995). Induction of L1 mRNA in PC12 cells by NGF is modulated by cell-cell contact and does not require the high affinity NGF receptor. *J. Neurosci.*, **15**, 2504–2512.

Ivy, G.O. and Killackey, H.P. (1981). The ontogeny of the distribution of callosal projection neurons in the rat parietal cortex. *J. Comp. Neurol.*, **195**, 367–389.

Jablonska, B., Geirdalski, M., Suicinska, E., Skangielkramska, J., and Kossut, M. (1995). Partial blocking of the NMDA receptors restricts plastic changes on adult mouse barrel cortex. *Behav. Brain Res.*, **66**, 207–216.

Jackson, C.A., Peduzzi, J.D., and Hickey, T.L. (1989). Visual cortex development in the ferret. I Genesis and migration of visual cortical neurons. *J. Neurosci.*, **9**, 1242–1253.

Jacobson, C.O. (1959). The localization of the presumptive cerebral regions in the neural plate of the axolotl larva. *J. Embryol. Exp. Morphal.*, **7**, 1–21.

Jacobson, M. (1960). Studies in the organisation of visual mechanisms in amphibians. Ph.D. thesis, Edinburgh University.

Jacobson, M. (1967). Retinal ganglion cells: Specification of central connections in larval *Xenopus laevis*. *Science*, **155**, 1106–1108.

Jacobson, M. and Levine, R.L. (1975). Plasticity in the adult frog brain: filling in the visual scotoma after excision or translocation of parts of the optic tectum. *Brain Res.*, **88**, 339–345.

Jeanprêtre, N, Clarke, P.G.H. and Gabriel, J.-P. (1996). Competitive exclusion between axons dependent on a single trophic substance: a mathematical analysis. *Math. Biosci.*, **133**, 23–54.

Jessell, T.M. (1988). Adhesion molecules and the hierarchy of neural development. *Neuron*, **1**, 3–13.

Jia, W.-G., Beaulieu, C., Huang, F.L., and Cynader, M.S. (1990). Protein kinase C immunoreactivity in kitten visual cortex is developmentally regulated and input-dependent. *Dev. Brain Res.*, **57**, 209–221.

Johnson, M.H. (1997). *Development cognitive neuroscience*. Blackwell, Oxford, UK.

Johnson, M.H., Dziurawiec, S., Ellis, H., and Morton, J. (1991). Newborn's preferential tracking of face-like stimuli and its subsequent decline. *Cognition*, **4**, 1–19.

Jones, E.G. (1985). *The thalamus*. Plenum Press, New York.

Jones, E.G. (1995). Cortical development and neuropathology in schizophrenia. In *Development of the cerebral cortex* (eds. G. Bock and G. Cardew). John Wiley and Sons, Chichester.

Joseph, S.R.H. and Willshaw, D.J. (1996). The role of activity in synaptic competition at the neuromuscular junction. *NIPS*, **8**, 96–102.

Jung, W., Castren, E., Odenthal, M., Vande Woude, G.F, Ishii, T., Dienes, H.P., Lindholm, D., and Schirmacher, P. (1994). Expression and functional interaction of hepatrocyte growth factor-scatter factor and its receptor c-met in mammalian brain. *J. Cell Biol.*, **126**, 485–494.

Kaas, J.H. and Guillery, R.W. (1973). The transfer of abnormal visual field representations from dorsal lateral geniculate nucleus to visual cortex in siamese cats. *Brain Res.*, **59**, 61–95.

Kass, J.H., Nelson, R.J., Sur, M., Lin, C.-S. and Merzenich, M.M. (1979). Multiple representations of the body within the primary somatosensory cortex of primates. *Science*, **204**, pp. 521–523.

Kageyama, G.H. and Robertson, R.T. (1993). Development of geniculocortical projections to visual cortex in rat: Evidence for early ingrowth and synaptogenesis. *J. Comp. Neurol.*, **335**, 123–148.

Kandel, E.R., Schwartz, J.H., and Jessell, T.M. (1991). *Principles of neural science.*, 3rd edn. Appleton and Lange, Prentice-Hall.

Kang, H. and Schumann, E.M. (1995). Long-lasting neurotrophin-induced enhancement of synaptic transmission in the adult hippocampus. *Science*, **267**, 1658–1662.

Kapfhammer, J.P. and Raper, J.A. (1987). Collapse of growth cone structure on contact with specific neurites in culture. *J. Neurosci.*, **7**, 201–212.

Karayiorgou, M. and Gogos, J.A. (1997). Dissecting the genetic complexity of schizophrenia. *Mol. Psychiatr.*, **2**, 211–223.

Karlstrom, R.O., Trowe, T., Klostermann, S., Baier, H., Brand, M., Crawford, A.D., Grunewald, B., Haffter, P., Hoffman, H., Meyer, S.U., Muller, B.K., Richter, S., van Eeden, F.J.M., Nusslein-Volhard, C. and Bonhoeffer, F. (1996). Zebrafish mutations affecting retinotectal axon pathfinding. *Development*, **123**, 427–438.

Karto, N., Artola, A., and Singer, W. (1991). Developmental changes in the susceptibility to long term potention of neurones in rat visual cortex slices. *Dev. Brain Res.*, **60**, 43–50.

Kasamatsu, T. and Pettigrew, J.D. (1976). Depletion of brain catecholamines: failure of ocular dominance shift after monocular occlusion in kittens. *Science*, **194**, 206–209.

Kato, N., Kawagachi, S., and Miyata, H. (1984). Geniculocortical projection to layer I of area 17 in kittens: orthograde and retrograde HRP studies. *J. Comp. Neurol.*, **225**, 441–447.

Kato, N., Astola, A., and Singer, W. (1991a). Developmental-changes in the susceptibility to long-term potentiation of neurons in rat visual-cortex slices. *Dev. Brain Res.*, **60**, 43–50.

Kato, N., Ferrer, J.M.R., and Price, D.J. (1991b). Regressive changes among corticocortical neurones projecting from the lateral suprasylvian cortex to area 18 of the kitten's visual cortex. *Neuroscience*, **43**, 291–306.

Kato, N., Ferrer, J.M.R., Price, D.J. and Blakemore, C. (1993). Effects of neonatal ablation of area 18 on corticocortical projections from area 17 to extrastriate visual areas in cats. *Behav. Brain Res.*, **54**, 205–210.

Katz, L.C. (1991). Specificity in the development of vertical connections in cat striate cortex. *Eur. J. Neurosci.*, **3**, 1–9.

Katz, L.C. and Callaway, E.M. (1992). Development of local circuits in mammalian visual cortex. *Annu. Rev. Neurosci.*, **15**, 31–56.

Kaufman, M.H. (1992). *The atlas of mouse development.* Academic Press Inc, San Diego, USA.

Keating, M.J. (1968). Functional interaction in the development of specific nerve connections. *J. Physiol.*, **198**, 75–77.

Kennedy, H. and Bullier, J. (1985). A double-labeling investigation of the afferent connectivity to cortical areas V1 and V2 of the macaque monkey. *J. Neurosci.*, **5**, 2815–2830.

Kennedy, H. and Dehay, C. (1997). The nature and nurture of cortical development. In *Normal and abnormal development of the cortex* (eds. A. Galaburda and Y. Christen), pp. 25–56. Springer–Verlag.

Kennedy, H., Bullier, J., and Dehay, C. (1989). Transient projections from STS to area 17 in the newborn monkey. *Proc. Natl. Acad. Sci. USA*, **86**, 8093–8097.

Kennedy, T.E., Serafini, T., De la Torre, J.R., and Tessier-Lavigne, M. (1994). Netrins are diffusible chemotropic factors for commissural axons in the embryonic spinal cord. *Cell*, **78**, 425–435.

Kerr, J.F., Wyllie, A.H., and Currie, A.R. (1972). Apoptosis: a basic biological phenomenon with wide-ranging implications in tissue kinetics. *Br. J. Cancer*, **26**, 239–257.

Keynes, R.J. and Cook, G.M.W. (1995). Axon guidance molecules. *Cell*, **83**, 161–169.

Kiang, N.Y.-S., Watanabe, T., Thomas, E.C., and Clarke, L.F. (1965). *Discharge patterns of single fibres in the cat's auditory nerve.* MIT Press, Cambridge, MA.

Kidd, K.K. (1997). Can we find genes for schizophrenia? *Am. J. Med. Genet.*, **74**, 104–111.

Killackey, H.P., Rhoades, R.W., and Bennett-Clarke, C.A. (1995). The formation of a cortical somatotopic map. *Trends Neurosci.*, **18**, 402–407.

Kilpatrick, T.J. and Bartlett, P.F. (1993). Cloning and growth of multipotential precursors: requirements for proliferation and differentiation. *Neuron*, **10**, 255–265.

Kimura, S., Hara, Y., Pineau, T., Fernandez-Salguero, P., Fox, C.H., Ward, J.M., and Gonzalez, F.J. (1996). The T/ebp null mouse: thyroid-specific enhancer binding protein is essential for the organogenesis of the thyroid, lung, ventral forebrain, and pituitary. *Genes Dev.*, **10**, 60–69.

Kincaid, A.E., Zheng, T., and Wilson, C.J. (1998). Connectivity and convergence of single corticostriatal neurons. *J. Neurosci.*, **18**, 4722–4731.

Kinnunen, A., Niemi, M., Kinnunen, T., Kaksonen, M., Nolo, R., and Rauvala, H. (1999). Heparan sulphate and HB-GAM (heparin-binding growth-associated molecule) in the development of the thalamocortical pathway of rat brain. *Eur. J. Neurosci.*, **11**, 491–502.

Kirkwood, A. and Bear, M.F. (1994a). Hebbian synapses in visual cortex. *J. Neurosci.*, **14**, 1634–1645.

Kirkwood, A. and Bear, M.F. (1994b). Homosynaptic long-term depression in the visual cortex. *J. Neurosci.*, **14**, 3404–3412.

Kirkwood, A., Dudek, S.M., Gold, J.T., Aizenman, C.D., and Bear, M.F. (1993). Common forms of synaptic plasticity in the hippocampus and neocortex *in vitro. Science*, **260**, 1518–1521.

Kirkwood, A., Lee, H-K, and Bear, M.F. (1995). Coregulation of long-term potentiation and experience-dependent synaptic plasticity in visual-cortex by age and experience. *Nature*, **375**, 328–331.

Klagsbrun, M. and Baird, A. (1991). A dual receptor system is required for basic fibroblast growth factor activity. *Cell*, **67**, 229–231.

Kleinschmidt, A., Bear, M.F., and Singer, W. (1987). Blockade of 'NMDA' receptors disrupts experience-dependent plasticity of kitten striate cortex. *Science*, **238**, 355–357.

Kliemann, W.A. (1987). Stochastic dynamic model for the characterization of the geometrical structure of dendritic processes. *Bulletin of Mathematical Biology*, **49**, 135–152.

Knudson, C.M., Tung, K.S., Tourtellotte, W.G., Brown, G.A., and Korsmeyer, S.J. (1995). Bax-deficient mice with lymphoid hyperplasia and male germ cell death. *Science*, **270**, 96–99.

Koester, S.E. and O'Leary, D.D.M. (1993). Connectional distinction between callosal and subcortical projecting cortical neurons is determined prior to axon extension. *Dev. Biol.*, **160**, 1–14.

Kolodkin, A.L., Levengood, D.V., Rowe, E.G., Tai, Y.T, Giger, R.J., and Ginty, D.D. (1997). Neuropilin is a semaphorin III receptor. *Cell*, **90**, 753–762.

Komuro, H. and Rakic, P. (1992). Specific role of N-type calcium channels in neuronal migration. *Science*, **257**, 806–809.

Komuro, H. and Rakic, P. (1993). Modulation of neuronal migration by NMDA receptors. *Science*, **260**, 95–97.

Komuro, H. and Rakic, P. (1996). Intracellular Ca^{2+} fluctuations modulate the rate of neuronal migration. *Neuron*, **17**, 275–285.

Kornack, D.R. and Rakic, P. (1995). Radial and horizontal deployment of clonally related cells in the primate neocortex: relationship to distinct mitotic lineages. *Neuron*, **15**, 311–321.

Kornberg, T. (1981). Engrailed: A gene controlling compartment and segment formation in Drosophila. *Proc. Natl. Acad. Sci. USA*, **78**, 1095–1099.

Kornblum, H.I., Hussain, R.J., Bronstein, J.M., Gall, C.M., Lee, D.C., and Seroogy, K.B. (1997). Prenatal ontogeny of the epidermal growth factor receptor and its ligand, transforming growth factor alpha, in rat brain. *J. Comp. Neurol.*, **380**, 243–261.

Korsching, S. (1993). The neurotrophic factor concept: a reexamination. *J. Neurosci.*, **13**, 2739–2748.

Korsmeyer, S.J., Shutter, J.R., Veis, D.J., Merry, D.E., and Oltvai, Z.N. (1993). BCL-2/Bax: a rheostat that regulates an anti-oxidant pathway and cell death. *Seminars in Cancer Biology*, **4**, 327–332.

Kostovic, I. and Rakic, P. (1980). Cytology and time of origin of intentitial neurones in the white matter in infant and adult human and monkey telencephalon. *J. Neurocytol.*, **9**, 219–242.

Kostovic, I. and Rakic, P. (1990). Developmental history of the transient subplate zone in the visual and somatosensory cortex of the macaque monkey and human brain. *J. Comp. Neurol.*, **297**, 441–470.

Kruger, L. (1969). Experimental analyses of the reptilian nervous system. *Ann. N.Y. Acad. Sci.*, **167**, 102–117.

Krumlauf, R. (1994). Hox genes in vertebrate development. *Cell*, **70**, 191–201.

Krumlauf, R., Marshall, H., Studer, M., Nonchev, S, Sham, M.H., and Lumsden, A. (1993). Hox homeobox genes and regionalisation of the nervous system. *Trends Neurosci.*, **24**, 1328–1340.

Kuhl, P.K., Williams, K.A., Lacerda, F., Stevens, K.N, and Lindblom, B. (1992). Linguistic experience alters phonetic perception in infants by 6 months of age. *Science*, **255**, 606–608.

Kuljis, R.O. and Rakic, P. (1990). Hypercolumns in the monkey visual cortex can develop in the absence of cues from the photoreceptors. *Proc. Natl. Acad. Sci. USA*, **87**, 5303–5306.

Lako, M., Lindsay, S., Bullen, P., Wilson, D.I., Robson, S.C., and Strachan, T. (1998). A novel mammalian Wnt gene, WNT8B, shows brain-restricted expression in early development, with sharply delimited expression boundaries in the developing forebrain. *Hum. Mol. Gen.*, **7**, 813–822.

LaMantia, A.-S., Colbert, M.C., and Linney, E. (1993). Retinoic acid induction and regional differentiation prefigure olfactory pathway formation in the mammalian forebrain. *Neuron*, **10**, 1035–1048.

Lamb, A.H. (1976). The projection patterns of the ventral horn to the hind limb during development. *Dev. Bio.*, **54**, 82–89.

Lamb, A.H. (1979). Evidence that some developing hindlimb motorneurones die for reason other than peripheral competition. *Dev. Biol.*, **71**, 8–21.

Lamb, A.H. (1980). Motorneurone counts in *Xenopus* frogs reared with one bilaterally innervated hindlimb. *Nature*, **284**, 347–350.

Lamb, A.H. (1981). Axon regeneration by developing limb motoneurones in *Xenopus laevis*. *Brain Res.*, **209**, 315–323.

Lamb, T. *et al.* (1993). Neural induction by the secreted polypeptide noggin. *Science*, **262**, 713–718.

Lance-Jones, C. and Landmesser, L. (1981). Pathway selection by chick lumbosacral motoneurons during normal development. *Proc. R. Soc. London B*, **214**, 1–18.

Landmesser, L. (1984). The development of specific motor pathways in the chick embryo. *Trends Neurosci.*, **7**, 336–339.

Langley, J.N. (1895). Note on regeneration of præ-ganglionic fibres of the sympathetic. *J. Physiol.*, **18**, 280–284.

Lavdas, A.A., Blue, M.E., Lincoln, J., and Parnavelas, J.G. (1997). Serotonin promotes the differentiation of glutamate neurons in organotypic slice cultures of the developing cerebral cortex. *J. Neurosci.*, **17**, 7872–7880.

Law, M.I. and Constantine-Paton, M. (1981). Anatomy and physiology of experimentally produced striped tecta. *J. Neurosci.*, **1**, 741–759.

Lawler, E.L., Lenstra, J.K., Rinnooy Kan, A.H.G., and Shmoys, D.B. (1986). The traveling salesman problem. Wiley, Chichester.

Lazzaro, D., Price, M., De Felice, and Di Lauro, R. (1991). The thyroid transcription factor TTF-1 is expressed at the onset of thyroid and lung morphogenesis and in restricted region in the foetal brain. *Development*, **113**, 1093–1104.

Lea, S.E.G. (1984). *Instinct, environment and behaviour*. Methuen, London and New York.

Le Douarin, N. (1982). *The neural crest*. Cambridge University Press, Cambridge.

Lee, S.M.K., Danielian, P.S., Fritzsch, B., and McMahon, A.P. (1997). Evidence that fgf8 signalling from the midbrain-hindbrain junction regulates growth and polarity in the developing midbrain. *Development*, **124**, 959–969.

Lein, P., Banker, G., and Higgins, D. (1992). Laminin selectively enhances axonal growth and accelerates the development of polarity by hippocampal neurons in culture. *Dev. Brain Res.*, **69**, 191–197.

Letourneau, P.C., Madsen, M., Palm, S.M., and Furcht, L.T. (1988). Immunoreactivity for laminin in the developing ventral longitudinal pathway of the brain. *Dev. Biol.*, **125**, 135–144.

Leussink, B., Brouwer, A., Khattabi, M.E., Poelmann, R.E. *et al.* (1995). Expression patterns of the paired-related homeobox genes mhox/prx1 and s8/prx2 suggest roles in development of the heart and the forebrain. *Mech. Dev.*, **52**, 51–64.

LeVay, S., Hubel, D.H., and Wiesel, T.N. (1975). The pattern of ocular dominance columns in macaque monkey visual cortex revealed by a reduced silver stain. *J. Comp. Neurol.*, **159**, 559–576.

LeVay, S., Stryker, M.P., and Shatz, C.J. (1978). Ocular dominance columns and their development in layer IV of the cat's visual cortex: a quantitative study. *J. Comp. Neurol.*, **179**, 223–244.

LeVay, S., Wiesel, T.N., and Hubel, D.H. (1980). The development of ocular dominance columns in normal and visually deprived monkeys. *J. Comp. Neurol.*, **191**, 1–51.

Levi-Montalcini, R. (1987). The nerve growth factor 35 years later. *Science*, **237**, 1154–1162.

Levi-Montalcini, R. and Angeletti, P.U. (1968). Nerve growth factor. *Physiol. Rev.*, **48**, 534–569.

Levine, E., Dreyfus, C., Black, I., and Plummer, M. (1995). Differential effects of NGF and BDNF on voltage-gated calcium currents in embryonic basal forebrain neurons. *J. Neurosci.*, **15**, 3084–3091.

Levine, R.L. and Jacobson, M. (1974). Deployment of optic nerve fibers is determined by positional markers in the frog's tectum. *Expl. Neurol.*, **43**, 527–538.

Levine, R.L. and Jacobson, M. (1975). Discontinuous mapping of retina onto tectum innervated by both eyes. *Brain Res.*, **98**, 172–176.

Levitt, P. (1984). A monoclonal antibody to limbic system neurons. *Science*, **223**, 229–301.

Levitt, P. and Rakic, P. (1980). Immunoperoxidase localisation of glial fibrillary acidic protein in radial glial cells and astrocytes of the developing rhesus monkey brain. *J. Comp. Neurol.*, **193**, 815–840.

Levitt, P., Ferri, R., and Eaglesen, K. (1995). *Molecular contributions to cerebral cortical specification in development of the cerebral cortex*. (eds. Bock, G.R. and Cardew). pp. 200–213. Wiley, New York.

Lewin, G.R. and Barde, Y.-A. (1996). Physiology of the neurotrophins. *Annu. Rev. Neurosci.*, **19**, 289–317.

Lewis, E. (1978). A gene complex controlling segmentation in Drosophila. *Nature*, **276**, 565–570.

Li, G.-H., Qin, C.-D., and Wang, Z.-S. (1992). Neurite branching pattern formation: Modeling and computer simulation. *J. Theor. Biol.*, **157**, 463–486.

Li, G.-H., Qin, C.-D., and Wang, Z.-S. (1995a). Computer model of growth cone behavior and neuronal morphogenesis. *J. Theor. Biol.*, **174**, 381–389.

Li, Y., Holtzman, D.M., Kromer, L.F., Kaplan, D.R., Chua-Couzens, J., Clary, D.O., Knuesel, B., and Mobley, W.C. (1995b). Regulation of TrkA and ChAt expression in developing rat basal forebain: evidence that both exogeneous and endogenous NGF regulate differentiation of cholinergic neurons. *J. Neurosci.*, **15**, 2888–2905.

Lichtman, J. (1977). The reorganization of synaptic connections in the rat submandibular ganglion during postnatal development. *J. Physiol.*, **273**, 155–177.

Lillien, L. (1998). Neural progenitors and stem cells: mechanisms of progenitor heterogeneity. *Curr. Opin. Neurobiol.*, **8**, 37–44.

Lindsay, R.M., Shooter, E.M., Radeke, M.J., Misko, T.P., Dechant, G.F., Thoenen, H., and Lindholm, D. (1990). Nerve growth factor regulates expression of the nerve growth factor gene in adult sensory neurons. *Eur. J. Neurosci.*, **2**, 389–396.

Lindsay, R.M., Wiegand, S.J., Altar, C.A., and DiStefano, P.S. (1994). Neurotrophic factors: from molecule to man. *Trends Neurosci.*, **17**, 182–190.

Linsker, R. (1986). From basic network principles to neural architecture: emergence of orientation columns. *Proc. Natl. Acad. Sci. USA*, **83**, 8779–83.

Linsker, R. (1989). How to generate ordered maps by maximising the mutual information between input & output signals. *Neural Comp.*, **1**, 402–411.

Lipton, S.A. and Kater, S.B. (1989). Neurotransmitter regulation of neuronal outgrowth, plasticity and survival. *Trends Neurosci.*, **12**, 265–270.

Liu, F., Hata, A., Baker, J.C., Doody, J., Carcamo, J., Harland, R.M., and Massague, J. (1996). A human Mad protein acting as a BMP-regulated transcription factor. *Nature*, **381**, 620–623.

Livingstone, M. (1996). Ocular dominance columns in New-World monkeys. *J. Neurosci.*, **16**, 2086–2096.

Livingstone, M. and Hubel, D. (1983). Specificity of cortico-cortical connections in monkey visual system. *Nature*, **304**, 531–534.

Livingstone, M. and Hubel, D. (1984). Anatomy and physiology of a color system in the primate visual cortex. *J. Neurosci.*, **4**, 309–356.

Livingstone, M. and Hubel, D. (1987). Connections between layer 4B of area 17 and the thick cytochrome oxidase stripes of area 18 in the squirrel monkey. *J. Neurosci.*, **7**, 3371–3377.

Livingstone, M. and Hubel, D. (1988). Segregation of form, color, movement, and depth: anatomy, physiology, and perception. *Science*, **240**, 740–749.

Lohof, A.M., Ip, N.Y., and Poo, M-m (1993). Potentiation of developing neuromuscular synapses by the neurotrophins NT-3 and BDNF. *Nature*, **363**, 350–353.

Lois, C., Garcia-Verdugo, J.M., and Alvarez-Buylla, A. (1996). Chain migration of neuronal precursors. *Science*, **271**, 978–981.

Lopresti, V., Macagno, E.R., and Levinthal, C. (1973). Structure and development of neuronal connections in isogenic organisms; cellular interactions in the development of the optic lamina of daphnia. *Proc. Natl. Acad. Sci. (Wash)*, **70**, 433–437.

Lotto, R.B. and Price, D.J. (1994). Evidence that molecules influencing axonal growth and termination in the developing geniculocortical pathway are conserved between divergent mammalian species. *Dev. Brain Res.*, **81**, 17–25.

Lotto, R.B. and Price, D.J. (1995). The stimulation of thalamic neurite outgrowth by cortical derived growth factors *in vitro*; the influence of cortical age and activity. *Eur. J. Neurosci.*, **7**, 318–328.

Lotto, R.B. and Price, D.J. (1996). Effects of subcortical structures on the growth of cortical neurites *in vitro*. *Neuroreport*, **7**, 1185–1188.

Lotto, R.B., Clausen, J.A., and Price, D.J. (1997). A role for neurotrophins in the survival of murine embryonic thalamic neurons. *Eur. J. Neurosci.*, **9**, 1940–1949.

Lotto, R.B., Aitkenhead, A., and Price, D.J. (1999). Effects of the thalamus on the development of cerebral cortical efferents *in vitro*. *J. Neurobiol.*, **39**, 186–196.

LoTurco, J.J., Owens, D.F., Heath, M.J.S., Davis, M.B.E., and Kriegstein, A.R. (1995). GABA and glutamate depolarize cortical progenitor cells and inhibit DNA synthesis. *Neuron*, **15**, 1287–1298.

Lu, S., Bogarad, L.D., Murtha, M.T., and Ruddle, F.H. (1992). Expression pattern of a murine homeobox gene, Dbx, displays extreme spatial restriction in embryonic forebrain and spinal cord. *Proc. Natl. Acad. Sci. USA*, **89**, 8053–8057.

Lubke, J. and Albus, K. (1992). Rapid rearrangement of intrinsic tangential connections in the striate cortex of normal and dark-reared kittens — lack of exuberance beyond the second postnatal week. *J. Comp. Neurol.*, **323**, 42–58.

Luhmann, H.J., Singer, W., and Martinez-Millan, L. (1990). Horizontal interactions in cat striate cortex: I. anatomical substriate and postnatal development. *Eur. J. Neurosci.*, **2**, 344–357.

Lumsden, A. (1990). The cellular basis of segmentation in the developing hindbrain. *Trends Neurosci.*, **13**, 329–335.

Lumsden, A.G.S. and Davies, A.M. (1983). Earliest sensory nerve fibres are guided to peripheral targets by attractants other than nerve growth factor. *Nature*, **306**, 786–788.

Lumsden, A.G.S. and Davies, A.M. (1986). Chemotropic effect of specific target epithelium in the developing mammalian nervous system. *Nature*, **323**, 538–539.

Lumsden, A. and Keynes, R. (1989). Segmental patterns of neuronal development in the chick hindbrain. *Nature*, **337**, 424–428.

Lund, R.D. and Mustari, M.J. (1977). Development of the geniculocortical pathway in rats. *J. Comp. Neurol.*, **173**, 289–306.

Luo, Y., Raible, D., and Raper, J.A. (1993). Collapsin: A protein in brain that induces the collapse and paralysis of neuronal growth cones. *Cell*, **75**, 217–227.

Luskin, M.B. and Shatz, C.J. (1985a). Neurogenesis of the cat's primary visual cortex. *J. Comp. Neurol.*, **242**, 611–631.

Luskin, M.B. and Shatz, C.J. (1985b). Studies of the earliest generated cells of the cat's visual cortex: cogeneration of subplate and marginal zones. *J. Neurosci.*, **5**, 1062–1075.

Luskin, M.B., Pearlman, A.L., and Sanes, J.R. (1988). Cell lineage in the cerebral cortex of the mouse studied *in vivo* and *in vitro* with a recombinant retrovirus. *Neuron*, **1**, 635–647.

Luskin, M.B., Parnavelas, J.G., and Barfield, J.A. (1993). Neurons, astrocytes, and oligodendrocytes of the rat cerebral cortex originate from separate progenitor cells: an ultrastructural analysis of clonally related cells. *J. Neurosci.*, **13**, 1730–1750.

Ma, Q., Kintner, C., and Anderson, D.J. (1996). Identification of neurogenin, a vertebrate neuronal differentiation gene. *Cell*, **87**, 43–52.

Maccioni, R. and Cambiazo, V. (1995). Role of microtubule-associated proteins in the control of microtubule assembly. *Physiol. Rev.*, **75**, 835–864.

Maden, M. (1982). Vitamin A and pattern formation of the regenerating limb. *Nature*, **295**, 672–675.

Maffei, L., Berardi, L. Domenici, L., Parisi, V., and Pizzorusso, T. (1992). Nerve growth factor (NGF) prevents the shift in ocular dominance distribution of visual cortical neurons in monocularly deprived rats. *J. Neurosci.*, **12**, 4651–4662.

Magnuson, T. and Faust, C. (1993). Genetic control of gastrulation in the mouse. *Curr. Opin. Genet. Dev.*, **3**, 491–498.

Magowan, G. and Price, D.J. (1996). Trophic and outgrowth-promoting effects of K^+-induced depolarization on developing thalamic cells in organotypic culture. *Neuroscience*, **74**, 1045–1057.

Mancini, J., DeSchonen, S.D., Deruelle, C., and Massoulier, A. (1994). A face recognition in children with early right or left brain-damage. *Dev. Med. Child Neurol.*, **36**, 156–166.

Maness, L.M., Kastin, A.J., Weber, J.T., Banks, W.A., Beckman, B.S., and Zadina, J.E. (1994). The neurotrophins and their receptors: structure, function, and neuropathology. *Neurosci. Behav. Rev.*, **18**, 143–159.

Mann, F., Zhukareva, V., Pimenta, A., Levitt, P., and Bolz, J. (1998). Membrane-associated molecules guide limbic and nonlimbic thalamocortical projections. *J. Neurosci.*, **18**, 9409–9419.

Marigo, V., Davey, R.A., Zuo, Y., Cunningham, J.M., and Tabin, C.J. (1996). Biochemical evidence that patched is the hedgehog receptor. *Nature*, **384**, 176–179.

Marin-Padilla, M. (1971). Early prenatal ontogenesis of the cerebral cortex (neocortex) of the cat (Felis domestica): a Golgi study. I. The primordial neocortical organization. *Z. Anat. Entwickl.-Gesch.*, **134**, 117–145.

Marin-Padilla, M. (1978). Dual origin of the mammalian neocortex and evolution of the cortical plate. *Anat. Embryol.*, **152**, 109–126.

Markram, H., Lubke, J., Forster, M., and Sakmann, B. (1997). *Science*, **275**, 213–215.

Martinou, J.-C., Dubois-Dauphin, M., Staple, J.K. *et al.* (1994). Overexpression of Bcl-2 in transgenic mice protects neurons from naturally occurring cell death and experimental ischemia. *Neuron*, **13**, 1017–1030.

Massague, J. (1996). TGFb signaling: receptors, transducers, and Mad proteins. *Cell*, **85**, 947–950.

Massague, J. and Polyak, K. (1995). Mammalian antiproliferative signals and their targets. *Curr. Opin. Gen. Dev.*, **5**, 91–96.

Mastick, G.S., Davis, N.M., Andrews, G.L., and Easter, S.S. Jr. (1997). Pax-6 functions in boundary formation and axon guidance in the embryonic mouse forebrainforebrain patterning defects in small eye mutant mice. *Development*, **124**, 1985–1997.

Matsubara, J., Cynader, M.S., and Swindale, N.V. (1987). Anatomical properties and physiological correlates of the intrinsic connections in cat area 18. *J. Neurosci.*, **7**, 1428–1446.

McAllister, K.A., Lo, D.C., and Katz, L.C. (1995). Neurotrophins regulate dendritic growth in developing visual cortex. *Neuron*, **15**, 791–803.

McAllister, K.A., Katz, L.C., and Lo, D.C. (1997). Opposing roles for endogenous BDNF and NT-3 in regulating cortical dendritic growth. *Neuron*, **18**, 767–778.

McArdle, J.J. (1975). Complex end-plate potentials at the regenerating neuromuscular junction of the rat. *Exp. Neurol.*, **49**, 629–645.

McCaig, C.D. and Rajnicek, A.M. (1991). Electrical fields, nerve growth and nerve regeneration. *Exp. Physiol.*, **76**, 473–494.

McConnell, S.K. (1988). Development and decision-making in the mammalian cerebral cortex. *Brain Res. Rev.*, **13**, 1–23.

McConnell, S.K. (1991). Specification of cerebral cortex during development. *Soc. Neurosci. Abstr.*, **17**, 1279.

McConnell, S.K. (1995). Strategies for the generation of neuronal diversity in the developing nervous system. *J. Neurosci.*, **15**, 6987–6998.

McConnell, S.K. and Kaznowski, C.E. (1991). Cell cycle dependence of laminar determination in developing neocortex. *Science*, **254**, 282–285.

McConnell, S.K., Ghosh, A., and Shatz, C.J. (1989). Subplate neurons pioneer the first axon pathway from the cerebral cortex. *Science*, **245**, 978–981.

McCulloch, W.S. and Pitts, W. (1943). A logical calculus of the ideas immanent in nervous activity. *Bull. Math. Biophysics*, **5**, 115–133.

McIntosh, H., Daw, N., and Parkinson, D. (1990). Gap-43 in the cat visual cortex during postnatal development. *Visual Neurosci.*, **4**, 585–593.

McMahan, U.J. (1990). The Agrin hypothesis. *Cold Spring Harbour Symp, Quant Biol*, **55**, 407–419.

Meakin, S.O. and Shooter, E.M. (1992). The nerve growth factor family of receptors. *Trends Neurosci.*, **15**, 323–331.

Meinhardt, H. (1982). *Models of biological pattern formation.* Academic Press, London.

Meisler, M.H. (1992). Insertional mutation of 'classical' and novel genes in transgenic mice. *Trends Genet.*, **8**, 341–344.

Meissirel, C., Dehay, C., Berland, M., and Kennedy, H. (1991). Segmentation of callosal and association pathways during development in the visual cortex of the primate. *J. Neurosci.*, **11**, 3297–3316.

Melzer, P., Crane, A.M, and Smith, C.B. (1993). Mouse barrel cortex functionally compensates for deprivation produced by neonatal lesion of the whisker follicles. *Eur. J. Neurosci.*, **5**, 1638–2652.

Melzer, P., Welker, E., Dorfl, J., and van der Loos, H. (1994). Maturation of the neuronal metabolic response to vibrissa stimulation in the developing whisker-to-barrel pathway of the mouse. *Dev. Brain Res.*, **77**, 227–250.

Menezes, J.R. and Luskin, M.B. (1994). Expression of neuron-specific tubulin defines a novel population in the proliferative layers of the developing telencephalon. *J. Neurosci.*, **14**, 5399–5416.

Merry, D.E. and Korsmeyer, S.J. (1997). Bcl-2 gene family in the nervous system. *Annu. Rev. Neurosci.*, **20**, 245–267.

Merry, D.E., Veis, D.J., Hickey, W.F., and Korsmeyer, S.J. (1994). Bcl-2 protein expression is widespread in the developing nervous system and retained in the adult PNS. *Development*, **120**, 301–311.

Messersmith, E.K., Leonardo, E.D., Shatz, C.J., Tessier-Lavigne, M., Goodwin, C.S., and Kolodkin, A.L. (1995). Semaphorin III can function as a selective chemorepellant to pattern sensory projections in the spinal cord. *Neuron*, **14**, 949–959.

Mesulam, M.-M. (1982). Principles of horseradish peroxidase neurohistochemistry and their applications for tracing neural pathways. In *Tracing neural connections with horseradish peroxidase* (ed. M.-M. Mesulam), pp. 1–155. Wiley, Chichester.

Metin, C. and Godement, P. (1996). The ganglionic eminence may be an intermediate target for corticofugal and thalamocortical axons. *J. Neurosci.*, **16**, 3219–3235.

Metin, C., Deleglise, D., Serafini, T., Kennedy, T.E., and Tessier-Lavigne, M. (1997). A role for netrin-1 in the guidance of cortical efferents. *Development*, **124**, 5063–5074.

Meyer, R.L. (1982). Tetrodotoxin blocks the formation of ocular dominance columns in goldfish. *Science*, **218**, 589–591.

Meyer, R.L. (1983). Tetrodotoxin inhibits the formation of refined retinotopography in goldfish. *Dev. Brain. Res.*, **6**, 293–298.

Meyer, R.L. and Sperry, R.W. (1973). Tests for neuroplasticity in the anuran retinotectal system. *Exp. Neurol.*, **40**, 525–539.

Meyer-Franke, A., Kaplan, M.R., Pfrieger, F.W., and Barres, B.A. (1995). Characterization of the signalling interactions that promote survival and growth of developing retinal ganglion cells in culture. *Neuron*, **15**, 805–819.

Miller, B., Chou, L., and Findlay, B.L. (1993). The early development of thalamocortical and corticothalamic projections. *J. Comp. Neurol.*, **335**, 16–41.

Miller, B., Sheppard, A.M., Bicknese, A.R., and Pearlman, A.L. (1995). Chondroitin sulfate proteoglycans in the developing cerebral cortex: the distribution of neurocan distinguishes forming afferent and efferent axonal pathways. *J. Comp. Neurol.*, **355**, 615–628.

Miller, K.D. (1994). A model for the development of simple cell receptive fields and the ordered orientation columns through the activity dependent competition between ON- and OFF- center inputs. *J. Neurosci.*, **14**, 409–441.

Miller, K.D. and MacKay, D.J.C. (1994). The role of constraints in Hebbian learning. *Neural Computation*, **6**, 100–126.

Miller, K.D., Keller, J.B., and Stryker, M.P. (1989). Ocular dominance column development: Analysis and simulation. *Science*, **245**, 605–615.

Miller, M.W. and Kuhn, P.E. (1995). Cell cycle kinetics in fetal rat cerebral cortex: effects of prenatal treatment with ethanol assessed by a cumulative labelling technique with flow cytometry. *Alcohol Clin. Exp. Res.*, **19**, 233–237.

Millet, S., Block-Gallego, E., Simeone, A., and Alvarado-Mallart, R.-M. (1996). The caudal limit of Otx2 gene expression as a marker of the midbrain/hindbrain boundary: a study using *in situ* hybridization and chick/quail homotopic grafts. *Development*, **122**, 3785–3797.

Minichiello, L. and Klein, R. (1996). TrkB and trkC neurotrophin receptors cooperate in promoting survival of hippocampal and cerebellar granule neurons. *Genes Dev.*, **10**, 2849–2858.

Mione, M.C., Danevic, C., Boardman, P., Harris, B., and Parnevelas, J. (1994). Lineage analysis reveals neurotransmitter (GABA or glutamate) but not calcium-binding protein homogeneity in clonally related neurons. *J. Neurosci.*, **14**, 107–123.

Mione, M.C., Cavanagh, J.F. R, Harris, B., and Parnavelas, J.G. (1997). Cell fate specification and symmetrical/asymmetrical divisions in the developing cerebral cortex. *J. Neurosci.*, **17**, 2018–2029.

Misson, J.P., Takahashi, T., and Caviness, V.S., Jr. (1991). Ontogeny of radial and other astroglial cells in murine cerebral cortex. *Glia*, **4**, 138–148.

Misson, J.-P., Edwards, M.A., Yamanoto, M., and Caviness, V.S., Jr. (1988). Identification of radial glial cells within the developing murine central nervous system: Studies based on a new immunohistochemical marker. *Dev. Brain Res.*, **44**, 95–108.

Mitchison, G. (1991). Neuronal branching patterns and the economy of cortical wiring. *Proc. R. Soc. B.*, **245**, 151–158.

Mitchison, T. and Kirschner, M.W. (1984). Microtubule assembly nucleated by isolated centrosomes. *Nature*, **312**, 232–237.

Mitchison, T. and Kirschner, M.W. (1988). Cytoskeletal dynamics and nerve growth. *Neuron*, **1**, 761–772.

Mitrofanis, J. and Guillery, R.W. (1993). New views of the thalamic reticular nucleus in the adult and developing brain. *Trends Neurosci.*, **16**, 240–245.

Miura, H., Yanazawa, M., Kato, K., and Kitamura, K. (1997). Expression of a novel aristaless related homeobox gene 'Arx' in the vertebrate telencephalon, diencephalon and floor plate. *Mech. Dev.*, **65**, 99–109.

Mogi, M., Harada, M., Kondo, T., Riederer, P., Inagaki, M., Minami, M., and Nagatsu, T. (1994). Interleukin-1 beta, interleukin-6, epidermal growth factor and transforming growth factor-alpha are elevated in the brain from Parkinsonian patients. *Neurosci. Lett.*, **180**, 147–150.

Molnar, Z. (1994). Multiple mechanisms in the establishment of thalamocortical innervation. Ph.D. thesis, University of Oxford.

Molnar, Z. (1998). *Development of thalamocortical connections*. Springer-Verlag.

Molnar, Z. and Blakemore, C. (1991). Lack of regional specificity for connections formed between thalamus and cortex in coculture. *Nature*, **351**, 475–477.

Molnar, Z. and Blakemore, C. (1995a). Guidance of thalamocortical innervation. In *Development of the cerebral cortex*, pp. 127–140, Chichester. (Ciba Foundation Symposium 193), John Wiley.

Molnar, Z. and Blakemore, C. (1995b). How do thalamic axons find their way to the cortex? *Trends Neurosci.*, **18**, 389–396.

Molnar, Z., Yee, K., Lund, R., and Blakemore, C. (1991). Development of rat thalamus and cerebral cortex after embryonic interruption of their connections. *Soc. Neurosci. Abstr.*, **17**, 305.3.

Morata, G. and Lawrence, P.A. (1975). Control of compartment development by the *engrailed* gene in *Drosophila*. *Nature*, **255**, 614–617.

Mountcastle, V.B., Talbot, W.H., Sakata, H., and Hyvarinen, J. (1969). Cortical neuronal mechanisms in flutter-vibration studied in unanaesthetised monkeys. Neuronal periodicity and frequency discrimination. *J. Neurophysiol.*, **32**, 452–484.

Mulderry, P. (1994). Neuropeptide expression by newborn and adult rat sensory neurons in culture: effects of nerve growth factor and other neurotrophic factors. *Neurosci.*, **59**, 673–688.

Murphy, K.C., Cardno, A.G., and McGuffin, P. (1996). The molecular genetics of schizophrenia. *J. Mol. Neurosci.*, **7**, 147–157.

Murray, A and Hunt, T. (1993). *The cell cycle*. Oxford University Press, Oxford, UK.

Murray, A.W. and Kirschner, M.W. (1989). Dominoes and clocks: the union of two views of the cell cycle. *Science*, **246**, 614–621.

Murtha, M.T., Leckman, J.F., and Ruddle, F.H. (1991). Detection of homeobox genes in development and evolution. *Proc. Natl. Acad. Sci. USA*, **88**, 10711–10715.

Muter, V., Taylor, S., and Vargha Khadem, F. (1997). A longitudinal study of early intellectual development in hemiplegic children. *Neurophsychologia*, **35**, 289–298.

Nadarajah, B., Jones, A.M., Evans, W.H., and Parnavalas, J.G. (1997). Differential expression of connexins during neocortical development and neuronal circuit formation. *J. Neurosci.*, **17**, 3096–3111.

Nadarajah, B., Makarenkova, H., Becker, D.L., Evans, W.H., and Parnavalas, J.G (1998). Basic FGF increases communication between cells of the developing neocortex. *J. Neurosci.*, **18**, 7881–7890.

Naegele, J.R., Jhaveri, S., and Schneider, G.E. (1988). Sharpening of topographical projections and maturation of geniculocortical axon arbors in the hamster. *J. Comp. Neurol.*, **277**, 593–607.

Nakajima, K., Mikoshiba, K., Miyata, T., Kudo, C., and Ogawa, M. (1997). Disruption of hippocampal development *in vivo* by CR-50 mAb against reelin. *Proc. Natl. Acad. Sci. USA*, **94**, 8196–8201.

Nakamoto, M., Cheng, H.-J., Friedman, G.C., McLaughlin, T., Hansen, M.J., Yoon, C.H., O'Leary, D.D.M., and Flanagan, J.G. (1996). Topographically specific effects of ELF-1 on retinal axon guidance *in vitro* and retinal axon mapping *in vivo*. *Cell*, **86**, 755–766.

Naruse, I. and Keino, H. (1995). Apoptosis in the developing CNS. *Prog. Neurobiol.*, **47**, 135–155.

Neuman, T., Keen, A., Zuber, M.X., Kristjansson, G.I., Gruss, P., and Nornes, H.O. (1993). Neuronal expression of regulatory helix-loop-helix factor Id2 gene in mouse. *Dev. Biol.*, **160**, 186–195.

Niazi, I.A. and Saxena, S. (1978). Abnormal hindlimb regeneration in tadpoles of the toad *Bufo andersonii* exposed to excess vitamin A. *Folia Biol.*, **26**, 3–8.

Nieuwkoop. P.D. and Albers, B. (1990). The role of competence in the craniocaudal segregation of the central nervous system. *Dev. Growth Differ.*, **32**, 23–31.

Norbeck, B.A. and Denburg, J.L. (1992). Molecular gradients along the proximodistal axis of embryonic insect legs: possible guidance cues of pioneer axon growth. *Development*, **116**, 467–479.

Nordlander, R.H. and Singer, M. (1978). The role of ependyma in regeneration of the spinal cord in the urodele amphibian tail. *J. Comp. Neurol.*, **180**, 349–374.

Norris, C.R. and Kalil, K. (1991). Guidance of callosal axons by radial glia in the developing cerebral cortex. *J. Neurosci.*, **11**, 3481–3492.

Novacek, M.J. (1992). Mammalian phylogeny—shaking the tree. *Nature*, **356**, 121–125.

Novak, N. and Bolz, J. (1993). Formation of specific efferent connections in organotypic slice cultures from rat visual cortex co-cultured with lateral geniculate nucleus and superior colliculus. *Eur. J. Neurosci.*, **5**, 15–24.

Nurcombe, V., Ford, M., and Bartlett, P.F. (1993). Developmental regulation of neural response to FGF-1 and FGF-2 by heparan sulfate proteoglycan. *Science*, **260**, 103–106.

Nurse, P. (1990). Universal control mechanism regulating onset of M-phase. *Nature*, **344**, 503–508.

Oakley, R.A., Lefcort, F.B., Clary, D.O., Reichardt, L.F. *et al.* (1997). Neurotrophin 3 promotes the differentiation of muscle spindle afferents in the absence of peripheral targets. *J. Neurosci.*, **17**, 4262–4274.

Obermayer, K., Ritter, H., and Schulten, K. (1990). A principle for the formation of the spatial structure of cortical feature maps. *Proc. Nat. Acad. Sci., USA*, **87**, 8345–8349.

O'Brien, R.A. D, Østberg, A.J.C., and Vrbova, G. (1978). Observations on the elimination of polyneural innervation in developing mammalian skeletal muscle. *J. Physiol.*, **282**, 571–582.

O'Connor, T.P. and Bentley, D. (1993). Accumulation of actin in subsets of pioneer growth cone filopodia in response to neural and epithelial guidance cues *in situ. J. Cell Biol.*, **123**, 935–948.

O'Keefe, J. and Nadel, L. (1978). *The hippocampus as a cognitive map.* Oxford University Press.

Olavaria, J. and Van Sluyters, R.C. (1985). Organization and postnatal development of callosal connections in the visual cortex of the rat. *J. Comp. Neurol.*, **239**, 1–26.

O'Leary, D.D.M. (1989). Do cortical areas emerge from a protocortex? *Trends Neurosci.*, **12**, 400–406.

O'Leary, D.D.M. and Koester, S.E. (1993). Development of projection neuron types, axon pathways, and patterned connections of the mammalian cortex. *Neuron*, **10**, 991–1006.

O'Leary, D.D.M. and Terashima, T. (1988). Cortical axons branch to multiple subcortical targets by interstitial axon budding; implications for target recognition and 'waiting periods'. *Neuron*, **1**, 901–910.

O'Leary, D.D.M., Stanfield, B.B., and Cowan, W.M. (1981). Evidence that the early postnatal restriction of the cells of origin of the callosal projection is due to the elimination of axonal collaterals rather than to the death of neurons. *Dev. Brain Res.*, **1**, 607–617.

O'Leary, D.D.M., Bicknese, A.R., De Carlos, J.A., Heffner, C.D., Koester, S.E., Kutka, L.J., and Terashima, T. (1990). Target selection by cortical axons: alternative mechanisms to establish axonal connections in the developing brain. *Cold Spring Harbor Symp. Quant. Biol.*, **55**, 453–468.

O'Leary, D.D.M., Yates, P.A., and McLaughlin, T. (1999). Molecular development of sensory maps: representing sights and smells in the brain. *Cell*, **96**, 255–269.

Oliver, G., Sosa-Pineda, B., Geisendorf, S., Spana, E.P., Doe, C.Q., and Gruss, P. (1993). Prox-1, a prospero-related homeobox gene expressed during mouse development. *Mech. Dev.*, **44**, 3–16.

Oltvai, Z.N., Milliman, C.L., and Korsmeyer, S.J. (1993). Bcl-2 heterodimerizes *in vivo* with a conserved homolog, Bax, that accelerates programmed cell death. *Cell*, **74**, 609–619.

Oppenheim, R.W. (1985). Naturally occurring cell death during neural development. *Trends Neurosci.*, **8**, 487–493.

Oppenheim, R.W. (1991). Cell death during development of the nervous system. *Annu. Rev. Neurosci.*, **14**, 453–501.

Oppenheim, R.W., Chu-Wang, I.-W., and Maderdrut (1978). Cell death of motoneurons in the chick embryo spinal cord. III. The differentation of motoneurons prior to their induced degeneration following limb-bud removal. *J. Comp. Neurol.*, **177**, 87–112.

O'Rourke, N.A., Dailey, M.E., Smith, S.J., and McConnell, S.K. (1992). Diverse migratory pathways in the developing cerebral cortex. *Science*, **258**, 299–302.

O'Rourke, N.A., Sullivan, D.P., Kaznowski, C.E., Jacobs, A.A., and McConnell, S.K. (1995). Tangential migration of neurons in the developing cerebral cortex. *Development*, **121**, 2165–2176.

O'Rourke, N.A., Chenn, A., and McConnell, S.K. (1997). Postmitotic neurons migrate tangentially in the cortical ventricular zone. *Development*, **124**, 997–1005.

Oumesmar, B.N., Vignais, L., and Baron-Van Evercooren, A. (1997). Developmental expression of platelet-derived growth factor alpha-receptor in neurons and glial cells of the mouse CNS. *J. Neurosci.*, **17**, 125–139.

Ozaki, H.S. and Wahlsten, D. (1992). Prenatal formation of the normal mouse corpus callosum—a quantitative study with carbocyanine dyes. *J. Comp. Neurol.*, **323**, 81–90.

Parker, A.J. and Hawken, M. (1985). Capabilities of monkey cortical neurons in spatial discrimination tasks. *J. Opt. Soc. Am. A*, **2**, 1101–1114.

Parker, A.J. and Newsome, W.T. (1998). Sense and the single neuron: probing the physiology of perception. *Annu. Rev. Neurosci.*, **21**, 227–277.

Parnavalas, J.G., Barfield, J.A., Franke, E., and Luskin, M.B. (1991). Separate progenitor cells give rise to pyramidal and nonpyramidal neurons in the rat telencephalon. *Cerebr. Cortex*, **1**, 1047–3211.

Pascalis, O. and De Schonen, S. (1994). Recognition memory in 3-day-old to 4-day-old human neonates. *Neuroreport*, **5**, 1721–1724.

Patel, N.H., Martin-Blanco, E., Coleman, K.G., Poole, S.J., Ellis, M.C., Kornberg, T.B. and Goodman, C.S. (1989). Expression of engrailed proteins in arthopods, annelids, and chordates. *Cell*, **58**, 955–968.

Patel, T., Gores, G.J., and Kaufmann, S.H. (1996). The role of proteases during apoptosis. *FASEB Journal*, **10**, 587–597.

Paxinos, G. and Watson, C. (1982). *The rat brain in sterotaxic coordinates*. Academic Press Inc., San Diego, USA.

Paxinos, G., Tork, I., Tecott, L.H., and Valentino, K.L. (1991). *Atlas of the developing rat brain*. Academic Press Inc., San Diego, USA.

Peng, X., Greene, L., Kaplan, D., and Stephens, R. (1995). Deletion of a conserved juxtamembrane sequence in Trk abolishes NGF-promoted neuritogenesis. *Neuron*, **15**, 395–406.

Pera, E.M. and Kessel, M. (1997). Patterning of the chick forebrain anlage by the prechordal plate. *Development*, **124**, 4153–4162.

Perrett, D.I. *et al.* (1982). Visual neurones responsive to faces in the monkey temporal cortex. *Exp. Brain Res.*, **47**, 329–342.

Perrone-Bizzozero, N.I., Sower, A.C., Bird, E.D. *et al.* (1996). Levels of the growth-associated protein gap-43 are selectively increased in association cortices in schizophrenia. *Proc. Natl. Acad. Sci. USA*, **93**, 14182–14187.

Peters, A. and Jones, E.G. (1984). *Cerebral cortex, volume 1: Cellular components of the cerebral cortex.* Plenum, New York.

Pettmann, B. and Henderson, C.E. (1998). Neuronal cell death. *Neuron*, **20**, 633–647.

Pimenta, A., Zhukareva, V., Barbe, M.F. *et al.*, (1995). The limbic system-associated membrane protein is an Ig superfamily member that mediates selective neuronal growth and axon targeting. *Neuron*, **14**, 1–15.

Pini, A. (1993). Chemorepulsion of axons in the developing mammalian central nervous system. *Science*, **261**, 95–98.

Pini, A. (1994). Growth cones say no. *Curr. Biol.*, **4**, 131–133.

Pinker, S. (1994). *The language instinct.* Allan Lane, The Penguin Press, England.

Pittman, R.N. (1985). Release of plasminogen activator and a calcium-dependent metalloprotease from cutured sympathetic and sensory neurons. *Dev. Biol.*, **110**, 91–101.

Pixley, S. and De Vellis, J. (1984). Transition between immature radial glia and mature astocytes studied with an antibody to vimentin. *Dev. Brain Res.*, **15**, 201–209.

Polleux, F., Giger, R.J., Ginty, D.D., Kolodkin, A.L., and Ghosh, A. (1998). Patterning of cortical efferent projections by semaphorin–neuropilin interactions. *Science*, **282**, 1904–1906.

Porter, F.D., Drago, J., Xu, Y., Cheema, S.S., Wassif, C. *et al.* (1997). Lhx2, a LIM homeobox gene, is required for eye, forebrain, and definitive erythrocyte development. *Development*, **124**, 2935–2944.

Porteus, M.H., Bulfone, A., Ciaranello, R.D., and Rubenstein, J.L.R. (1991). Isolation and characterisation of a novel cDNA clone encoding a homeodomain that is developmentally regulated in the ventral forebrain. *Neuron*, **7**, 221–229.

Porteus, M.H., Bulfone, A., Liu, J.-K., Puelles, L., Lo, L.-C., and Rubenstein, J.L.R. (1994). DLX-2, MASH-1, and MAP-2 expression and bromodeoxyuridine incorporation define molecularly distinct cell populations in the embryonic mouse forebrain. *J. Neurosci.*, **14**, 6370–6383.

Pousset, F. (1994). Developmental expression of cytokine genes in the cortex and hippocampus of the rat central nervous system. *Dev. Brain Res.*, **81**, 143–146.

Presson, J., Fernald, R.D., and Max, M. (1985). The organization of retinal projections to the diencephalon and pretectum in the Cichlid fish, *Haplochromis burtoni. J. Comp. Neurol.*, **235**, 360–374.

Prestige, M.C. (1967). The control of cell number in the lumber ventral horns during the development of *Xenopus laevis* tadpoles. *J. Embryol. Exp. Morph.*, **18**, 359–387.

Prestige, M.C. (1970). Differentation, degeneration and the role of the periphery. Quantitative considerations. In *The Neurosciences: second study programme* (ed. F. Schmidt), Rockfeller University Press, New York.

Prestige, M.C. and Willshaw, D.J. (1975). On a role for competition in the formation of patterned neural connexions. *Proc. R. Soc. London B*, **190**, 77–98.

Price, D.J. (1986). The postnatal development of clustered intrinsic connections in area 18 of the visual cortex in kittens. *Dev. Brain Res.*, **24**, 31–38.

Price, D.J. (1991). The development of visual cortical afferents. In *Vision and Visual Dysfunction;* vol. 11, *Development and Plasticity of the Visual System* (ed. J. Cronly-Dillon), chapter 17, pp. 337–352. Macmillan Press.

Price, D.J. (1995). Lesions of area 17 in newborn kittens cause selective changes in the development of area 18. *Neuroreport*, **7**, 201–204.

Price, D.J. and Blakemore, C (1985a). The postnatal development of the association projection from visual cortical area 17 to area 18 in the cat. *J. Neurosci.*, **5**, 2443–2452.

Price, D.J. and Blakemore, C (1985b). Regressive events in the postnatal development of association projections in the visual cortex. *Nature*, **316**, 721–724.

Price, D.J. and Ferrer, J.M.R. (1993). The incidence of bifurcation among corticocortical connections from area 17 in the developing visual cortex of the cat. *Eur. J. Neurosci.*, **5**, 223–231.

Price, D.J. and Lotto, R.B. (1996). Influences of the thalamus on the survival of subplate and cortical plate cells in cultured embryonic mouse brain. *J. Neurosci.*, **16**, 3247–3255.

Price, D.J. and Thurlow, L. (1988). Cell lineage in the rat cerebral cortex: a study using retroviral mediated gene transfer. *Development*, **104**, 473–482.

Price, D.J. and Zumbroich, T.J. (1989). Postnatal development of corticocortical efferents from area 17 in the cat's visual cortex. *J. Neurosci.*, **9**, 600–613.

Price, D.J., Zumbroich, T.J., and Blakemore, C. (1988). Development of stimulus selectivity and functional organization in the suprasylvian visual cortex of the cat. *Proc. R. Soc. London B*, **233**, 123–163.

Price, D.J., Ferrer, J.M.R., Blakemore, C., and Kato, N. (1994a). Functional organisation of corticocortical projections from area 17 to area 18 in the cat's visual cortex. *J. Neurosci.*, **14**, 2732–2746.

Price, D.J., Ferrer, J.M.R., Blakemore, C., and Kato, N. (1994b). Postnatal development and plasticity of corticocortical projections from area 17 to area 18 in the cat's visual cortex. *J. Neurosci.*, **14**, 2747–2762.

Price, D.J., Lotto, R.B., Warren, N., Magowan, G., and Clausen, J.A. (1995). The roles of growth factors and neural activity in the development of the neocortex. In *Development of the cerebral cortex* (eds. G. Bock and G. Cardew). John Wiley and Sons, Chichester.

Price, D.J., Aslam, S., Tasker, L., and Gillies, K. (1997). The fates of the earliest generated cells in the developing murine neocortex. *J. Comp. Neurol.*, **377**, 414–422.

Price, M. (1993). Members of the Dlx- and Nkx2-gene families are regionally expressed in the developing forebrain. *J. Neurobiol.*, **24**, 1385–1399.

Price, M., Lemaistre, M., Pischetola, M., Di Lauro, R., and Duboule, D. (1991). A mouse gene related to distal-less shows a restricted expression in the developing forebrain. *Nature*, **351**, 748–751.

Price, M., Lazzaro, D., Pohl, T., Mattei, M.-G., Ruther, U., Olivo, J.-C., Duboule, D., and Di Lauro, R. (1992). Regional expression of the homeobox gene Nkx-2.2 in the developing mammalian forebrain. *Neuron*, **8**, 241–255.

Puelles, L. and Rubenstein, J.L.R. (1993). Expression patterns of homeobox and other putative regulatory genes in the embryonic mouse forebrain suggest a neuromeric organisation. *Trends Neurosci.*, **16**, 472–479.

Purves, D. (1994). *Neural Activity and the Growth of the Brain.* Cambridge University Press, New York.

Purves, D. and Lichtman, J.W. (1985). Elimination of the synapses in the developing nervous system. *Science*, **210**, 153–157.

Purves, D. and Lichtman, J.W. (1985). *Principles of Neural Development.* Sinauer Associates, Sunderland, M.A.

Purves, D., Snider, W.D., and Voyrodic, J.T. (1988). Trophic regulation of nerve cell morphology and innervation in the autonomic nervous system. *Nature*, **336**, 123–128.

Qian, X., Goderie, S.K., Shen, Q., Stern, J.H., and Temple, S. (1998). Intrinsic programs of patterned cell lineages in isolated vertebrate CNS ventricular zone cells. *Development*, **125**, 3143–3152.

Quartz, S. and Sejnowski, T.J. (1997). The neural basis of cognitive development: A constructivist manifesto. *Behav. Brain Sci.*, **20**, 537–596.

Raczkowski, D. and Rosenquist, A.C. (1983). Connections of the multiple visual cortical areas with the lateral posterior-pulvinar complex and adjacent thalamic nuclei in the cat. *J. Neurosci.*, **3**, 1912–1942.

Raedler, E. and Raedler, A. (1978). Autoradiographic study of early neurogenesis in rat neocortex. *Anat. Embryol.*, **154**, 267–284.

Raedler, T.J., Knable, M.B., and Weinberger, D.R. (1998). Schizophrenia as a developmental disorder of the cerebral cortex. *Curr. Opin. Neurobiol.*, **8**, 157–161.

Raff, M. (1992). Social controls on cell survival and cell death. *Nature*, **356**, 397–400.

Raff, M. (1998). Cell suicide for beginners. *Nature*, **396**, 119–122.

Rager, G. and von Oeynhausen, B. (1979). Ingrowth and ramification of retinal fibres in the developing optic tectum of the chick embryo. *Exp. Brain Res.*, **33**, 65–78.

Rakic, P. (1972). Mode of cell migration to the superficial layers of fetal monkey neocortex. *J. Comp. Neurol.*, **145**, 61–84.

Rakic, P. (1974). Neurons in the rhesus monkey visual cortex: systematic relationship between time of origin and eventual deposition. *Science*, **183**, 425–427.

Rakic, P. (1976a). Prenatal genesis of connections subserving ocular dominance in the rhesus monkey. *Nature*, **261**, 467–471.

Rakic, P. (1976b). Differences in the time of origin and in eventual distribution of neurons in areas 17 and 18 of the visual cortex in the rhesus monkey. *Exp. Brain Res. Suppl.*, **1**, 244–248.

Rakic, P. (1977). Prenatal development of the visual system in the rhesus monkey. *Phil. Trans. R. Soc. Lond. B. Biol. Sci.*, **278**, 245–260.

Rakic, P. (1983). Geniculo-cortical connections in primates: normal and experimentally altered development. *Prog. Brain Res.*, **58**, 393–404.

Rakic, P. (1988). Specification of cerebral cortical areas. *Science*, **241**, 170–176.

Rakic, P. (1995). Radial versus tangential migration of neuronal clones in the developing cerebral cortex. *Proc. Natl. Acad. Sci. USA*, **92**, 11323–11327.

Rakic, P. (1997). Intra- and extracellular control of neuronal migration: relevance to cortical malformations. In *Normal and abnormal development of the cortex* (eds. A. Galaburda and Y. Christen). Springer-Verlag.

Rakic, P., Bourgeois, J.P., Eckenhoff, M.F., Zecevic, N., Goldman-Rakic, P.S. (1986). Concurrent overproduction of synapses in diverse regions of the primate cerebral-cortex. *Science*, **232**, 232–235.

Rakic, P., Cameron, R.S., and Komuro, H. (1994). Recognition, adhesion, transmembrane signalling, and cell motility in guided neuronal migration. *Curr. Opin. Neurobiol.*, **4**, 63–69.

Rankin, E.C.C and Cook, J.E. (1986). Topographic refinement of the regenerating retinotectal projection of the goldfish in standard laboratory conditions: a quantitative WGA-HRP study. *Exp. Brain Res.*, **63**, 409–420.

Rashevsky, N. (1938). *Mathematical biophysics*. University of Chicago Press, Chicago.

Rasmussen, C.E. and Willshaw, D.J. (1993). Presynaptic and postsynaptic competition in models for the development of neuromuscular connections. *Biol. Cybern.*, **68**, 409–419.

Rauschecker, J.P. and Singer, W. (1979). Changes in the circuitry of the kitten's visual cortex are gated by postsynaptic activity. *Nature*, **280**, 58–60.

Redfern, P.A. (1970). Neuromuscular transmission in newborn rats. *J. Physiol.*, **209**, 701–709.

Reh, T.A. and Constantine-Paton, M. (1983). Retinal ganglion cell terminals change their projection sites during larval development of Rana Pipiens. *J. Neurosci.*, **4**, 442–457.

Reh, T.A. and Constantine-Paton, M. (1985). Eye-specific segregation requires neural activity in three-eyed Rana pipiens. *J. Neurosci.*, **5**, 1132–1143.

Reid, C.B., Liang, I., and Walsh, C. (1995). Systematic widespread clonal organisation in cerebral cortex. *Neuron*, **15**, 299–310.

Reinoso, B.S. and O'Leary, D.D.M. (1990). Correlation of geniculocortical growth into the cortical plate with the migration of their layer 4 and 6 target cells. *Soc. Neurosci. Abstr.*, **16**, 493.

Reith, A.D. and Bernstein, A. (1991). Molecular-basis of mouse developmental mutants. *Genes and Development*, **5**, 1115–1123.

Rennie, S., Lotto, R.B., and Price, D.J. (1994). Growth-promoting interactions between the murine neocortex and thalamus in organotypic co-cultures. *Neuroscience*, **61**, 547–564.

Reynolds, B.A. and Weiss, S. (1992). Generation of neurons and astrocytes from isolated cells of the adult mammalian central nervous system. *Science*, **255**, 1707–1710.

Ribchester, R.R. (1993). Co-existence and elimination of convergent motor nerve terminals in reinnervated and paralysed adult rat skeletal muscle. *J. Physiol.*, **466**, 421–441.

Ribchester, R. and Barry, J.A. (1994). Spatial versus consumptive competition at polyneuronally innervated neuromuscular junctions. *Exp. Physiol.*, **79**, 465–494.

Ribchester, R.R. and Taxt, T. (1983). Motor unit size and synaptic competition in rat lumbrical muscles reinnervated by active and inactive motor axons. *J. Physiol.*, **344**, 89–111.

Ribchester, R.R. and Taxt, T. (1984). Repression of inactive motor nerve terminals in partially denervated rat muscle after regeneration of active motor axons. *J. Physiol.*, **347**, 497–511.

Richards, L.J., Koester, S.E., Tuttle, R., and O'Leary, D.D.M. (1997). Directed growth of early cortical axons is influenced by a chemoattractant released from an intermediate target. *J. Neurosci.*, **17**, 2445–2456.

Riddle, D.R., Lo, D.C., and Katz, L.C. (1995). NT-4-mediated rescue of lateral geniculate neurons from effects of monocular deprivation. *Nature*, **378**, 189–191.

Rio, C., Rieff, H.I., Qi, P.M., and Corfas, G. (1997). Neuregulin and erbB receptors play a critical role in neuronal migration. *Neuron*, **19**, 39–50.

Riss, W., Halpern, M., and Scalia, F. (1969). The quest for clues to forebrain evolution – the study of reptiles. *Brain Behav. Evol.*, **2**, 1–15.

Rivera-Pomar, R. and Jackle, H. (1996). From gradients to stripes in Drosophila embryogenesis: filling in the gaps. *Trends Genet.*, **12**, 478–483.

Roberts, G.W., Royston, M.C., and Götz, M. (1995). Pathology of cortical development and neuropsychiatric disorders. In *Development of the cerebral cortex* (eds. G. Bock and G. Cardew). John Wiley and Sons, Chichester.

Rodieck, R.W. (1967). Maintained acivity of cat retinal ganglion cells. *J. Neurophysiol.*, **30**, 1043–1071.

Rodriguez-Tebar, A., Dechant, G., and Barde, Y.A. (1990). Binding of brain-derived neurotrophic factor to the nerve growth factor receptor. *Neuron*, **4**, 487–492.

Rodriguez-Tebar, A., Dechant, G., Gotz, R., and Barde, Y.A. (1992). Binding of neurotrophin-3 to its neuronal receptors and interactions with nerve growth factor and brain-derived neurotrophic factor. *EMBO J.*, **11**, 917–922.

Roger, M. (1998). Experimental evidence that there is an early commitment of neocortical cells to develop area-specific connectivity. In *Proc. Eur. Res. Conf. on Brain development and cognition in human infants: development and functional specialization of the cortex*, p. 37, San Feliu de Guixols, Spain.

Rose, J.E., Galambos, R., and Hughes, J.R. (1959). Microelectrode studies of the cochlear nuclei of the cat. *Bull. John Hopkins Hosp.*, **104**, 211–251.

Rose, J.E. and Mountcastle, V.B. (1959). Touch and kinesthesis. In *Handbook of Physiology* (eds. W.H. Field and V.E. Hall), vol. 1. American Physiological Society, Washington D.C.

Ross, C.A. and Pearlson, G.D. (1996). Schizophrenia, the heteromodal association neocortex and development: potential for a neurogenetic approach. *Trends Neurosci.*, **19**, 171–176.

Roth, S. and Marchase, R.B. (1976). An *in vitro* assay for retinotectal specificity. In *Neuronal recognition* (ed. S. Barondes), pp. 227–248. Plenum, New York.

Royaux, I., Lambert de Rouvroit, C., D'Arcangelo, G., *et al.* (1997). Genomic organization of the mouse reelin gene. *Genomics*, **46**, 240–250.

Rubenstein, J.L.R. and Beachy, P.A. (1998). Patterning of the embryonic forebrain. *Curr. Opin. Neurobiol.*, **8**, 18–26.

Rubenstein, J.L.R., Shimamura, K., Martinez, S., and Puelles, L. (1998). Regionalization of the prosencephalic neural plate. *Annu. Rev. Neurosci.*, **21**, 445–477.

Ruit, K.G. and Snider, W.D. (1991). Administration or deprivation of nerve growth factor during development permanently alters neuronal geometry. *J. Comp. Neurol.*, **314**, 106–131.

Ruiz i Altaba, A. (1994). Pattern formation in the vertebrate neural plate. *Trends Neurosci.*, **17**, 233–243.

Rusoff, A. (1984). Paths of axons in the visual system of perciform fish and implications of these paths for rules governing axonal growth. *J. Neurosci.*, **4**, 1414–1428.

Ryle, G. (1967). *The concept of mind*. Hutchison, London.

Sadler, M. and Berry, M. (1984). Remodelling during development of the Purkinje cell dendritic tree in the mouse. *Proc. R. Soc. London B*, **221**, 349–368.

Salin, P.A. and Bullier, J. (1995). Corticocortical connections in the visual system: structure and function. *Physiol. Rev.*, **75**, 107–154.

Salinas, P.C. and Nusse, R. (1992). Regional expression of the Wnt-3 gene in the developing mouse forebrain in relationship to diencephalic neuromeres. *Mech. Dev.*, **39**, 151–160.

Sanides, D. (1978). The retinotopic distribution of visual callosal projections in the suprasylvian visual areas compared to the classical visual areas (17, 18, 19) in the cat. *Exp. Brain Res.*, **33**, 435–443.

Sasai, Y. *et al.* (1994). *Xenopus* chordin: a novel dorsalizing factor activated by organizer-specific homeobox genes. *Cell*, **79**, 779–790.

Sasaki, H., Hui, C., Nakafuku, M., and Kondoh, H.A. (1997). Binding site for Gli proteins is essential for HNF-3b floor plate enhancer activity in transgenics and can respond to Shh *in vitro*. *Development*, **124**, 1313–1322.

Sauer, F.C. (1935). Mitosis in the neural tube. *J. Comp. Neurol.*, **62**, 377–405.

Saunders, J.W.J. (1966). Death in embryonic systems. *Science*, **154**, 604–612.

Saunders, J.W. Jr. and Gasseling, M.F. (1968). Ectodermal-messenchymal interactions in the origin of limb symmetry. In *Epithelial–Mesenchymal Interactions* (eds. R. Fleischmajer and R. Billingham), pp. 78–97. Williams & Wilkins, Baltimore.

Saxen, L. (1989). Neural induction. *Int. J. Dev. Biol.*, **33**, 21–48.

Schall, J.D., Ault, S.J., Vitek, D.J., and Leventhal, A.G. (1988). Experimental induction of an abnormal ipsilateral visual field representation in the geniculocortical pathway of normally pigmented cats. *J. Neurosc.,* **8**, 2039–2048.

Schambra, U.B., Lauder, J.M., and Silver, J. (1992). *Atlas of the prenatal mouse brain.* Academic Press Inc., San Diego, USA.

Schendel, S.L., Xie, Z., Montal, M.O., Matsuyama, S., Montal, M., and Reed, J.C. (1997). Channel formation by antiapoptotic proein Bcl-2. *Proc. Natl. Acad. Sci. USA,* **94**, 5113–5118.

Schiffmann, S.N., Bernier, B., and Goffinet, A.M. (1997). Relin mRNA expression during mouse brain development. *Eur. J. Neurosci.,* **9**, 1055–1071.

Schlagger, B.L. and O'Leary, D.D.M. (1992). Potential of visual cortex to develop an array of functional units unique to somatosensory cortex. *Science,* **252**, 1556–1560.

Schlagger, B.L. and O'Leary, D.D.M. (1994). Early development of the somatotopic map and barrel patterning. *J. Comp. Neurol.,* **346**, 80–96.

Schmahl, W. (1983). Developmental gradient of cell cycle in the telencephalic roof of the fetal NMRI-mouse. *Anat. Embryol,* **167**, 355–364.

Schmechel, D.E. and Rakic, P. (1979). Arrested proliferation of radial glial cells during midgestation in rhesus monkey. *Nature,* **227**, 303–305.

Schmidt, J.T. (1978). Retinal fibres alter tectal positional markers during expansion of the half retinal projection in goldfish. *J. Comp. Neurol.,* **177**, 279–300.

Schmidt, J.T. (1980). Long term potentiation and activity dependent retinotopic sharpening in the regenerating retinotectal projection of goldfish: common sensitive period and sensitivity to NMDA blockers. *J. Neurosci.,* **10**, 233–246.

Schmidt, J.T. and Edwards, D.L. (1983). Activity sharpens the map during the regeneration of the retinotectal projection in goldfish. *Brain Res.,* **269**, 29–39.

Schmidt, J.T., Cicerone, C.M., and Easter, S.S. (1978). Expansion of the half retinal projection to the tectum in goldfish: an electrophysiological and anatomical study. *J. Comp. Neurol.,* **177**, 257–278.

Schnell, L., Schneider, R., Kolbeck, R., Barde, Y.A., and Schwab, M.E. (1994). Neurotrophin-3 enhances sprouting of corticospinal tract during development and after adult spinal cord lesion. *Nature,* **367**, 170–173.

Scholes, J. (1979). Nerve fibre topography in the retinal projection to the tectum. *Nature,* **278**, 620–624.

Scholes, J. (1981). Ribbon optic nerves and axonal growth patterns in the retinal projection to the tectum. In *Development of the nervous system* (eds D.R. Garrod and J.D. Feldman). Cambridge University Press, Cambridge, UK.

Schultze, B. and Korr, H. (1981). Cell kinetic studies of different cell types in the developing and adult brain of the rat and the mouse: a review. *Cell Tissue Kinet.,* **14**, 309–325.

Schwartz, E.L. (1977). The development of specific visual connections in the monkey and the goldfish: Outline of a geometric theory of receptotopic structure. *J. Theor. Biol.,* **69**, 655–683.

Schwartz, M.L., Rakic, P., and Goldmanrakic, P.S. (1991). Early phenotype expression of cortical neurons—evidence that a subclass of migrating neurons have callosal axons. *Proc. Natl. Acad. Sci. USA*, **88**, 1354–1358.

Seeger, M., Tear, G., Ferres-Marco, D., and Goodman, C.S. (1993). Mutations affecting growth core guidance in Drosophila: genes necessary for guidance towards or away from the midline. *Neuron*, **10**, 409–426.

Segal, R.A. and Greenberg, M.E. (1996). Intracellular signaling pathways activated by neurotrophic factors. *Annu. Rev. Neurosci.*, **19**, 463–489.

Sejnowski, T.J. (1977a). Storing covariance with nonlinearly interacting neurons. *J. Math. Biol.*, **4**, 303–321.

Sejnowski, T.J. (1977b). Statistical constraints on synaptic plasticity. *J. Theor. Biol.*, **69**, 385–389.

Sejnowski, T.J., Koch, C., and Churchland, P.S. (1988). Computational neuroscience. *Science*, **241**, 1299–1306.

Seniuk-Tatton, N.A., Henderson, J.T., and Roder, J.C. (1995). Neurons express ciliary neurotrophic factor mrna in the early postnatal and adult rat brain. *J. Neurosci. Res.*, **41**, 663–676.

Serafini, T., Kennedy, T.E., Galko, M.J., Mirzayan, C., Jessell, T.M., and Tessier-Lavigne, M. (1994). The netrins define a family of axon outgrowth-promoting proteins homologous to C. Elegans UNC-6. *Cell*, **78**, 409–424.

Serafini, T., Colamarino, S.A., Leonardo, E.D., Wang, H., Beddington, R., Skarnes, W.C., and Tessier-Lavigne, M. (1996). Netrin-1 is required for commissural axon guidance in the developing vertebrate nervous system. *Cell*, **87**, 1001–1014.

Sergent, J. *et al.* (1992). Functional neuroanatomy of face and object processing. *Brain*, **115**, 15–36.

Shah, N.M., Marchionni, M.A., Isaacs, I., Stroobant, P., and Anderson, D.J. (1994). Glial growth factor restricts mammalian neural crest stem cells to a glial fate. *Cell*, **77**, 349–360.

Sharma, S.C. (1972). The retinal projection in adult goldfish: An experimental study. *Brain Res.*, **39**, 213–223.

Shatz, C.J. (1977a). A comparison of visual pathways in Boston and Midwestern Siamese cats. *J. Comp. Neurol.*, **171**, 205–228.

Shatz, C.J. (1977b). Anatomy of interhemispheric connections in the visual system of Boston Siamese and ordinary cats. *J. Comp. Neurol.*, **173**, 497–518.

Shatz, C.J. (1996). Emergence of order in visual system development. *Proc. Natl. Acad. Sci. USA*, **93**, 602–608.

Shatz, C.J. and Luskin, M.B. (1986). The relationship between the geniculocortical afferents and their cortical target cells during development of the cat's primary visual cortex. *J. Neurosci.*, **6**, 3655–3668.

Shatz, C.J. and Stryker, M.P. (1978). Ocular dominance in layer IV of the cat's visual cortex and the effects of monocular deprivation. *J. Physiol.*, **281**, 267–283.

Shatz, C.J., Chun, J.J.M., and Luskin, M.B. (1988). The role of the subplate in the development of the mammalian telencephalon. In *Development and maturation of the cerebral cortex* (eds. A. Peters and E.G. Jones). Plenum, New York.

Shatz, C.J., Ghosh, A., McConnell, S.K., Allendoerfer, K.L., Friauf, E., and Antonini, A. (1991). Subplate neurons and the development of neocortical connections. In *Development of the visual system* (eds. D.M.K. Lam and C.J. Shatz). MIT Press, Cambridge, Massachusetts.

Shawert, W. and Behringer, R.R. (1995). Requirement for Lim1 in head-organizer function. *Nature*, **374**, 425–430.

Sheldon, M., Rice, D.S., D'Arcangelo, G., and Yoneshima, H., *et al.* (1997). Scrambler and yotari disrupt the disabled gene and produce a reeler-like phenotype in mice. *Nature*, **389**, 730–733.

Sheng, H.Z., Bertuzzi, S., Chiang, C., Shawlot, W., Taira, M., Dawid, I., and Westphal, H. (1997). Expression of murine Lhx5 suggests a role in specifying the forebrain. *Dev. Dyn.*, **208**, 266–277.

Shepherd, G.M. (1994). *Neurobiology; 3rd Edition.* Oxford University Press, New York.

Sheppard, A.M. and Pearlman, A.L. (1997). Abnormal reorganization of preplate neurons and their associated extracellular matrix: an early manifestation of altered neocortical development in the reeler mutant mouse. *J. Comp. Neurol.*, **378**, 173–179.

Sheppard, A.M., Hamilton, S.K., and Pearlman, A.L. (1991). Changes in the distribution of extracellular matrix components accompany early morphogenetic events of mammalian cortical development. *J. Neurosci.*, **11**, 3928–3942.

Shering, A.F. and Lowenstein, P.R. (1994). Neocortex provides direct synaptic input to interstitial neurons of the intermediate zone of kittens and white matter of cats: A light and electron microscopic study. *J. Comp. Neurol.*, **347**, 433–443.

Sherk, H. (1978). Area 18 cell responses in cat during reversible inactivation of area 17. *J. Neurophysiol.*, **41**, 204–215.

Sherman, S.M., Hoffman, K.P., and Stone, J. (1972). Loss of a specific cell type from the dorsal lateral geniculate nucleus in visually deprived cats. *J. Neurophysiol.*, **35**, 532–541.

Shi, R. and Borgens, R.B. (1995). Three-dimensional gradients of voltage during development of the nervous system as invisible coordinates for the establishment of embryonic pattern. *Dev. Dyn.*, **202**, 101–114.

Shimamura, K. and Rubenstein, J.L.R. (1997). Inductive interactions direct early regionalization of the mouse forebrain. *Development*, **124**, 2709–2718.

Shimamura, K., Hartigan, D.J., Martinez, S., Puelles, L., and Rubenstein, J.L.R. (1995). Longitudinal organisation of the anterior neural plate and neural tube. *Development*, **121**, 3923–3933.

Shoen, S.W., Leutrnecker, B., Kreutzberg, G.W., and Singer, W. (1990). Ocular dominance plasticity and developmental changes of 5′-nucleotidase distributions in the kitten visual cortex. *J. Comp. Neurol.*, **296**, 379–392.

Sidman, R.L., Miale, I.L., and Feder, N. (1959). Cell proliferation and migration in the primitive ependymal zone: an autoradiographic study of histogenesis in the nervous system. *Exp. Neurol.*, **1**, 322–333.

Silos-Santiago, I., Fagan, A., Garber, M., Fritzsch, B., and Barbacid, M. (1997). Severe sensory deficits but normal CNS development in newborn mice lacking TrkB and TrkC tyrosine protein kinase receptors. *Eur. J. Neurosci.*, **9**, 2045–2056.

Silver, J. and Robb, R.M. (1979). Studies on the development of the eyecup and optic nerve in normal mice and in mutants with congenital optic nerve aplasia. *Dev. Biol.*, **68**, 175–190.

Simeone, A., Acampora, D., Gulisano, M., Stornaiolo, A, and Boncinelli, E. (1992a). Nested expression domains of four homeobox genes in the developing rostral brain. *Nature*, **358**, 687–690.

Simeone, A., Gulisano, M., Acampora, D., Stornaiolo, A., *et al.* (1992b). Two vertebrate homeobox genes related to the *Drosophila* empty spiracles genes are expressed in the embryonic cerebral cortex. *EMBO J.*, **11**, 2541–2550.

Singer, M., Norlander, R., and Egar, M. (1979). Axonal guidance during embryogenesis and regeneration in the spinal cord of the newt: The blueprint hypothesis of neuronal pathway patterning. *J. Comp. Neurol.*, **185**, 1–22.

Skaliora, I., Singer, W., Betz, H., and Puschel, A.W. (1998). Differential patterns of semaphorin expression in the developing rat brain. *Eur. J. Neurosci.*, **10**, 1215–1229.

Slack, J.M.W. (1991). *From egg to embryo: determinative events in early development*. Cambridge University Press, Cambridge, UK.

Smallheiser, N.R. and Crain, S.M. (1984). The possible role of 'sibling neurite bias' in the coordination of neurite extension, branching and survival. *J. Neurobiol.*, **15**, 517–529.

Smart, I.H.M and Smart, M. (1982). Growth patterns in the lateral wall of the mouse telencephalon: I autoradiographic studies of the histogenesis of the isocortex and adjacent areas. *J. Anat.*, **134**, 273–298.

Smart, I.H.M. (1983). Three dimensional growth of the mouse isocortex. *J. Anat.*, **137**, 683–694.

Smith, A. (1984). *The mind*. London, Hodder and Stoughton.

Snider, W.D. (1994). Functions of neurotrophins during nervous system development: What are knockouts teaching us? *Cell*, **77**, 627–638.

Snider, W.D. and Johnson, E.M. (1989). Neurotrophic molecules. *Ann. Neurol.*, **26**, 489–506.

Sommer, L., Ma, Q., and Anderson, D.J. (1996). Neurogenins, a novel family of atonal-related bHLH transcription factors, are putative mammalian neuronal determination genes that reveal progenitor cell heterogeneity in the developing CNS and PNS. *Mol. Cell. Neurosci.*, **8**, 221–241.

Spemann, H. (1938). *Embryonic development and induction*. Reprinted by Garland Publishing 1988.

Sperry, R.W. (1943). Visuomotor co-ordination in the newt (*Triturus viridescens*) after regeneration of the optic nerve. *J. Comp. Neurol.*, **79**, 33–55.

Sperry, R.W. (1944). Optic nerve regeneration with return of vision in anurans. *J. Neurophysiol.*, **7**, 57–69.

Sperry, R.W. (1945). Restoration of vision after crossing of optic nerves and after contralateral transplantation of the eye. *J. Neurophysiol.*, **8**, 15–28.

Sperry, R.W. (1951). Mechanisms of neural maturation. In *Handbook of experimental psychology* (ed. S.S. Stevens), p. 236–280. Wiley, New York.

Sperry, R.W. (1963). Chemoaffinity in the orderly growth of nerve fiber patterns and connections. *Proc. Nat. Acad. Sci., USA*, **50**, 703–710.

Sperry, R.W. (1965). Embryogenesis of behavioural nerve nets. In *Organogenesis* (eds. R. De Haan and H. Ursprung), p. 161–186. Holt, Rinehart and Winston: New York.

Stahl, B., Muller, B., Boxberg, Yv., Cox, E.C., and Bonhoeffer, F. (1990). Biochemical characterisation of a putative axonal guidance molecule of the chick visual system. *Neuron*, **5**, 735–743.

Stahl, N. and Yancopoulos, G.D. (1994). The tripartite CNTF receptor complex: activation and signaling involves components shared with other cytokines. *J. Neurobiol.*, **25**, 1454–1466.

Stanfield, B.B., O'Leary, D.D.M., and Fricks, C. (1982). Selective collateral elimination in early postnatal development restricts cortical distribution of pyramidal tract axons. *Nature*, **298**, 371–373.

Steller, H. (1995). Mechanisms and genes of cellular suicide. *Science*, **267**, 1445–1448.

Stent, G.S. (1973). A physiological mechanism for Hebb's postulate of learning. *Proc. Nat. Acad. Sci. USA*, **70**, 997–1001.

Stent, G.S. (1991). Strength and weakness of the genetic approach to the development of the nervous system. *Annu. Rev. Neurosci.*, **4**, 163–194.

Stewart, B.W. (1994). Mechanisms of apoptosis: integration of genetic, biochemical and cellular indicators. *J. Natl. Cancer. Inst.*, **86**, 1286–1295.

Stewart, C.E.H. and Rotwein, P. (1996). Growth, differentiation, and survival: multiple physiological functions for insulin-like growth factors. *Physiol. Rev.*, **76**, 1005–1026.

Stewart, G.R. and Pearlman, A.L. (1987). Fibronectin-like immunoreactivity in the developing cerebral cortex. *J. Neurosci.*, **7**, 3325–3333.

Stewart, R., Erskine, L., and McCaig, C.D. (1995). Calcium channel subtypes and intracellular calcium stores modulate electric field-stimulated and -oriented nerve growth. *Dev. Biol.*, **171**, 340–351.

Stirling, R.V. and Summerbell, D. (1979). The segregation of axons from the segmental nerve roots to the chick wing. *Nature*, **278**, 640–642.

Stone, J. (1983). *Parallel processing in the visual system*. Plenum Press, New York.

Stout, R.P. and Gradziadei, P.P.C. (1980). Influence of the olfactory placode on the development of the brain in *Xenopus laevis* (Daudin). *Neurosci.*, **5**, 2175–2186.

Stoykova, A. and Gruss, P. (1994). Roles of Pax-genes in developing and adult brain as suggested by expression patterns. *J. Neurosci.*, **14**, 1395–1412.

Stoykova, A., Fritsch, R., Walther, C., and Gruss, P. (1996). Forebrain patterning defects in small eye mutant mice. *Development*, **122**, 3453–3465.

Stratford, D., Horton, C., and Maden, M. (1996). Retinoic acid is required for the initiation of outgrowth in the chick limb bud. *Curr. Biol.*, **6**, 1124–1133.

Straznicky, C., Gaze, R.M., and Keating, M.J. (1980). The retinotectal projections from surgically rounded-up half-eyes in *Xenopus*. *J. Embryol. exp. Morph.*, **58**, 79–91.

Straznicky, C., Gaze, R.M., and Keating, M.J. (1981). The development of the retinotectal projections from compound eyes in *Xenopus*. *J. Embryol. exp. Morph.*, **62**, 13–35.

Straznicky, C., Gaze, R.M., and Horder, T.J. (1979). Selection of appropriate medial branch of the optic tract by fibres of ventral retinal origin during development and in regeneration: An autoradiographic study in *Xenopus*. *J. Embryol. exp. Morph.*, **50**, 253–267.

Straznicky, K. and Gaze, R.M. (1971). The growth of the retina in *Xenopus laevis*: an autodioradiographical study. *J. Embryol. Exp. Morph.*, **26**, 67–79.

Straznicky, K. and Gaze, R.M. (1972). The development of the tectum in *Xenopus laevis*: an autoradiographical study. *J. Embryol. Exp. Morph.*, **28**, 87–115.

Straznicky, K. and Tay, D. (1982). Retinotectal map formation in dually innervated tecta: a regeneration study in Xenopus with one compound eye following bilateral optic nerve section. *J. Comp. Neurol.*, **206**, 119–130.

Stryker, M.P. and Harris, W. (1986). Binocular impulse blockade prevents the formation of ocular dominance columns in cat visual cortex. *J. Neurosci.*, **6**, 2117–2133.

Stuermer, C.A.O. (1990). Retinotopic organization of the developing rentinotectal projection in the zebrafish embryo under TTX-induced neural-impulse blockade. *J. Neurosci.*, **10**, 3615–3626.

Suda, Y., Matsua, I., Kuratani, S., and Aizawa, S. (1996). Otx1 function overlaps with Otx2 in development of mouse forebrain and midbrain. *Genes to Cells*, **1**, 1031–1044.

Suddath, R.L., Christison, G.W., Torrey, E.F., Casanove, M.F., and Weinberger, D.R. (1990). Anatomical abnormalities in the brains of monozygotic twins discordant for schizophrenia. *N. Engl. J. Med.*, **322**, 789–794.

Suga, N. (1978). Specialization of the auditory system for reception and processing of species-specific sounds. *Fed. Proc.*, **37**, 2342–2354.

Summerbell, D. (1983). The effect of local application of retinoic acid to the anterior margin of the developing chick limb. *J. Embryol. Exp. Morph.*, **78**, 269–289.

Summerbell, D. and Stirling, V. (1981). The innervation of dorsoventrally reversed chick wings: evidence that motor axons do not actively seek out their appropriate targets. *J. Embryol Exp. Morph.*, **61**, 233–247.

Sur, M., Garraghty, P.E., and Roe, A.W. (1988). Experimentally induced visual projections in auditory thalamus and cortex. *Science*, **242**, 1434–1441.

Swindale, N.V. (1979). How ocular dominance stripes may be formed. In *Developmental neurobiology of vision*, vol. 27, p. 267–273. Plenum Press, New York.

Swindale, N.V. (1980). A model for the formation of ocular dominance stripes. *Proc. R. Soc. London B*, **208**, 243–264.

Swindale, N.V. (1982). A model for the formation of orientation columns. *Proc. R. Soc. London B*, **215**, 211–230.

Swindale, N.V. (1988). Role of visual experience in promoting segregation of eye dominance patches in the visual cortex of the cat. *J. Comp. Neurol.*, **267**, 472–488.

Swindale, N.V. (1990). Theory of self-organising of cortical maps: mathematical framework. *Neural Networks*, **3**, 625–40.

Swindale, N.V. (1991). Coverage and design of the striate cortex. *Biol. Cybern.*, **65**, 415–424.

Swindale, N.V. (1996). The development of topography in the visual cortex: a review of models. *Network*, **7**, 161–247.

Tagashira, S., Ozaki, K., Ohta, M., and Itoh, N. (1995). Localisation of fibroblast growth factor-9 in the rat brain. *Mol. Brain Res.*, **30**, 233–241.

Taghert, P.H., Bastiani, M.J., Ho, R.K., Goodman, C.S. (1982). Guidance of pioneer growth cones: Filopodial contacts and coupling revealed with an antibody to lucifer yellow. *Dev. Bio.*, **94**, 391–399.

Takahashi, T., Misson, J.P., and Caviness, V.S. (1990). Glial process elongation and branching in the developing murine neocortex: A quantitative immunohistochemical analysis. *J. Comp. Neurol.*, **302**, 15–28.

Takahashi, T., Nowakowski, R.S., and Caviness, V.S., Jr. (1992a). Cytogenesis in the secondary proliferative population of the murine cerebral wall. *Soc. Neurosci. Abstr.*, **22**, 20.6.

Takahashi, T., Nowakowski, R.S., and Caviness, V.S., Jr. (1992b). BUdr as an S-phase marker for quantitative studies of cytokinetic behaviour in the murine cerebral ventricular zone. *J. Neurocytol.*, **21**, 185–197.

Takahashi, T., Nowakowski, R.S., and Caviness, V.S., Jr. (1993). Cell cycle parameters and patterns of nuclear movement in the neocortical proliferative zone of the fetal mouse. *J. Neurosci.*, **13**, 820–833.

Takahashi, T., Nowakowski, R.S., and Caviness, V.S., Jr. (1994). Mode of cell proliferation in the developing mouse neocortex. *Proc. Natl. Acad. Sci. USA*, **91**, 375–379.

Takahashi, T., Nowakowski, R.S., and Caviness, V.S., Jr. (1995a). The cell cycle of the pseudostratified ventricular-epithelium of the murine cerebral wall. *J. Neurosci.*, **15**, 6046–6057.

Takahashi, T., Nowakowski, R.S., and Caviness, V.S., Jr. (1995b). Early ontogeny of the secondary proliferative population of the embryonic murine cerebral wall. *J. Neurosci.*, **15**, 6058–6068.

Takahashi, T., Nowakowski, R.S., and Caviness, V.S., Jr. (1996). Interkinetic and migratory behavior of a cohort of neocortical neurons arising in the early embryonic murine cerebral wall. *J. Neurosci.*, **16**, 5762–5776.

Takeuchi, A. and Amari, S. (1979). Formation of topographic maps and columnar microstructures in nerve fields. *Biol. Cybern.*, **35**, 63–72.

Talbot, S.A. and Marshall, W.H. (1941). Physiological studies on neural mechanisms of visual location and discrimination. *Am. J. Ophthal.*, **24**, 1255–1264.

Talbot, W.H., Darian-Smith, I., Kornhuber, H.H., and Mountcastle, V.B. (1968). The sense of flutter-vibration: comparison of the human capacity with response patterns of mechanoreceptive afferents from the monkey hand. *J. Neurophysiol.*, **31**, 301–334.

Tanaka, E.M. and Sabry, J. (1995). Making the connection: cytoskeletal rearrangements during growth cone guidance. *Cell*, **83**, 171–176.

Tanebe, Y. and Jessell, T.M. (1996). Diversity and pattern in the developing spinal cord. *Science*, **274**, 1115–1123.

Tao, W. and Lai, E. (1992). Telencephalon-restricted expression of BF-1, a new member of the HNF-3/fork head gene family, in the developing rat brain. *Neuron*, **8**, 957–966.

Taxt, T. (1983). Motor unit numbers, motor unit sizes and innervation of single muscle fibres in hyperinnervated adult mouse soleus muscle. *Acta Physiol. Scand.*, **117**, 571–580.

Temple, S. (1989). Division and differentiation of isolateral CNS blast cells in microculture. *Nature*, **340**, 471–473.

Tessier-Lavigne, M. and Goodman, C.S. (1996). The molecular biology of axon guidance. *Science*, **274**, 1123–1132.

Tessier-Lavigne, M., Placzek, M., Lumsden, A.G.S., Dodd, J., and Jessell, T.M. (1988). Chemotropic guidance of developing axons in the mammalian central nervous system. *Nature*, **336**, 775–778.

Thoenen, H. and Edgar, D. (1985). Neurotrophic factors. *Science*, **229**, 238–242.

Thomaidou, D., Mione, M.C., Cavanagh, J.F.R, and Parnavelas, J.G. (1997). Apoptosis and its relation to the cell cycle in the developing cerebral cortex. *J. Neurosci.*, **17**, 1075–1085.

Thomas, P. and Beddington, R. (1996). Anterior primitive endoderm may be responsible for patterning the anterior neural plate in the mouse embryo. *Curr. Biol.*, **6**, 1487–1496.

Thompson, W.J., Kuffler, D.P. and Jansen, J.K.S. (1979). The effect of prolonged, reversible block of nerve impulses on the elimination of polyneuronal innervation of new-born rat skeletal muscle fibres. *Neurosci.*, **4**, 271–281.

Thompson, W.J. (1983). Synapse elimination in neonatal rat muscle is sensitive to pattern of muscle use. *Nature*, **302**, 614–616.

Thong, I.G. and Dreher, B. (1986). The development of the corticotectal pathway in the albino rat. *Dev. Brain Res.*, **25**, 227–238.

Tickle, C., Summerbell, D., and Wolpert, L. (1975). Positional signalling and specification of digits in chick limb morphogenesis. *Nature*, **254**, 199–202.

Tickle, C., Alberts, B., Wolpert, L., and Lee, J. (1982). Local application of retinoic acid to the limb bud mimics the action of the polarising region. *Nature*, **296**, 564–566.

Toledo-Aral, J., Brehm, P., Halegoua, S., and Mandel, G. (1995). A single pulse of nerve growth factor triggers long-term neuronal excitability through sodium channel induction. *Neuron*, **14**, 607–611.

Ton, C.C.T., Hirovenen, H., Miwa, H., Weil, M.W., Monaghan, A.P., Jordan, T., van Heyningen, V., Hastie, N.D., Meijers-Heijboer, H., Drechsler, M., Royer-Pokora, B., Collins, F., Swaroop, A., Strong, L.C., and Saunders, G.F. (1991). Positional cloning and characterisation of a paired box and homeobox containing gene from the aniridia region. *Cell*, **67**, 1059–1074.

Tootell, R.L., Silverman, M.S., and De Valois, R.L. (1981). Spatial frequency columns in primary visual cortex. *Science*, **214**, 813–815.

Tootell, R.B.H., Silverman, M.S., Switkes, E., and De Valois, R.L. (1982). Deoxyglucose analysis of retinotopic organization in primate striate cortex. *Science*, **218**, 902–904.

Torii, M.A., Matsuzaki, F., Osumi, N., Kaibuchi, K., Nakamura, S., Casarosa, S., Guillemot, F., and Nakafuku, M. (1999). Transcription factors Mash-1 and Prox-1 delineate early steps in differentiation of neural stem cells in the developing central nervous system. *Development*, **126**, 443–456.

Tovee, M.J. (1995). What are faces for? *Curr. Biol.*, **5**(5), 480–482.

Tovee, M.J. (1998). Face processing: Getting by with a little help from its friends. *Curr. Biol.*, **8**, 317–320.

Treanor, J.J.S., Goodman, L., deSauvage, F., Stone, D.M., Poulsen, K.T., Beck, C.D., Gray, C., Armanini, M.P., Pollock, R.A., Hefti, F., Phillips, H.S., Goddard, A., Moore, M.W., BujBello, A., Davies, A.M., Asai, N., Takahashi, M., Vandlen, R., Henderson, C.E., and Rosenthal, A. (1996). Characterization of a multicomponent receptor for GDNF. *Nature*, **382**, 80–83.

Treisman, F., Harris, E., and Desplan, C. (1991). The paired box encodes a second DNA-binding domain in the Paired homeodomain protein. *Genes Dev.*, **5**, 594–604.

Trisler, G.D. and Schneider, M.D. (1981). A topographic gradient of molecules in retina can be used to identify neuron position. *Proc. Natl. Acad. Sci. USA*, **78**, 2145–2149.

Trowe, T., Klostermann, S. Baier, H., Granato, M., Crawford, A.D., Grunewald, B., Hoffmann, H., Karlstrom, R.O., Meyer, S.U., Muller, B., Richter, S., Nusslein-Volhard, C. and Bonhoeffer, F. (1996). Mutations disrupting the ordering and topographic mapping of axons in the retinotectal projection of the zebrafish, *Danio rerio*. *Development*, **123**, 439–450.

Ts'o, D, Gilbert, C.D., and Wiesel, T. (1986). Relationships between horizontal interactions and functional architecture in cat striate cortex as revealed by cross-correlation analysis. *J. Neurosci.*, **6**, 1160–1170.

Turing, A.M. (1952). The chemical basis of morphogenesis. *Phil. Trans. R. Soc. London Ser. B*, **237**, 37–72.

Turner, D. and Cepko, C. (1987). Cell lineage in the rat retina: a common progenitor for neurons and glia persists late in development. *Nature*, **328**, 131–136.

Tuttle, R. and O'Leary, D.D.M. (1993). Cortical connections in cocultures. *Curr. Biol.*, **3**, 70–72.

Tuttle, R., Schlagger, B., Braisted, J.E., and O'Leary, D.D.M. (1995). Maturation-dependent upregulation of growth-promoting molecules in developing cortical plate controls thalamic and cortical neurite growth. *J. Neurosci.*, **15**, 3039–3052.

Tuttle, R., Nakagawa, Y., Johnson, J.E., and O'Leary, D.D.M. (1999). Defects in thalamocortical axon pathfinding correlate with altered cell domains in Mash-1-deficient mice. *Development*, **126**, 1903–1916.

Tuzi, N.L. and Gullick, W.J. (1994). Eph, the largest known family of purative growth factor receptors. *Br. J. Cancer*, **69**, 417–21.

Uwanogho, D., Rex, M., Cartwright, E.J., Pearl, G., Healy, C., *et al.* (1995). Embryonic expression of the chicken Sox2, Sox3 and Sox11 genes suggests an interactive role in neuronal development. *Mech. Dev.*, **49**, 23–36.

Uylings, H.B.M., Van Eden, C.G., Parnavelas, J.G., and Kalsbeek, A. (1990). The prenatal and postnatal development of rat cerebral cortex. In *The cerebral cortex of the rat* (eds. B. Kolb and R.C. Tees). MIT Press, Cambridge, MA.

Vaccarino, F.M., Schwartz, M.L., Raballo, R., Nilsen, J., Rhee, J., Zhou, M., Doetschman, T., Coffin, J.D., Wyland, J.J., and Hung, Y.-T.E. (1999). Changes in cerebral cortex size are governed by fibroblast growth factor during embryogenesis. *Nature Neurosci.*, **2**, 246–253.

Valverde, F., Lopez-Mascaraque, L., Santacana, M., and De Carlos, J.A. (1995a). Persistence of early-generated neurons in the rodent subplate: assessment of cell death in neocortex during early postnatal period. *J. Neurosci.*, **15**, 5014–5024.

Valverde, F., Facal-Valverde, M.V., Santacana, M., and Heredia, M. (1995b). Development and differentiation of early generated cells of sublayer VIb in the somatosensory cortex of the rat: a correlated Golgi and autoradiographic study. *J. Comp. Neurol.*, **290**, 118–140.

van den Heuvel, M. and Ingham, P.W. (1996). Smoothened encodes a receptor-like serpentine protein required for hedgehog signaling. *Nature*, **382**, 547–551.

van der Kooy, D., McConnell, S.K., and Kaznowski, C.E. (1992). Neocortex development and the cell cycle. *Science*, **256**, 849–850.

van der Loos, H. (1976). Neuronal circuitry and its development. *Prog. Brain Res.*, **45**, 259–278.

van der Loos, H. and Dorfl, J. (1978). Does the skin tell the somatosensory cortex have to construct a map of the periphery. *Neurosci. Lett.*, **7**, 23–30.

van der Loos, H. and Woolsey, T.A. (1973). Somatosensory cortex: Structured alterations following early injury to sense organs. *Science*, **179**, 395–398.

van Essen, D.C. and Maunsell, J.H.R. (1983). Hierarchical organisation and functional streams in the visual cortex. *Trends Neurosci.*, **6**, 370–375.

van Huizen, F., Strosberg, A.D., and Cynader, M.S. (1988). Cellular and sub-cellular localization of muscarinic acetylcholine receptors during postnatal development of cat visual cortex using immunocytochemical procedures. *Dev. Brain Res.*, **44**, 296–301.

van Ooyen, A. and Willshaw, D.J. (1999). Competition for neurotrophic factor in the development of nerve connections. *Proc. R. Soc. London*, **266**, 883–892.

van Pelt, J. and Verwer, R.W.H. (1986). Topological properties of binary trees grown with order-dependent branching probabilities. *Bulletin of Mathematical Biology*, **48**, 197–211.

van Pelt, J., Dityatev, A., and Uylings, H. (1997). Natural variability in the number of dendritic segments: Model-based inferences about branching during neurite outgrowth. *J. Comp. Neurol.*, **387**, 325–340.

Vargha Khadem, F. (1998). Compensation of function after hemispherectomy in childhood. *Eur. J. Neurosci.*, **S10**, 12 404.

Vargha Khadem, F., Carr, L.J., Isaacs, E., Brett, E., Adams, C., and Mishkin, M. (1997). Onset of speech after left hemispherectomy in a nine-year-old boy. *Brain*, **120**, 159–182.

Varmus, H. (1988). Retroviruses. *Science*, **240**, 1427–1435.

Vaux, D.L. and Strasser, A. (1996). The molecular biology of apoptosis. *Proc. Natl. Acad. Sci. USA*, **93**, 2239–2244.

Vercelli, A., Assal, F., and Innocenti, G.M. (1992). Emergence of callosally projecting neurons with stellate morphology in the visual cortex of the kitten. *Exp. Brain Res.*, **90**, 346–358.

Vicario-Abejon, C., Johe, K.K., Hazel, T.G., Collazo, D., and McKay, R.D.G. (1995). Functions of basic fibroblast growth factor and neurotrophins in the differentiation of hippocampal neurons. *Neuron*, **15**, 105–114.

Vitalis, T., Cases, O., Callebert, J., Launey, J., Price, D.J., Seif, I., and Gaspar, P. (1998). Effects of monoamine oxidase A inhibition on barrel formation in the mouse somatosensory cortex. Determination of a sensitive developmental period. *J. Comp. Neurol.*, **393**, 169–184.

Voigt, T. (1989). Development of glial cells in the cerebral wall of ferrets: Direct tracing of their transformation from radial glia into astrocytes. *J. Comp. Neurol.*, **289**, 74–88.

von der Malsburg, C. (1973). Self-organization of orientation sensitive cells in the striate cortex. *Kybernetik*, **14**, 85–100.

von der Malsburg, C. (1979). Development of ocularity domains and growth behaviour of axon terminals. *Biol. Cybern.*, **32**, 49–62.

von der Malsburg, C. and Willshaw, D.J. (1976). A mechanism for producing continuous neural mappings: ocularity dominance stripes and ordered retino-tectal projections. *Exp. Brain Res.*, **1**, 463–469.

von der Malsburg, C. and Willshaw, D.J. (1977). How to label nerve cells so that they can interconnect in an ordered fashion. *Proc. Natl. Acad. Sci. USA*, **74**, 5176–5178.

von der Malsburg, C. and Willshaw, D.J. (1981). Differential equations for the development of topological nerve fibre projections. *SIAM-AMS Proceedings*, **13**, 39–47.

Waechter, R.V. and Jaensch, B. (1972). Generation time of the matrix cells during embryonic brain development: an autoradiographic study in rats. *Brain Res.*, **46**, 235–250.

Wahle, P. and Meyer, G. (1987). Morphology and quantitative changes of transient NPY-ir neuronal populations during early post-natal development of the cat's visual cortex. *J. Comp. Neurol.*, **261**, 165–192.

Walicke, P. and Baird, A. (1988). Neurotrophic effects of basic and acidic fibroblast growth factors are not mediated through glial cells. *Brain Res.*, **468**, 71–79.

Walicke, P., Cowan, W.M., Ueno, N., Baird, A., and Guillemin, R. (1986). Fibroblast growth factor promotes survival of dissociated hippocampal neurons and enhances neurite extension. *Proc. Natl. Acad. Sci. USA*, **83**, 3012–3016.

Walsh, C. and Cepko, C.L. (1988). Clonally related cortical cells show several migration patterns. *Science*, **241**, 1342–1345.

Walsh, C. and Cepko, C.L. (1992). Widespread dispersion of neuronal clones across functional regions of the cerebral cortex. *Science*, **255**, 434–440.

Walter, J., Henke-Fahle, S., and Bonheoffer, F. (1987). Avoidance of posterior tectal membranes by temporal retinal axons. *Development*, **101**, 909–913.

Walther, C. and Gruss, P. (1991). Pax-6, a murine paired box gene, is expressed in the developing CNS. *Development*, **113**, 1435–1449.

Ware, C.B., Horowitz, M.C., and Renshaw B.R. *et al.* (1995). Targeted disruption of the low-affinity leukemia inhibitor factor receptor gene causes placental, skeletal, neural and metabolic defects, and results in perinatal death. *Development*, **121**, 1283–1299.

Ware, M.L., Fox, J.W., Gonzalez, J.L., Davis, N.M., *et al.* (1997). Aberrant splicing of a mouse disabled homolog, mdab1, in the scrambler mouse. *Neuron*, **19**, 239–249.

Warren, N. and Price, D.J. (1997). Roles of Pax-6 in murine diencephalic development. *Development*, **124**, 1573–1582.

Warren, N., Caric, D., Pratt, T., Clausen, J.A., Asavaritikrai, P., Mason, J.O., Hill, R.E., and Price, D.J. (1999). The transcription factor, Pax6, is required for cell proliferation and differentiation in the developing cerebral cortex. *Cerebral Cortex*, **9**, 627–635.

Watanabe, D., Yoshimura, R., Khalil, M., Yoshida, K, Kishimoto, T., *et al.* (1996). Characteristic localization of gp130 (the signal-transducing receptor component used in common for IL-6/IL-11/CNTF/LIF/OSM) in the rat brain. *Eur. J. Neurosci.*, **8**, 1630–1640.

Wegner, M., Drolet, D.W., and Rosenfeld, M.G. (1993). POU-domain proteins: structure and function of developmental regulators. *Curr. Opin. Cell Biol.*, **5**, 488–498.

Weisblat, D.A. and Shankland, M. (1985). Cell lineage and segmentation in the leech. *Phil. Trans. R. Soc. London Ser. B*, **312**, 39–56.

Weisblat, D.A., Sawyer, R.T., , and Stent, G.S. (1978). Cell lineage analysis by intracellular injection of a tracer enzyme. *Science*, **202**, 1295–1298.

Weiss, P. (1937a). Further experimental investigations on the phenomenon of homologous response in transplanted amphibian limbs. I. Functional observations. *J. Comp Neurosci.*, **66**, 181–209.

Weiss, P. (1937b). Further experimental investigations on the phenomenon of homologous response in transplanted amphibian limbs. II. Nerve regeneration and the innervation of transplanted limbs. *J. Comp. Neurosci.*, **66**, 481–536.

Weiss, P. (1939). *Principles of development.* Holt, New York.

Weiss, P. (1958). Cell contact. *Int. Rev. Cytol.*, **7**, 391–423.

Weisskopf, M. and Innocenti, G.M. (1991). Neurons with callosal projections in visual areas of newborn kittens—an analysis of their dendritic phenotype with respect to the fate of the callosal axon and of its target. *Exp. Brain Res.*, **86**, 151–158.

Weliky, M. and Katz, L.C. (1997). Disruption of orientation tuning in visual cortex by artificially correlated neuronal activity. *Nature*, **386**, 680–685.

Wessells, N.K. (1977). *Tissue interactions and development.* Benjamin-Cummings, Menlo Park, CA.

Wetts, R. and Fraser, S.E. (1988). Multipotential precursors can give rise to all major cell types of the frog retina. *Science*, **239**, 1142–1145.

Whitelaw, V.A. and Cowan, J.D. (1981). Specificity and plasticity of retinotectal connections: a computational model. *J. Neurosci.*, **1**, 1369–1387.

Whitman, C.O. (1978). The embryology of *Clepsine*. *Q. J. Microsc. Sci.*, **18**, 215–315.

Whitman, C.O. (1987). A contribution to the history of the germ layers in *Clepsine*. *J. Morphol.*, **1**, 105–182.

Wichterle, H., Garcia-Verdugo, J.M., and Alvarez-Buylla, A. (1997). Direct evidence for homotypic, glia-independent neuronal migration. *Neuron*, **18**, 779–791.

Wiesel, T.N. (1982). Postnatal development of the visual cortex and the influence of environment. *Nature*, **299**, 583–591.

Wiesel, T.N. and Hubel, D.H. (1963). Single-cell responses in striate cortex of kittens deprived of vision in one eye. *J. Neurophysiol.*, **26**, 1003–1017.

Wiesel, T.N. and Hubel, D.H. (1965). Comparison of the effects of unilateral and bilateral eye closure on cortical unit responses in kittens. *J. Neurophysiol.*, **26**, 1003–1017.

Wilkinson, D.G., Bhatt, S., Cook, M., Boncinelli, E., and Krumlauf, R. (1989). Segmental expression of Hox-2 homeobox-containing genes in the developing mouse hindbrain. *Nature*, **341**, 405–409.

Williams, B.P. and Price, J. (1995). Evidence for multiple precursor cell types in the embryonic rat cerebral cortex. *Neuron*, **14**, 1181–1188.

Williams, R.W. and Rakic, P. (1988). Elimination of neurons from the rhesus-monkeys lateral geniculate-nucleus during development. *J. Comp. Neurol.*, **272**, 424–436.

Willshaw, D.J. (1981). The establishment and the subsequent elimination of polyneural innervation of developing muscle: theoretical considerations. *Proc. R. Soc. London B*, **212**, 233–252.

Willshaw D.J. and Dayan, P.S. (1990). Optimal plasticity from matrix memories: What goes up must come down. *Neural Computation*, **1**, 85–93.

Willshaw, D.J. and von der Malsburg, C. (1976). How patterned neural connexions can be set up by self-organisation. *Proc. R. Soc. London B*, **194**, 431–445.

Willshaw, D.J. and von der Malsburg, C. (1979). A marker induction mechanism for the establishment of ordered neural mappings: its application to the retinotectal problem. *Phil. Trans. R. Soc. London Ser. B*, **287**, 203–243.

Wilson, S.W., Placzek, M., and Furley, A.J. (1993). Border disputes: do boundaries play a role in growth-cone guidance? *Trends Neurosci.*, **16**, 316–323.

Windrem, M.S. and Finlay, B.L. (1991). Thalamic ablations and neocortical development: alterations of cortical cytoarchitecture and cell number. *Cerebr. Cortex*, **1**, 230–240.

Winfree, A.T. (1970). An integrated view of the re-setting of a circadian clock. *J. Theor. Biol.*, **28**, 327–374.

Winfree, A.T. (1972). Oscillatory glycolysis in yeast: the pattern of resetting by oxygen. *Archs. Biochem. Biophys.*, **148**, 388–401.

Winslow, J.W., Moran, P., Valverde, J., Shih, A., and Yuan J.Q. (1995). Cloning of an AL-1, a ligand for an Eph-related tyrosine kinase receptor involved in axon bundle formation. *Neuron*, **14**, 973–981.

Wise, S.P. and Jones, E.G. (1978). Developmental studies of thalamocortical and commisural connections in the rat somatic sensory cortex. *J. Comp. Neurol.*, **178**, 187–208.

Wisniewski, K.E., Kida, E., Kuchna, I., Wierzba-Bobrowicz, T., and Dambska, M. (1997). Regulators of neuronal survival (Bcl-2, Bax, c-Jun) in prenatal and postnatal human frontal and temporal lobes in normal and down syndrome brain. In *Normal and abnormal development of the cortex* (eds. A.M. Galaburda and Y. Christen). Springer-Verlag, Berlin Heidelberg.

Wizenmann, A., Thanos, S., Boxberg, Y.V., and Bonhoeffer, F. (1993). Differential reaction of non-crossing rat retinal axons on cell membrane preparations from the chiasm midline: An *in vitro* study. *Development*, **117**, 725–735.

Wolpert, L. (1969). Positional information and the spatial pattern of cellular differentiation. *J. Theor. Biol.*, **25**, 1–47.

Wolpert, L. (1971). Positional information and pattern formation. *Curr. Top. Devel. Biol.*, **6**, 183–223.

Wolter, K.G., Hsu, Y.T., Smith, C.L., Nechushtan, A., Xi, X.G., and Youle, R.J. (1997). Movement of bax from the cytosol to mitochondria during apoptosis. *J. Cell Biol.*, **139**, 1281–1292.

Wong, M.L. and Licinio, J. (1994). Localisation of stem cell factor mRNA in adult rat hippocampus. *Neuroimmunomodulation*, **1**, 181–187.

Woo, K. and Fraser, S.E. (1995). Order and coherence in the fate map of the zebrafish nervous system. *Development*, **121**, 2595–2609.

Woo, T.U., Beale, J.M., and Finlay, B.L. (1991). Dual fate of subplate neurons in a rodent. *Cerebr. Cortex*, **1**, 433–443.

Wood, J.G., Martin, S., and Price, D.J. (1992). Evidence that the earliest generated cells of the murine cerebral cortex form a transient population in the subplate and marginal zone. *Dev. Brain Res.*, **66**, 137–140.

Woolsey, C.N. (1952). Pattern of localisation in sensory and motor areas of cerebral cortex. In *The biology of mental health and disease*. Hoeber, New York.

Woolsey, T.A. and van der Loos, H. (1970). The structural organization of layer IV in the somato-sensory region (SI) of mouse cerebral cortex. The description of a cortical field composed of discrete cytoarchitectonic units. *Brain Res.*, **17**, 205–242.

Wright, D.E., Zhou, L., Kucera, J., and Snider, W.D. (1997). Introduction of a neurotrophin-3 transgene into muscle selectively rescues proprioceptive neurons in mice lacking endogenous neurotrophin-3. *Neuron*, **19**, 503–517.

Xu, Y., Baldassare, M., Fisher, P., Rathbun, G., Oltz, E.M., Yancopoulos, G.D., Jessell, T.M., and Alt, F.W. (1993). LH-2: A LIM/homeodomain gene expressed in developing lymphocytes and neural cells. *Proc. Natl. Acad. Sci. USA*, **2**, 227–231.

Xuan, S., Baptista, C.A., Balas, G., Tao, W., Soares, V.C., and Lai, E. (1995). Winged helix transcription factor BF-1 is essential for the development of the cerebral hemispheres. *Neuron*, **14**, 1141–1152.

Yamakumi, H., Minami, M., and Satoh, M. (1996). Localisation of mRNA for leukaemia inhibitory factor receptor in the adult rat brain. *J. Neuroimmunol.*, **70**, 45–53.

Yamamoto, N., Kurotani, T., and Toyama, K. (1989). Neural connections between the lateral geniculate nucleus and visual cortex *in vitro*. *Science*, **245**, 192–194.

Yamamoto, N., Yamada, K., Kurotani, T., and Toyama, K. (1992). Laminar specificity of extrinsic cortical connections studied in coculture preparations. *Neuron*, **9**, 217–228.

Yang, E. and Korsmeyer, S.J. (1996). Molecular thanatopsis: a discourse on the BCL2 family and cell death. *Blood*, **88**, 386–401.

Ye, P., Carson, J., and D'Ercole, A.J. (1995). *In vivo* actions of insulin-like growth factor-1 (IGF-1) on brain myelination: studies of IGF-1 and IGF binding protein-1 (IGFBP-1) transgenic mice. *J. Neurosci.*, **15**, 7344–7356.

Yodzis, P. (1989). *Introduction to Theoretical Ecology*. Harper & Row, New York.

Yoon, M. (1971). Reorganization of retinotectal projection following surgical operations on the optic tectum in goldfish. *Exp. Neurol.*, **33**, 395–411.

Yoon, M. (1972). Transposition of the visual projection from the nasal hemiretina onto the foreign rostral zone of the optic tectum in goldfish. *Exp. Neurol.*, **37**, 451–462.

Yoon, M.G. (1980). Retention of the topographic addresses by reciprocally translated tectal re-implant in adult goldfish. *J. Physiol.*, **308**, 197–215.

Yoshida, M., Suda, Y., Matsua, I., Miyamoto, N., Takeda, N., Kuratani, S., and Aizawa, S. (1997). Emx1 and Emx2 functions in development of dorsal telencephalon. *Development*, **124**, 101–111.

Yuan, J. (1997). Transducing signals of life and death. *Curr. Opin. Cell Biol.*, **9**, 247–251.

Yuasa, S., Kitoh, J., and Kawamura, K. (1994). Interactions between growing thalamocortical afferent axons and the neocortical primordium in normal and reeler mutant mice. *Anat. Embryol.*, **190**, 137–154.

Zacco, A., Cooper, V., Chantler, P.D., Fisher-Hyland, S., Horton, H.L., and Levitt, P. (1990). Isolation, biochemical characterization and ultrastructural analysis of the limbic system-associated membrane protein (LAMP), a protein expressed by neurons comprising functional neural circuits. *J. Neurosci.*, **10**, 73–90.

Zeki, S. and Shipp, S. (1988). The functional logic of cortical connections. *Nature*, **335**, 311–317.

Zhang, L.I., Tao, H.W., Holt, C.E., Harris, W.A., and Poo, M.-M. (1998). A critical window for cooperation and competition among developing retinotectal synapses. *Nature*, **395**, 37–44.

Zheng, J.G., Felder, M., Conner, J.A., and Poo, M.-M. (1994). Turning of growth cones induced by neurotransmitters. *Nature*, **368**, 140–144.

Zheng, J.Q., Wan, J.J., and Poo, M.-M. (1996). Essential role of filopodia in chemotropic turning of nerve growth cone induced by a glutamate gradient. *J. Neurosci.*, **16**, 1140–1149.

Zumbroich, T.J., Blakemore, C., and Price, D.J. (1988a). Stimulus selectivity and its postnatal development in the cat's suprasylvian visual cortex. *Prog. Brain Res.*, **75**, 211–230.

Zumbroich, T.J., Price, D.J., and Blakemore, C. (1988b). Development of spatial and temporal selectivity in the suprasylvian visual cortex of the cat. *J. Neurosci.*, **8**, 2713–2728.

Glossary of terms and list of abbreviations

Terms relating to the basic biological and neurobiological vocabulary are not included. In the description of each term, italicisation indicates a cross reference.

Amblyopia: lack of visual acuity caused by disuse of the eye.

Ambystoma: a genus of tailed amphibians in the salamandroid suborder; in the larval stage it is called axolotl.

AMPA: α-amino-3-hydroxy-5-methyl-4-isoxazole proprionic acid.

Antennapedia: a *homeobox*-containing gene that regulates segmental identity in *Drosophila*.

anterior: refers to the part of the animal that points to the front; ie, when the animal is walking. Opposite of *posterior*.

AP5: 2-amino-5-phosphono-valerate.

apoptosis: programmed cell death that involves the activation of specific intracellular pathways.

astrotactin: an adhesion molecule implicated in neuronal migration.

Bax: a gene product involved in *apoptosis*; has a pro-apoptotic effect.

Bcl-2: a gene product involved in *apoptosis*; has an anti-apoptotic effect.

BCM: Bienenstock-Cooper-Munro model.

BDNF: Brain-derived neurotrophic factor; a member of the *neurotrophin* family of proteins that promote nerve growth and survival.

Betz cells: nerve cells of the motor cortex with giant perikarya.

BMP: bone morphogenetic protein.

bromodeoxyuridine (BrdU): a *thymidine* analogue identifiable with a monoclonal antibody used to label cells in S-phase.

cadherin: a member of the class of Cell Adhesion Molecules (CAM) whose action is dependent on calcium; contrast with *N-CAM*.

Caenorhabditis elegans (C. elegans): a species of nematode which has been useful for the study of the roles of genes in development.

Cajal–Retzius cells: the earliest generated nerve cells in cortical neurogenesis found in the *preplate* and the *cortical marginal zone*.

CAM: cell adhesion molecule

carbocyanine dyes: lypophilic fluorescent dyes used to trace axonal connections particularly in post mortem material. One example is *DiI*.

caudal: towards the tail; specifically following the *neuraxis* irrespective of tissue folds. Opposite of *rostral*.

ced: genes in *Caenorhabditis elegans* involved in regulating *apoptosis*.

Cerberus: secreted protein involved in *induction* of *rostral* parts of the nervous system.

chemotropism: directed movement of cells or their processes towards the source of a diffusible chemical.

commitment: property of a cell or tissue region which causes it to follow a particular developmental path. Two different levels of commitment can be distinguished, namely *specification* and *determination*.

compartment: a term defined in *Drosophila* embryology to mean a multicellular region within which the progeny of every cell are confined.

complex cells: nerve cells in mammalian visual cortex that, in distinction to *simple cells*, are responsive to oriented bars of light in a manner that is unpredictable from the arrangement of the component subregions in their *receptive field*.

compound eye in Xenopus: a surgically constructed eye made, in the embryo, by replacing a portion of the eye rudiment by a similar sized portion from another eye rudiment.

conserved: describes a feature that has remained relatively unchanged throughout evolution.

cortical plate: a region of the developing *telencephalon* that forms layers 2 to 6 of the cerebral cortex.

critical period: a period during early postnatal development during which the structure of the nervous system is highly susceptible to environmental perturbation.

cytochrome oxidase (CO): an enzyme complex responsible for the reduction of oxygen that is used as a marker of subregions within the mammalian visual cortex.

cytokines: intercellular signalling molecules, originally identified in the immune system, that play a role in nerve growth and survival.

determination: describing a high level of *commitment* in which cells or tissues follow their normal path of development when subject to an array of different environments. Contrast with *specification*.

diencephalon: one of the two major subdivisions of the *prosencephalon*.

DiI and *DiO: carbocyanine* dyes.

dorsal: one of the four directions specifying the axes in the plane perpendicular to the *neuraxis*; towards the back and opposite of *ventral*.

Drosophila melanogaster: fruit fly that was used to unravel basic genetic concepts and more recently has been used to study genes that *regulate* development.

E(n): embryonic day n.

ECM: extracellular matrix.

engrailed: A *Drosophila homeobox* gene involved in segmentation.

ephrins: a family of membrane ligands acting on *receptor tyrosine kinases* some of which are expressed in graded form.

Epidermal Growth Factor (EGF): A family of proteins mediating a variety of interactions involving particularly epidermal and epithelial cells.

fasciclin: a member of the *semaphorin* family now renamed *G-Sema I.*

fate: as applied to a differentiating cell it describes what structures this cell will give rise to.

fate map: a map of the embryo at any developmental stage that describes what each part of the embryo will become.

feature map: shows how the population of nerve cells in a sensory structure responds to one particular aspect of the external world. This is shown in the form of a map of the structure showing the distribution of optimal stimuli.

fibroblast growth factor (FGF): a family of signalling molecules.

fibronectin: adhesive *glycoprotein* mediating attachment to the extracellular matrix.

5-HT: 5-hydroxy-tryptamine.

G1 phase: gap phase 1, during cell cycle.

G2 phase: gap phase 2, during cell cycle.

GABA: gamma-aminobutyric acid.

ganglionic eminence: embryonic forerunner of the striatum.

GDNF: glial cell line-derived *neurotrophic factor.*

glycoprotein: a carbohydrate linked to a protein; important components of cell membranes.

glycosaminoglycans (GAGs): a group of polysaccharides that form part of the extracellular matrix.

G-Sema: a member of the *semaphorin* family originally named *fasciclin I.*

haptotaxis: the ability of a growth cone or cell to migrate up a gradient of adhesivity.

Hebb rule: The proposal that a synaptic connection is strengthened by the coincident activity in the presynaptic and postsynaptic neurons.

homeobox: a short length of DNA within a particular class of *regulatory* gene that encodes the *homeodomain.*

homeodomain: a region within a regulatory protein allowing binding to the DNA and thereby allowing the protein to influence the transcription of other genes.

homeotic gene: a gene that *regulates* the identity of a cell or group of cells.

horseradish peroxidase (HRP): An electron dense enzyme used in axonal tracing.

Hox genes: *homeobox* genes in mice that are related to the *Antennapedia* gene in *Drosophila.*

imaginal disc: a group of undifferentiated cells in insect larvae that develop into a specific adult structure.

induction: effect on the developmental pathway of one group of cells by an external agent.

intermediate zone: the territory in the developing *telencephalon* that lies between the *ventricular zone* and the *cortical plate*.

internal capsule: the region of the *telencephalon* through which the thalamocortical and the corticothalamic axons grow.

knock-out: the disruption of a specific gene usually involving its replacement by an inactive form.

laminin: an adhesive *glycoprotein* mediating cell adhesion.

lateral: one of the four directions specifying the axes in the plane perpendicular to the *neuraxis*; away from the midline and opposite of *medial*.

LGN: lateral geniculate nucleus.

limbic system-associated protein (LAMP): a cell adhesion molecule expressed in specific regions of the developing cortex.

lineage: a description of the ancestry of a cell.

LTD: long term depression.

LTP: long term potentiation.

M phase: mitosis phase, during cell cycle.

MAM Ac: methylazoxymethanol acetate.

map: either a *fate map* or a plot (usually in two dimensions) of the variation of optimal stimuli over a sensory surface, such as a *feature map*.

marginal zone: the most superficial component of the developing cerebral cortex that develops into cortical layer I.

medial: one of the four directions specifying the axes in the plane perpendicular to the *neuraxis*; towards the midline and opposite of *lateral*.

mesencephalon: the midbrain; one of the three divisions of the vertebrate brain, with the *prosencephalon* and the *rhombencephalon*.

morphogen: a molecule that directs *morphogenesis*.

morphogenesis: the process by which embryonic form and structure are achieved.

morphogenetic field: a group of cells whose position and fate are defined with respect to certain boundaries.

mosaicism: describes the property of a cell or group of cells which follow the same developmental pathway regardless of the experimental manipulation applied to it or them.

N-CAM (Neural Cell Adhesion Molecule): a member of the class of Cell Adhesion Molecules (CAMs) whose action does not require calcium and thought to be involved in the development of the nervous system; contrast with *cadherin*.

necrosis: cell death caused by injury or the effect of toxic substances.

nerve growth factor (NGF): a protein promoting the growth and survival of some neurons; the first member of the *neurotrophin* family to be described, another example of which is *BDNF*.

netrin: a protein that guides growth cones during development of the central nervous system.

neural constructivism: the view that the development of neural structures proceeds through a dynamic interaction with the environment involving simultaneous generation of new structure and the removal of old structure; has been used as the opposite of *selectionism.*

neural crest cells: the cells from the *dorsal* most portion of the *neural tube* that migrate *laterally* and *ventrally* to give rise to a variety of cell types in the peripheral and autonomic nervous system.

neural plate: a strip of ectoderm above the *notochord* that lies along the *neuraxis* of the early embryo and develops into the main parts of the nervous system.

neural tube: formed by the folding of the *neural plate* along the *neuraxis* of the embryo.

neuraxis: the central axis of the embryo, running from *rostral* to *caudal.*

neuregulins: growth factors that have been implicated in glial-guided neuronal migration.

neurogenins: transcription factors expressed in cortical *stem cells.*

neuromere: a *segment* of the *neural tube* of vertebrates.

neurotrophic factor: any substance that promotes the growth and survival of neurons.

neurotrophins: a family of soluble ligands (eg, *NGF, BDNF*) that are released by neurons and bind with identified receptors (eg, *Trk*) and promote nerve growth and survival.

NGF: nerve growth factor.

NN: a form of *Xenopus compound eye* made up of two halves of nasal origin.

NMDA: N-methyl-D-aspartate.

NT-3 and *NT-4: neurotrophins* 3 and 4.

ocularity dominance: expresses the fact that cells in visual cortex with binocular innervation may respond better to stimuli through one eye than the other.

P(n) postnatal day n.

pattern formation: the establishment of an ordered spatial arrangement of differentiated cells or connections between nerve cells.

PKC: protein kinase C.

pluripotent: describes a cell that has the potential to develop into a variety of tissues.

PMLS: posteromedial lateral suprasylvian cortex.

posterior: refers to the part of the animal that points to the back; ie, when the animal is walking. Opposite of *anterior.*

positional information: the spatial distribution of information available to a cell, available intracellularlly or extracellularly, that can influence its development.

postmitotic cell: a cell that has undergone mitosis but commonly used to describe a cell (eg, a neuron) that will not divide during the life time of the organism.

potency: the developmental potential of a nucleus, cell or tissue. Different levels are recognised, eg *pluripotency.*

precursor cell: a cell which will differentiate into a specific cell type.

preplate: a population of cells around the edge of the *telencephalon.*

progenitor cells: cells that have not undergone their final division.

prosencephalon: the forebrain; one of the three divisions of the vertebrate brain, with the *mesencephalon* and the *rhombencephalon.* Its major subdivisions are the *telencephalon* and the *diencephalon.*

prosomere: a *neuromere* in the *prosencephalon.*

proteoglycan: large molecules in the extracellular matrix composed of a core protein and *glycosaminoglycans.*

PVE: pseudostratified *ventricular* epithelium.

RAGS: repulsive axon guidance signal.

reaction-diffusion: describes a class of models of the interaction of two *morphogens,* an activator and an inhibitor, which interact to form spatially distributed morphogenetic patterns.

receptive field of a nerve cell: the portion of the sensory space which evokes a response in the cell in question.

receptor tyrosine kinases: the largest class of enzyme-linked receptors (that includes most of the growth factor receptors) which phosphorylates selected intracellular proteins.

reeler: a naturally-occurring mutation in mice resulting in defective migration of cortical cells.

reelin: a large extracellular matrix-like protein that is mutated in *reeler* mice.

regulation: originally used in embryology to indicate that the developmental pathway of a particular cell or cells can be altered by experimental manipulation; more specifically, that cell fates can be altered relatively late in development to compensate for an earlier perturbation. Now used more generally to describe a process of control; for example by one (*regulatory*) gene on another.

regulatory genes: genes that control the expression of other genes.

repulsive guidance molecule (RGM): a freely moving molecule that causes repulsion of growth cones.

retinoic acid: a *morphogen* that controls *pattern formation* in chick and amphibian limbs.

rhombencephalon: the hindbrain; one of the three divisions of the brain, with the *prosencephalon* and the *mesencephalon.*

rhombomere: a *neuromere* in the *rhombencephalon.*

rostral: literally 'resembling a beak'; the direction along the *neuraxis* towards the head; opposite of *caudal.*

S phase: synthesis phase, during cell cycle.

selectionism: the idea that the nervous system develops by an initial production of structure followed by the selective pruning away of cells and synapses. Has been used as the opposite of *neural constructivism*.

semaphorin: a family of proteins that act as *repulsive guidance molecules*.

segment: a repetitive body unit.

simple cells: in contrast to *complex cells*, these are neurons of visual cortex with spatially segregated excitatory and inhibitory subregions of their *receptive field*, knowledge of which enables the optimal stimulus of the cell to be predicted.

sonic hedgehog: an example of a diffusible *morphogen* that induces patterning in the nervous system.

specification: describes a low level of *commitment* of a cell to a particular fate that can be reversed if environmental conditions are changed.

SPP: secondary proliferative population.

stereotropism: relates to the idea that physical cues in the substratum direct neural growth.

stem cells: cells that reproduce themselves and give rise to differentiated progeny; originally defined as cells that divide throughout the life of the organism and now includes cells that divide for a limited period of time (for example, *progenitor cells* in the *ventricular* zone).

subventricular zone (SVZ): a layer that is deep to the ventricular zone in the *telencephalon* from which the majority of cortical glial cells are thought to derive.

telencephalon: one of the two major subdivisions of the *prosencephalon*.

tetrodotoxin (TTX): a naturally occurring toxin that blocks sodium channels and thereby prevents nerve impulse propagation.

Transforming Growth Factor-α (TGF α): A member of the *Epidermal Growth Factor (EGF)* family of proteins.

Transforming Growth Factor-β (TGF β): A superfamily of proteins involved in a wide variety of interactions during development.

topographic map: refers to the ordered two-dimensional representation of a sensory surface on structures to which the sensory surface projects. Contrast with *feature map*.

totipotent: describes a nucleus or cell that is capable of developing into any of the tissues of the organism.

transcription factor: a protein that interacts with the *regulatory* elements of a gene to influence transcription.

transfate: to change the fate of a cell.

Transforming Growth Factor-α (TGF-α): A member of the *Epidermal Growth Factor (EGF)* family of proteins.

Transforming Growth Factor-β (TGF-β): A superfamily of proteins involved in a wide variety of interactions during development.

transgenic: describes an organism in which an exogeneous gene has been incorporated into the genome.

tritiated thymidine: radioactive-labelled thymidine for studying cell proliferation and migration.

Trk receptors: a family of high-affinity *receptor tyrosine kinases* responsive to the *neurotrophins*.

trophic response: a response of a cell that promotes its growth or its survival.

TT: a form of *Xenopus compound eye* made up of two halves of temporal origin.

tumour necrosis factor receptor: receptors that induce cell death.

V1–V5: areas of visual cortex in primate, labelled 1–5.

VC: visual cortex.

ventral: one of the four directions specifying the axes in the plane perpendicular to the *neuraxis*; towards the chest and opposite of *dorsal*.

ventricular zone (VZ): a region of the *telencephalon* containing neural *progenitors*.

VV: a form of *Xenopus compound eye* made up of two halves of *ventral* origin.

Xenopus laevis: an amphibian resembling a frog or a toad that is used widely in developmental studies owing to the relative ease with which its development can be followed from initial fertilisation onwards.

X, Y and *W cells:* different types of cell found in the retina and *LGN*.

zinc finger: a DNA-binding element found in many *transcription factors*.

Zone of Polarising Activity (ZPA): a region in the limb bud in chick and other vertebrates that specifies the *anterior-posterior* axis of the limb.

Index